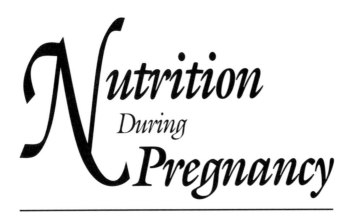

Nutrition During Pregnancy

Part I
WEIGHT GAIN
Part II
NUTRIENT SUPPLEMENTS

Subcommittee on Nutritional Status and Weight Gain During Pregnancy
Subcommittee on Dietary Intake and Nutrient Supplements
During Pregnancy
Committee on Nutritional Status During Pregnancy and Lactation
Food and Nutrition Board
Institute of Medicine
National Academy of Sciences

NATIONAL ACADEMY PRESS
Washington, D.C. 1990

National Academy Press • 2101 Constitution Avenue, N.W. • Washington, D.C. 20418

NOTICE: The project that is the subject of this report was approved by the Governing Board of the National Research Council, whose members are drawn from the councils of the National Academy of Sciences, the National Academy of Engineering, and the Institute of Medicine. The members of the committee responsible for the report were chosen for their special competences and with regard for appropriate balance.

This report has been reviewed by a group other than the authors according to procedures approved by a Report Review Committee consisting of members of the National Academy of Sciences, the National Academy of Engineering, and the Institute of Medicine.

The Institute of Medicine was chartered in 1970 by the National Academy of Sciences to enlist distinguished members of the appropriate professions in the examination of policy matters pertaining to the health of the public. In this, the Institute acts under both the Academy's 1863 congressional charter responsibility to be an adviser to the federal government and its own initiative in identifying issues of medical care, research, and education. Dr. Samuel O. Thier is president of the Institute of Medicine.

This study was supported by project no. MCJ 116011 from the Maternal and Child Health Program (Title V, Social Security Act), Health Resources and Services Administration, U.S. Department of Health and Human Services.

Library of Congress Cataloging-in-Publication Data

Institute of Medicine (U.S.). Subcommittee on Nutritional Status and
Weight Gain During Pregnancy.
    Nutrition during pregnancy : part I, weight gain : part II,
nutrient supplements / Subcommittee on Nutritional Status and Weight
Gain During Pregnancy, Subcommittee on Dietary Intake and Nutrient
Supplements During Pregnancy, Committee on Nutritional Status During
Pregnancy and Lactation, Food and Nutrition Board, Institute of
Medicine, National Academy of Sciences.
        p.   cm.
    Includes bibliographical references.
    ISBN 0-309-04138-4
    1. Pregnancy—Nutritional aspects. 2. Pregnant women—Weight
gain. I. Institute of Medicine (U.S.). Subcommittee on Dietary
Intake and Nutrient Supplements during Pregnancy. II. Title.
    [DNLM: 1. Nutrition—in pregnancy. 2. Weight Gain—in pregnancy.
WQ 175 I617n]
    RG559.I57 1990
    618.2'4—dc20
    DNLM/DLC   90-5661
    for Library of Congress   CIP

Copyright © 1990 by the National Academy of Sciences

Printed in the United States of America

SUBCOMMITTEE ON NUTRITIONAL STATUS AND WEIGHT GAIN DURING PREGNANCY

JANET C. KING (*Chair*), Department of Nutritional Sciences, University of California, Berkeley, California
NANCY F. BUTTE, Children's Nutrition Research Center, Department of Pediatrics, Baylor College of Medicine, Houston, Texas
RONALD A. CHEZ, Department of Obstetrics and Gynecology, University of South Florida School of Medicine, Tampa, Florida
JERE D. HAAS, Division of Nutritional Sciences, Cornell University, Ithaca, New York
JOEL C. KLEINMAN, Division of Analysis, National Center for Health Statistics, Hyattsville, Maryland
MICHAEL S. KRAMER, McGill University, Montreal, Quebec, Canada
SALLY A. LEDERMAN, Center for Population and Family Health, School of Public Health, and Institute of Human Nutrition, Columbia University, New York, New York

SUBCOMMITTEE ON DIETARY INTAKE AND NUTRIENT SUPPLEMENTS DURING PREGNANCY

LINDSAY ALLEN (*Chair*), Department of Nutritional Sciences, University of Connecticut, Storrs, Connecticut
GERTRUD S. BERKOWITZ, Departments of Obstetrics, Gynecology, and Reproductive Science, and Community Medicine, Mount Sinai Medical Center, New York, New York
PETER DALLMAN, Department of Pediatrics, University of California, San Francisco, California
K. MICHAEL HAMBIDGE, Department of Pediatrics, School of Medicine, University of Colorado, Denver, Colorado
AVANELLE KIRKSEY, Department of Foods and Nutrition, School of Consumer and Family Science, Purdue University, West Lafayette, Indiana
JENNIFER R. NIEBYL, Department of Obstetrics and Gynecology, University of Iowa College of Medicine, Iowa City, Iowa
JOHN W. SPARKS, Department of Pediatrics, School of Medicine, University of Colorado, Denver, Colorado

Staff

CAROL WEST SUITOR, Program Officer
MARIAN M. F. MILLSTONE, Research Assistant
WILHELMENA TAMALE, Senior Secretary

iv

FOOD AND NUTRITION BOARD

RICHARD J. HAVEL (*Chair*), Cardiovascular Research Institute, University of California School of Medicine, San Francisco, California
DONALD B. McCORMICK (*Vice Chair*), Department of Biochemistry, Emory University School of Medicine, Atlanta, Georgia
EDWIN L. BIERMAN, Division of Metabolism, Endocrinology, and Nutrition, University of Washington School of Medicine, Seattle, Washington
EDWARD J. CALABRESE, Environmental Health Program, Division of Public Health, University of Massachusetts, Amherst, Massachusetts
DORIS H. CALLOWAY, University of California, Berkeley, California
DeWITT GOODMAN, Institute of Human Nutrition, Columbia University, New York, New York
M.R.C. GREENWOOD, University of California, Davis, California
JOAN D. GUSSOW, Department of Nutrition Education, Teachers College, Columbia University, New York, New York
JOHN E. KINSELLA, Institute of Food Science, Cornell University, Ithaca, New York
LAURENCE N. KOLONEL, Cancer Center of Hawaii, University of Hawaii, Honolulu, Hawaii
REYNALDO MARTORELL, Food Research Institute, Stanford University, Stanford, California
WALTER MERTZ, Human Nutrition Research Center, Agricultural Research Service, U.S. Department of Agriculture, Beltsville, Maryland
MALDEN C. NESHEIM, Office of the Provost, Cornell University, Ithaca, New York
JOHN LISTON (*Ex Officio*), Division of Food Science, School of Fisheries, College of Ocean and Fishery Sciences, University of Washington, Seattle, Washington
ARNO G. MOTULSKY (*Ex Officio*), Center for Inherited Diseases, University of Washington, Seattle, Washington
ROY M. PITKIN (*Ex Officio*), Department of Obstetrics and Gynecology, School of Medicine, University of California, Los Angeles, California

Staff

SUSHMA PALMER, Director (until September 1, 1989)
ALVIN G. LAZEN, Interim Director (beginning September 5, 1989)
FRANCES M. PETER, Deputy Director
SHIRLEY ASH, Financial Specialist
UTE HAYMAN, Administrative Assistant

Preface

In the quest for a favorable outcome of pregnancy, namely, delivery of a full-term, healthy infant of appropriate size, pregnant women have long directed their attention to weight gain and dietary intake. However, despite many reports on the subject published since the early 1970s, consensus has not been reached regarding recommendations for gestational weight gain. Furthermore, many women and health care providers in the United States have become concerned about the adequacy of the usual dietary intake of nutrients during pregnancy. Consequently, vitamin-mineral supplementation during pregnancy has become widespread. Recognizing a need to examine these issues carefully, the Bureau of Maternal and Child Health and Resources Development of the U.S. Department of Health and Human Services (DHHS) asked the National Academy of Sciences to conduct a study of maternal nutrition. In response, the Committee on Nutritional Status During Pregnancy and Lactation was formed in the Food and Nutrition Board, Institute of Medicine, and subcommittees were appointed to focus on specific aspects of the overall charge. The first two of the committee's reports are presented in this volume as Part I, Nutritional Status and Weight Gain, and Part II, Dietary Intake and Nutrient Supplements. These reports are preceded by an overall summary (Chapter 1). The third report of the committee, to be published within the year, will focus on nutrition during lactation.

The major objective of the Subcommittee on Nutritional Status and Weight Gain During Pregnancy was to evaluate the scientific evidence and formulate recommendations for desirable weight gains during pregnancy.

vii

The Subcommittee on Dietary Intake and Nutrient Supplements During Pregnancy evaluated the scientific evidence and formulated recommendations on vitamin, mineral, and protein supplementation during gestation. Both subcommittees were asked specifically to consider the justification for special recommendations for pregnant adolescents, women over age 35, and women of black, Hispanic, and Southeast Asian origin. The approaches to the study are described in detail in the separate introductions to the two parts of the report.

This volume should be widely used both by researchers and students seeking a fuller knowledge of pregnancy and by health care providers seeking guidance for practice. Therefore, we have included some discussions of value to both these groups as well as some that will be less relevant to one or the other.

Both subcommittees benefited from advice and suggestions provided by the Committee on Nutritional Status During Pregnancy and Lactation, from the sharing of information between the subcommittees, and from the assistance provided by the Food and Nutrition Board and its Subcommittee on the Tenth Edition of the Recommended Dietary Allowances. The committee and subcommittees appreciate the support provided by the Food and Nutrition Board staff headed by Dr. Sushma Palmer (until September 1989) and including Drs. Virginia Laukaran and Chessa Lutter (prior to August 1988), Dr. Carol West Suitor (beginning August 1988), Mrs. Frances Peter, Ms. Marian Millstone, Ms. Wilhelmena Tamale, Ms. Sandra Johnson (until November 1989), and Ms. Janie Marshall.

Many people made important contributions to this combined report by giving presentations, providing the subcommittees with data or special written reports or analyses, sharing their views during workshops, commenting on drafts, or otherwise serving as resource persons. In particular, the committee and subcommittees wish to thank Dr. Judith Brown, University of Minnesota; Dr. Neville Coleman, Bronx Veterans' Administration Medical Center; Dr. Catherine Cowell, Bureau of Nutrition, City of New York; Dr. Jan Dodds, Bureau of Nutrition, New York State; Dr. J. V. G. A. Durnin, University of Glasgow; Dr. Jan Ekstrand, University of Iowa; Dr. Virginia Ernster, University of California, San Francisco; Dr. J. David Erickson, Centers for Disease Control; Dr. J. M. Gertner, New York Hospital; Dr. J.-P. Habicht, Cornell University; Dr. Suzanne Harris, Food and Consumer Services, U.S. Department of Agriculture (USDA); Mr. Jay Hirshman, Food and Nutrition Service, USDA; Dr. Frank Hytten, retired; Ms. Patricia Jensen, Santa Clara County Department of Health, California; Ms. Heidi Kalkwarf, Cornell University; Dr. Susan Krebs-Smith, Human Nutrition Information Service, USDA; Ms. Lynn Kuba, Childbirth Educator, Fairfax County, Va.; Ms. Alice Lenihan, National Association of WIC (Supplemental Food Program for Women, Infants, and Children) Directors; Ms.

Brenda Lisi, Food and Nutrition Service, USDA; Ms. Ruth Lubic, Maternity Center Association, New York City; Ms. Shelly Marks, Harbor University of California at Los Angeles Medical Center; Dr. Richard Naeye, Pennsylvania State University College of Medicine; Dr. Godfrey Oakley, Centers for Disease Control; Dr. James Olson, Iowa State University; Dr. Theresa Scholl, School of Osteopathic Medicine, University of Medicine and Dentistry of New Jersey; Dr. Rita Thomas, Bristol-Myers; Dr. Bea van den Berg, University of California, Berkeley; Dr. Honor Wolfe, Wayne State University School of Medicine; Dr. Jose Villar, National Institute of Child Health and Human Development; Dr. Catherine Woteki, National Center for Health Statistics; Dr. Ray Yip, Centers for Disease Control; and Ms. Colette Zyrkowski, Centers for Disease Control. The committees extend special thanks to Ms. Elizabeth Brannon of the Office of Maternal and Child Health, DHHS, for encouragement, facilitating searches for data, and identifying resource people and materials.

ROY M. PITKIN, *Chair*
Committee on Nutritional Status
During Pregnancy and Lactation

Contents

PART II
DIETARY INTAKE AND NUTRIENT SUPPLEMENTS

APPENDIXES

1

Summary

In the 20 years since publication of the Food and Nutrition Board's landmark report *Maternal Nutrition and the Course of Pregnancy* (NRC, 1970), the fields of nutrition and obstetrics have changed greatly. These changes, many of them stimulated by the report itself and the work of successor committees of the board and of the Institute of Medicine, include expanded private and governmental research efforts, enhanced teaching of perinatal nutrition to students in the health care professions, and a resurgence of interest in applied nutrition by clinicians in obstetrics and pediatrics. Also during the period, the Supplemental Food Program for Women, Infants, and Children (WIC) was established in the U.S. Department of Agriculture; the reports *Preventing Low Birthweight* (IOM, 1985) and *Prenatal Care* (IOM, 1988) were published by the Institute of Medicine; the National Commission for the Prevention of Infant Mortality was established; and the report *Caring for Our Future: The Content of Prenatal Care* was released by the Public Health Service (DHHS, 1989). All these events have underscored the importance of nutrition during pregnancy and the perinatal period.

Greater visibility of maternity services in the United States has also drawn attention to many gaps and weaknesses in knowledge about maternal nutrition and about how recent findings should be applied in prenatal care. To address these deficiencies, the Food and Nutrition Board (FNB) established the Committee on Nutritional Status During Pregnancy and Lactation late in 1987 to conduct a detailed assessment of the published data. The committee addressed its task by forming three subcommittees:

Nutritional Status and Weight Gain During Pregnancy, Dietary Intake and Nutrient Supplements During Pregnancy, and Nutritional Status During Lactation. The parent committee, in addition to coordinating the work of its subcommittees, has maintained close liaison with the FNB's Subcommittee on the Tenth Edition of the Recommended Dietary Allowances in order to maintain consistency in the work of the two groups.

In general, the committee found few well-designed studies and little scientific evidence regarding many important issues. For this reason, areas needing further research are underscored in this publication. Careful attention to the information in these reports should help stimulate both research and practice toward a common goal of improving the health and well-being of mothers and children in the United States.

This publication includes two reports. Part I is a critical evaluation of the data concerning nutritional status and weight gain during pregnancy. Part II contains an examination of the evidence on the need for nutrient supplements during pregnancy. A second publication covering nutrition during lactation will be released in late 1990. Each of these reports responds to specific requests from the Bureau of Maternal and Child Health and Resources Development of the U.S. Department of Health and Human Services, which funded the study. The committee anticipates that material presented in the three reports will serve as a basis for additional publications that provide a comprehensive, practical approach for delivering nutritional care curing pregnancy and lactation.

PART I: NUTRITIONAL STATUS AND WEIGHT GAIN

The overall goals of the Subcommittee on Nutritional Status and Weight Gain During Pregnancy were to analyze the scientific evidence pertaining to weight gain during pregnancy and to formulate recommendations for healthy gestational weight gain. The subcommittee was asked to address the following questions:

• How do nutritional status prior to pregnancy and dietary intake during gestation influence the pattern and total amount of weight gain?

• Which, if any, anthropometric measurements are useful in assessing nutritional status during pregnancy?

• How should weight gain recommendations be modified for pregnant women of black, Hispanic, and Southeast Asian origin and for those under age 20 or over age 35?

Part I deals only to a limited extent with nutritional care during pregnancy. It does not include many other elements of prenatal nutrition services, such as the evaluation and improvement of the nutritional quality of diet (briefly covered in Part II of this volume), and the importance of access to a regular and adequate supply of nutritious foods, development of sound eating practices for the family, dietary adjustments for mothers with acute and chronic medical conditions, and breastfeeding promotion and education. Although the subcommittee limited its review to its charge, it recognized that such a broad spectrum of nutrition services is an important part of comprehensive maternal health care.

The subcommittee began its work by tracing trends in selected aspects of prenatal care, maternal nutritional status, and the course and outcomes of pregnancy (e.g., fetal growth, birth weight, postpartum weight retention). It then undertook its major effort—an extensive critical review of the scientific literature. Epidemiologic and clinical evidence pertaining to determinants of weight gain and effects of weight gain on maternal and child health were examined. This included consideration of total gain, pattern of gain, and composition of the added tissue. The practicality and usefulness of anthropometric measurements in the clinical setting were assessed. The subcommittee paid close attention to new analyses from the 1980 National Natality Survey, which provides the only recent nationally representative U.S. data on weight gain during pregnancy, infant birth weight, and an assortment of maternal characteristics.

Most of the literature reviewed pertained to women living in industrialized nations. Data were more complete for whites than for nonwhites. The conclusions and recommendations presented in this report relate to healthy women in the United States; they have not been evaluated with respect to women in less developed countries or women who have recently emigrated from those countries to the United States.

The subcommittee took particular care in clarifying its definitions and in examining the strengths and limitations of study methods. For example, the term *prepregnancy nutritional status* can have many meanings. The subcommittee agreed that prepregnancy weight for height is the simplest and most useful index for evaluating prepregnancy nutritional status in the clinical setting, while recognizing that this is an indirect measure of energy stores only. The measurements are relatively easy to make, and the approach provides a systematic method for distinguishing between women who weigh more because of their greater height and those whose greater weight reflects extra fat or lean body mass. Much more complex methods are required for defining other aspects of nutritional status. However, weight for height is applicable to most studies that address gestational weight gain.

The meaning of *gestational weight gain* also received the subcommittee's attention. Comparisons among studies are complicated by the many different methods used to compute gestational weight gain. In this report, three types of gestational weight gain are discussed in detail, namely:

- *total weight gain* (weight just before delivery minus weight just before conception);
- *net weight gain* (total weight gain minus the infant's birth weight); and
- *rate per week* (weight gained over a specified period divided by the duration of that period in weeks).

Attention is also given to different methods of comparing weight gain with standards in both clinical and research settings.

The subcommittee considered gestational weight gain in relation to clinical care and to several maternal and infant outcomes, especially to birth weight. The emphasis on birth weight reflects its importance for child mortality, morbidity, and physical and mental performance. There is a relative lack of studies relating gestational weight gain to other important maternal and child health outcomes.

A central question is whether or not gestational weight gain is causally associated with pregnancy outcomes such as fetal growth and postpartum retention of adipose tissue. Potential causal relationships were examined by applying standard epidemiologic terms and concepts to characterize the relationships between maternal factors, nutritional intervention, gestational weight gain, and maternal and child health.

Factors that investigators have linked with gestational weight gain include maternal prepregnancy weight for height, prepregnancy weight, maternal height, ethnic background, age and parity, cigarette smoking, socioeconomic status, and energy intake. Analyses of data from the 1980 National Natality Survey made it possible to examine whether specified maternal characteristics are independently associated with weight gain. For example, the association between smoking and gestational weight gain can be tested while holding constant prepregnancy weight for height, ethnic origin, and other factors. However, even this large, relatively representative data set was not big enough for an examination of all the relationships of interest, such as the association of Hispanic origin with weight gain in obese women.

For certain analyses of data from the 1980 National Natality Survey, the subcommittee used a gestational duration of 39 to 41 weeks and a live birth weight of 3 to 4 kg as an operational definition of *favorable pregnancy outcome* (recognizing that a small percentage of such infants may have serious birth defects or other health problems). The use of this range for birth weight represents a balance between the benefits of increased fetal growth for the infant, on the one hand, and the possible risks to the mother and infant of complicated labor and delivery with high birth weight (>4 kg), on the other.

Historical Perspective

Between the 1960s and 1980s, it gradually became common to recommend a gestational weight gain averaging 11 kg (24 lb) or more, rather than the 8 to 9 kg (18 to 20 lb) or less recommended previously. This change was accompanied by a 50% increase in gestational weight gain. Between 1971 and 1980, mean birth weight increased by approximately 60 g for whites and 30 g for blacks, low birth weight (<2.5 kg) prevalence was reduced by about 20% for whites and 7% for blacks, and the high birth weight prevalence increased by 30% for whites and by 15% for blacks. Several factors that may also have contributed to fetal growth or gestational weight gain during the period include increased prepregnancy weight, increased height, decreased smoking during pregnancy, increased participation in the WIC program, and earlier prenatal care.

Conclusions on Weight Gain During Pregnancy

Assessment of Weight and Weight Gain

Prepregnancy weight-for-height and serial weight measurements are the only anthropometric measurements with documented clinical value for assessment of gestational weight gain. In the clinical setting, it is difficult for different individuals or even for the same person to obtain reproducible measurements of skinfold thicknesses. Even those skinfold thickness measurements that are reliable are not useful clinically, because there are no properly validated equations that use skinfold thicknesses to predict the total body composition of pregnant women, nor are there reference standards for skinfold thickness measurements validated against fetal outcomes.

Body mass index (BMI), defined as weight/height^2, is a better indicator of maternal nutritional status than is weight alone. The subcommittee used metric units (kilograms and meters) to calculate the BMIs used in this report. Weight for height expressed as a percentage of a standard is also usable. Since none of the weight-for-height classification schemes has been validated against pregnancy outcome, any cutoff points will be arbitrary for women of reproductive age. However, the subcommittee agreed on the following weight-for-height categories:

- underweight: BMI <19.8
- normal weight: BMI 19.8 to 26.0
- overweight: BMI >26.0 to 29.0
- obese: BMI >29.0

The cutoff points generally correspond to 90, 120, and 135% of the 1959

Metropolitan Life Insurance Company's weight-for-height standards (Metropolitan Life Insurance Company, 1959)—the standards which have been in most common use in the United States.

Although specific weight gain grids have substantial limitations, most are useful in the clinical setting because they permit visual tracking of weight gain by week of gestation. That is, they provide the practitioner with a visual impression of the progress of weight gain and simplify detection of an abnormal change in weight over time. Studies indicate that after the first trimester, the typical pattern of weight gain is one of gradual, steady increments, but definitive studies have not yet been conducted to determine what rates of gain are most desirable for favorable maternal and fetal outcomes and whether the optimal pattern of gain varies over the second and third trimesters. The subcommittee concluded that heavy emphasis should be placed on identifying major deviations in the rate of gain that may signal problems and warrant further assessment, as opposed to deviations related to errors in measurement or recording or to common shifts in weight related to fluid changes, contents of bladder and bowel, clothing, and time of day. Deviations from the expected pattern of weight gain may be entirely unrelated to nutrient intake and energy balance but, rather, may be related to such factors as those listed above.

Gestational weight gain is normally attributable to increases in both lean and fat tissue of the mother and the fetus as well as to water retention. Most methods for assessing body composition (e.g., underwater weighing and total body water) are based on assumptions that have not been validated for pregnant women and that may not be applicable because they do not distinguish between the added maternal and fetal tissues. As a result, different methods yield inconsistent results when applied in a research setting to the same population of pregnant women. Smooth, progressive weight gain generally represents a gain of lean and fat tissue, whereas erratically high weight gain is likely to represent excessive fluid retention. The clinical determination of ankle or leg edema (which worsens on standing) or generalized edema (which is not dependent on body position) can be useful in identifying extra fluid retention. However, it provides insufficient quantitative information about the amount of fluid that has been gained.

Determinants of Gestational Weight Gain

Prepregnancy weight for height is a determinant of gestational weight gain. On average, women who are overweight at conception (i.e., women whose BMI exceeds 26.0) gain less weight during pregnancy than do thinner women. However, there is wide variation in weight gain by women with normal pregnancies within each prepregnancy weight-for-height category. The variation is highest among obese women (BMI >29.0).

Some of the other maternal characteristics associated with an increased risk of low gestational weight gain (less than 7 kg, or 16 lb) occur in combination, e.g., low family income, black race, young age, unmarried status, and low educational level. These characteristics are also associated with shortened gestational duration. Studies using analytic methods to control for gestational duration and other factors suggest that black women are more likely to have low weight gain than are white women, but the reason for this difference is not known. Some ethnic groups with small average body size (e.g., Southeast Asians) have been reported to have low average weight gains, but the clinical significance of this has not been established.

In studies of groups of women in the United States and elsewhere, energy intake is a determinant of gestational weight gain, but the reported relationship is weak. Changes in energy intake during pregnancy are difficult to detect because they are relatively small, on average, and current dietary assessment methods are rather imprecise. Variation in energy intake during pregnancy is determined largely by body size and the level of physical activity, not by gestational weight gain. Furthermore, energy intake may erroneously appear to be relatively unimportant for gestational weight gain if women expend less energy by decreasing their physical activity. Overall, however, there is no question that restriction of energy intake can limit weight gain or that excessive energy intake leads to extra fat storage.

The impact of food supplementation on gestational weight gain (and fetal growth) appears to depend on the prior energy deficit of the woman and the extent to which the supplement makes up for the deficit between usual energy intake and requirements. That is, the impact is greater in women with low prepregnancy weight for height or in women whose food intake has been restricted.

Consequences of Gestational Weight Gain

Wide variation is seen in weight gains among women giving birth to live, optimally grown (i.e., 3 to 4 kg at 39 to 41 weeks of gestation) infants. For example, in the United States in 1980, the 15th and 85th percentiles of weight gain were 7.3 and 18.2 kg (16 and 40 lb), respectively, for normal-weight women who delivered babies with these characteristics. This wide variation indicates that many factors in addition to weight gain during pregnancy contribute to a favorable outcome. Nevertheless, a large body of evidence indicates that gestational weight gain, particularly during the second and third trimesters, is an important determinant of fetal growth. Low gestational weight gain is associated with an increased risk of giving birth to a growth-retarded infant. This has important adverse consequences for subsequent somatic growth and, possibly, neurobehavioral development, and it increases the risk of infant mortality. (More direct evidence also indicates a link between low weight gain and fetal and infant mortality.) The effect of first-trimester weight gain or weight loss on fetal growth is less clear, because the weight change is usually small, and because very few studies have included women in this trimester of pregnancy.

The effect of gestational weight gain on fetal growth is modified by the mother's prepregnancy weight for height. Several epidemiologic studies, including the 1980 National Natality Survey, have convincingly demonstrated that the effect of a given weight gain (or rate of weight gain) is greatest in thin women and least in overweight and obese women. However, prepregnancy weight for height is a determinant of fetal growth above and beyond the effect of gestational weight gain: women who are thinner before pregnancy tend to have babies that are smaller than those of their heavier counterparts with the *same* gestational weight gain. Since higher birth weights generally present lower risks for the infants, desirable weight gains for thin women are higher than those for normal-weight women, whereas desirable weight gains for overweight and obese women are lower. Among obese women, the measured effect of weight gain on birth weight is weak.

Most epidemiologic evidence suggests that maternal age does not modify the effect of weight gain on fetal growth. Very young adolescents (less than 2 years postmenarche) may, however, give birth to smaller infants for a given weight gain than do older women. Although the limited data indicate no clear modification of the effect by racial or ethnic background, black infants tend to be smaller than white infants for the same gestational weight gain of the mothers. Young girls and black women should therefore strive for weight gains toward the upper end of the ranges otherwise recommended for women with similar weights for height.

Data concerning the effect of changes in maternal body composition on fetal growth are meager and inconclusive. Studies suggest that increases in maternal fat, lean tissue, and body water may each be associated with increased fetal growth.

Very high gestational weight gain is associated with an increased rate of high birth weight which in turn is associated with some increase in the risk of fetopelvic disproportion, operative delivery (forceps or cesarean delivery), birth trauma, and asphyxia and mortality. These associations appear to be more pronounced in short women, i.e., <157 cm (62 in.). A lower ceiling on weight gain may therefore be preferable in short women at any given weight for height.

Energy supplementation of pregnant women whose usual energy intake is low relative to their needs may result in slightly higher average birth weights and decreased incidence of intrauterine growth retardation, although concurrent increases in gestational weight gain have not always been observed.

Several, but not all, reports suggest that low rates of gestational weight gain are associated with a shorter mean gestational duration and an increased risk of preterm delivery. Difficulties in determining the length of gestation and assessing weight gain patterns prevent firm inferences, however.

Gestational weight gain does not seem to be an important determinant of spontaneous abortion (miscarriage), congenital anomalies, maternal mortality, pregnancy-induced hypertension and preeclampsia, or volume or composition of milk produced during lactation. However, a sharp increase in weight accompanied by generalized edema and an elevated blood pressure remain the hallmarks of preeclampsia, a complication of pregnancy that requires immediate attention.

On average, each successive birth adds about 1 kg (2.2 lb) of postpartum body weight above that normally gained with age. This gain is likely to be surpassed, however, in women with high gestational weight gains.

In women carrying multiple fetuses, mean gestational weight gain appears to be greater by an amount larger than that accounted for by the weight of the additional fetuses and support tissues. In twin pregnancies, increased maternal weight gain also appears to be associated with increased birth weight.

Clinical Recommendations

The following recommendations are based largely on observational studies of weight gains in large groups of women and an attempt to balance the benefits of increased fetal growth with the risks of complicated labor and delivery and of postpartum maternal weight retention. In the absence of definitive data regarding optimal gestational weight gain, the subcommittee concluded that the target range for desirable maternal weight gain should be based on prepregnancy weight for height and should include the mean weight gain for women delivering full-term babies weighing between 3 and 4 kg. However, because the observed range for such mothers is too broad to be useful clinically, the subcommittee used its judgment in setting narrower target ranges by weight-for-height categories.

Measurement

Health care providers should adopt specific, reliable procedures for obtaining and recording weight and height and should implement them consistently in classifying women according to weight for height, setting weight gain goals, and monitoring weight gain over the course of pregnancy. Attention should be directed to the following elements:

TABLE 1-1 Recommended Total Weight Gain Ranges for Pregnant Women,[a] by Prepregnancy Body Mass Index (BMI)[b]

Weight-for-Height Category	Recommended Total Gain	
	kg	lb
Low (BMI < 19.8)	12.5–18	28–40
Normal (BMI of 19.8 to 26.0)	11.5–16	25–35
High[c] (BMI > 26.0 to 29.0)	7–11.5	15–25

[a] Young adolescents and black women should strive for gains at the upper end of the recommended range. Short women (<157 cm, or 62 in.) should strive for gains at the lower end of the range.
[b] BMI is calculated using metric units.
[c] The recommended target weight gain for obese women (BMI > 29.0) is at least 6.0 kg (15 lb).

• **Prior to conception use consistent and reliable procedures to accurately measure and record in the medical record the woman's weight and height without shoes.** These are the preferred bases for calculating prepregnancy weight for height.
• **Determine the woman's prepregnancy BMI.** The table in Appendix C simplifies this calculation. The weight-for-height classifications shown in Table 1-1 are recommended.
• **Measure height and weight at the first prenatal visit carefully by procedures that have been rigorously standardized at the site of prenatal care.** The initial weight measurement can be compared with prepregnancy weight and provides the baseline for monitoring weight change over the course of pregnancy. Measurement of height is recommended because objective data on height are often not recorded in the medical record.
• **Use consistent, reliable procedures to measure weight at each subsequent visit.**
• **Estimate the woman's gestational age from the onset of her last menstruation,** preferably supplemented by estimates based on the obstetric clinical examination and, perhaps, by early ultrasound examination.
• **Record weight in a table and plot it on a chart included in the obstetric record,** which should show the week of gestation on the horizontal axis and weight on the vertical axis. The subcommittee developed provisional charts (see Appendix B) showing the recommended target gain as the end points and the recommended rate of gain as the slope. Until a weight gain chart has been validated, the subcommittee favors use of these provisional charts. A notation should be made if gestational age is uncertain, since this can markedly affect placement of the woman's current

weight on the chart. The charts are not meant to imply that the weight gain of all women of the designated BMI group should fall on the dashed line. Rather, the rate of gain should approximately parallel that shown by the dashed line.

Counseling

During pregnancy a woman may be particularly receptive to guidance regarding behaviors that may influence her health and that of her developing fetus. The subcommittee recommends that women receive guidance regarding a healthy diet that will promote adequate weight gain. Sound dietary guidelines can be found in publications by federal agencies (e.g., DHHS/USDA/March of Dimes Birth Defects Foundation, 1982; USDA, 1979, 1989), by state agencies (e.g., Corruccini, 1977), and by private sources (e.g., American Red Cross, 1984; Dimperio, 1988).

• **Set a weight gain goal together with the pregnant woman, preferably beginning at the comprehensive initial prenatal examination, and explain to her why weight gain is important.** This goal is best identified as a range of desirable total gestational weight gain and the rate of such gain. The subcommittee emphasizes use of a range rather than a single target weight, because a wide range of gestational weight gains is compatible with desirable pregnancy outcomes, because there is no method available for establishing the ideal gestational weight gain for an individual woman, and because a range rather than a single number may help alleviate excessive concern about weight gain during pregnancy. All women should be encouraged to gain enough weight to achieve at least the lower limit of weight specified for their weight-for-height category in Table 1-1. To help the woman achieve her weight gain goal, she should be given appropriate counseling or referred (e.g., to a social worker, dietitian, or WIC) to promote consumption of a wholesome, balanced diet consistent with ethnic, cultural, and financial considerations.

• **Base the recommended range of total weight gain and pattern of gain mainly on prepregnancy weight for height.** The subcommittee recommends that women of normal prepregnancy weight for height carrying a single fetus aim for a weight gain of between 11.5 and 16 kg (25 and 35 lb). This range is higher than that recommended in previous Food and Nutrition Board reports, which recommended a range of 9 to 11.5 kg (20 to 25 lb). The basis of this higher recommendation is the reduced risk of delivering an infant with intrauterine growth retardation with higher weight gains. However, the risk of maternal weight retention postpartum and fetal macrosomia may increase with higher weight gains in this range.

A slightly higher target range of 13 to 18 kg (28 to 40 lb) is recommended for women with a low prepregnancy BMI (<19.8). For those with a high BMI (>26.0 to 29.0), the recommended range is lower—7 to 11.5 kg (15 to 25 lb). Short women should try to reach the lower end of the target weight gain range for their weight for height, and black and very young women should strive to gain weight at the upper end of the target range. Setting a realistic range for target weight at 40 weeks of gestation can be more of a problem if there is a question about the accuracy of prepregnancy weight. An appropriate approach for handling this situation is to determine gestational age and then focus on the rate of weight gain.

The subcommittee set a 6.8-kg (15-lb) lower limit on gestational weight gain by extremely obese women (BMI >29.0), but it recognizes that many obese women with good pregnancy outcomes do gain less weight. Obese women should be encouraged to consume moderate amounts of nutritious food and a sufficient quantity of essential nutrients. All obese women should receive an individual dietary assessment and nutritional counseling.

The recommended target total weight gain at term for women carrying twins is 16 to 20.5 kg (35 to 45 lb). There are insufficient data at this time to warrant different target gains based on prepregnancy BMI in a twin gestation.

- **For women with a normal prepregnancy BMI, recommend gain at the rate of approximately 0.4 kg (~1 lb) per week in the second and third trimesters of pregnancy.** Underweight women (BMI <19.8) should strive to gain weight at a somewhat higher rate, i.e., 0.5 kg (or slightly more than 1 lb) per week, and overweight women (BMI 26.0 to 29.0) should strive to gain weight at a somewhat lower rate of 0.3 kg (0.66 lb) per week. The target rate for extremely obese women should be determined on an individual basis.

Monitoring Progress

Periodic prenatal care provides health care workers with opportunities for identifying potential problems and intervening early when indicated. The monitoring of weight gain is a key part of this process.

- **Monitor the prenatal course to identify any abnormal pattern of gain that may indicate a need to intervene. Assess the pattern of gain at each visit relative to the established weight gain goal and the course leading to that goal.** A slightly lower or higher rate of weight gain than that recommended is not cause for alarm, as long as there is a progressive increase in weight that approximately equals the recommended rate of gain. Reasons for marked or persistent deviations from the expected pattern of gain should be investigated. In particular, gains of less than 0.5 kg (1 lb) *per month* for obese women and less than 1 kg (2 lb) *per month* for women of normal weight require further evaluation. Gains greater than 3 kg (6.5 lb) per month may also benefit from evaluation, especially after week 20 of gestation, but they should not be viewed as a reason to curb food intake sharply. Possible reasons for deviations from the normal pattern of gain include, in addition to inadequate or excessive food intake, measurement or recording errors, differences in clothing or time of day, accumulation of fluid, and multiple gestations. Health care providers are encouraged to assess the extent to which inaccuracies in measurement may have contributed to a seemingly abnormal rate of weight gain and to take corrective action.

• **When abnormal gain appears to be real, rather than a result of an error in measurement or recording, try to determine the cause and then develop and implement corrective actions jointly with the woman.** For example, if a multiple gestation is identified, it would be advisable to revise the weight gain goal upward and support efforts to increase weight accumulation. If it appears that a lower than recommended weight gain is the result of an inadequate food supply or inappropriate self-restriction, corrective measures should be taken promptly. If evidence indicates that the abnormally high weight gain probably resulted from overeating, it would still be appropriate to revise the total weight gain goal upward to allow for the recommended rate of weight gain, but in this case it would be desirable to provide counseling to moderate food intake. Physical activity patterns should also be evaluated, and women should be encouraged to undertake or continue appropriate levels of activity.

Research Recommendations

The following research needs were identified during the literature review and subsequent discussions. These are not presented in order of priority. The subcommittee encourages investigators to give careful consideration to methodologic problems related to estimates of gestational weight gain, prepregnancy weight for height, and gestational duration (discussed in Chapter 4) when designing studies and interpreting results.

Epidemiologic Research

• Examine the effect of gestational weight gain (and the pattern of gain) on preterm delivery.
• Examine the relationships between weight gain and maternal health.
• Investigate the relationship between high gestational weight gain and subsequent maternal obesity.
• Identify the effects of overall gestational weight gain, weight gain patterns, and composition of gained tissue on pregnancy outcomes within specific ethnic groups and among very young women and women over age 35.

• Identify the characteristics of women who would benefit from increased energy intake.

• Examine the effects of energy intake and weight gain on maternal and perinatal outcomes in markedly or moderately obese women.

• Explore the use of different measures of gestational weight gain (e.g., net weight gain and rate of weight gain) in research on gestational weight gain and pregnancy outcomes.

Basic Research

• Determine the incremental dietary energy needs for pregnancy by measuring energy stores and expenditures over the course of gestation.

• Identify appropriate animal models to use in investigations of the role of nutrition in human pregnancy, considering the number of fetuses, type of placentation, maturity of the fetus at delivery, body composition, and physiologic adaptations such as plasma volume expansion.

• Investigate the influence of energy intake and prepregnancy weight-for-height status on patterns of gain of fat, lean, water, and total weight by using longitudinal studies beginning before conception and continuing throughout gestation. This requires research to develop new methods or modify existing ones for measuring body composition accurately during pregnancy.

• Identify the hormonal and biochemical determinants of weight gain pattern and composition.

Applied Research

• Develop and validate protocols and standards for use in the clinical setting. For example, establish cutoff values for prepregnancy BMIs as they relate to gestational weight gain and maternal and fetal outcomes.

• Develop a clinically useful weight gain chart and validate it against outcome data.

• Improve methods of prenatal nutritional surveillance for public health purposes. For example, include prepregnancy weight and height on birth certificates and standardize assessment and reporting instruments used in government programs such as WIC.

• Test recommended ranges of gestational weight gain against outcomes.

• Test the effectiveness of specific interventions that are used to improve weight gain.

PART II: DIETARY INTAKE AND NUTRIENT SUPPLEMENTS

In the United States, vitamin and mineral supplementation is common, especially among pregnant women. The Subcommittee on Dietary Intake and Nutrient Supplements During Pregnancy and the parent committee consider food as the optimal vehicle for delivering nutrients and nutrient supplementation as an intervention. As with other types of intervention, a recommendation to supplement the diet with special vitamin, mineral, or protein preparations should be based on evidence of a benefit as well as a lack of harmful effects.

In addressing the advisability of supplementation, the subcommittee first reviewed biochemical, anthropometric, clinical, and dietary methods for measuring the adequacy of specific nutrients during pregnancy. It then identified nutrients that can be provided in adequate amounts by dietary means and those for which supplementation may be desirable. Special attention was directed toward protein, folate, iron, zinc, calcium, and vitamins that might exert toxic effects if taken in high doses. Evidence was sought concerning special recommendations for pregnant women of black, Hispanic, and Southeast Asian origin and for women in their teens or over age 35. Evidence regarding the potential value of periconceptional multivitamin supplements in the prevention of neural tube defects was evaluated. The interaction of diet with use of tobacco, alcohol, and caffeine was also reviewed. In view of the widespread use of marijuana, the epidemic of cocaine use among women of childbearing years, and cocaine's major adverse effects on health, the consideration of nonfood substances was enlarged to include those illegal drugs.

Specific recommendations for nutrition counseling and other services to help improve maternal and family food intakes are beyond the scope of this report. Among the many sources of information on these topics are the National Center for Education in Maternal and Child Health in Washington, D.C., Cooperative Extension's Expanded Food and Nutrition Education Program (operated at the county level), state WIC programs, state departments of health, the American Red Cross, and the American College of Obstetricians and Gynecologists.

Methodology

To determine whether nutrient supplements should be recommended during pregnancy, the subcommittee examined several lines of evidence. These included the results of controlled experimental studies of nutrient requirements of women, laboratory studies and functional tests of nutrient status, epidemiologic studies linking diet or supplement use with various pregnancy outcomes, dietary intake data, and in some cases, studies in which animal models were used to examine the effects of nutrient deficiency or excess.

In its initial deliberations, the subcommittee determined that it would limit its review to trace elements and vitamins for which a human requirement has been established and to calcium, magnesium, and protein. Protein is not an ingredient of vitamin-mineral preparations but is available in special powders and formulas as a dietary supplement. Essential micronutrients excluded from consideration were phosphorus, sodium, chloride, and potassium—all of which are widely available in foods but are not ordinarily included in multivitamin-mineral preparations.

Limitations in the Data

Maternal physiologic changes during pregnancy affect the results of laboratory tests and of tests reflecting how well the body is functioning (e.g., enzyme activity and cellular uptake of nutrients). Reference standards and cutoff points for laboratory and functional tests are affected by normal pregnancy to degrees that vary with the stage of gestation.

Review of dietary intake data provides one method of determining which nutrients warrant close attention. Less likely candidates for routine supplementation are nutrients consumed at levels close to the 1989 Recommended Dietary Allowance (RDA) for pregnant women, especially if there is no evidence that a sizable segment of the pregnant population has intake falling substantially below the RDA. On the other hand, average nutrient intakes lower than the RDA were viewed as inadequate evidence to support routine supplementation of pregnant women with that nutrient. Because the RDAs for most minerals and vitamins include a wide margin of safety, the needs of many pregnant women can be met with intakes below the RDA. Moreover, estimates of nutrient intake based on dietary intake data are imprecise and tend to underestimate total food and nutrient intake. The data indicate that, on average, dietary intake by pregnant women is less than the RDA for eight nutrients: vitamins B_6, D, E, and folate; iron; zinc; calcium; and magnesium.

Since nutrient supplements typically contain multiple nutrients, there is the potential for nutrient-nutrient interactions during absorption and metabolism. An increase in the concentration of one nutrient may adversely affect the availability, absorption, or utilization of other nutrients provided by the supplement and by diet.

The use of such substances as tobacco, alcohol, caffeine or coffee, marijuana, and cocaine may affect maternal nutrition in two general ways.

The substance may increase the actual need for one or more nutrients by a variety of mechanisms, for example, by increasing urinary excretion, or it may lead to undesirable changes in food and nutrient intake.

Criteria Used in Formulating Recommendations

The subcommittee decided to recommend routine supplementation only if the usual dietary intake of the nutrient is likely to be low enough to limit the production of compounds essential for body function or to adversely affect the health of the mother, fetus, or newborn and if supplementation poses no known dangers for the mother or fetus. Data on nutrient interactions were considered in formulating recommendations for specific nutrients and combinations of nutrients. In the subcommittee's view, dietary supplements should not replace dietary counseling or a well-balanced diet. Improvement of diet quality through use of nutritious foods is strongly preferred to supplementation. Foods supply energy and essential nutrients not found in supplements, and there is less risk of undesirable nutrient-nutrient interactions when nutrients are provided by foods. Nonetheless, certain situations may warrant use of a multivitamin-mineral supplement, as described later in this chapter.

Conclusions

The subcommittee concluded that evaluation of a pregnant woman's dietary pattern by a food history or food frequency questionnaire, augmented by questions about special problems or conditions that might affect her dietary adequacy or needs, may provide the best information on which to assess the need for nutrient supplementation. Except for tests for hemoglobin (or hematocrit) and, possibly, serum ferritin, it is impractical to use other laboratory and functional tests to assess nutrient status in routine prenatal care.

After an in-depth review of dietary intake data for women in the United States and evidence from clinical, metabolic, and epidemiologic studies, the subcommittee concluded that iron is the only known nutrient for which requirements cannot be met reasonably by diet alone. To meet the increased need for iron during the second and third trimesters of pregnancy, the average woman needs to absorb approximately 3 mg of iron per day in addition to the amount of iron usually absorbed from food. Evidence from iron absorption studies indicates that low-dose supplements (e.g., 30 mg of ferrous iron daily) can provide this amount of extra iron.

Two lines of evidence contributed to the conclusion that supplementation with iron is advisable: need for iron is high in relation to usual dietary supply, and iron-supplemented pregnant women have higher hemoglobin levels than do unsupplemented women. Iron meets the subcommittee's criterion that intake is likely to be low enough to limit the production of a compound—hemoglobin—that is essential for body function. Evidence that iron deficiency adversely affects maternal and fetal health is only suggestive. Because iron at low doses poses no known dangers to the mother or fetus, the subcommittee concluded that in populations that commonly have iron deficiency, the potential benefits of iron supplementation outweigh the risks. Low-dose iron supplements offer distinct advantages over higher-dose ones: less potential for undesirable nutrient-nutrient interactions, more efficient absorption, and less risk of causing gastrointestinal distress.

Pregnant women can meet the physiologic requirements for folate from diet by following dietary guidelines such as those provided in the publications listed at the end of this chapter (American Red Cross, 1984; Corruccini, 1977; DHHS/USDA/March of Dimes Birth Defects Foundation, 1982; Dimperio, 1988; USDA, 1979, 1989). Folate deficiency now appears to be very rare among pregnant women in the United States. The extent to which the common practice of folate supplementation has contributed to the rarity of this deficiency is unknown. In the past, particularly during the 1950s and 1960s, folate deficiency was identified in some women in industrialized nations, including the United States and the United Kingdom. Pending further research, the subcommittee considers it prudent to supplement the diet with low amounts of folate if there is any question of adequacy of intake of this nutrient.

Evidence is not sufficient to conclude that routine supplementation with other nutrients is warranted, although clearly there are situations requiring special consideration. For example, certain dietary practices that restrict or prohibit the consumption of an important source of nutrients, such as avoidance of all animal foods or of vitamin D-fortified milk, increase the risk of inadequate nutrient intake. In such cases, if diet quality cannot be improved through better food selection, selective supplementation may be desirable. There is evidence that women carrying more than one fetus and those who use cigarettes, alcohol, or illicit drugs have increased requirements for certain nutrients. Furthermore, adolescents and drug users often follow dietary practices that lead to low intakes of a number of nutrients.

Because protein is abundant in usual diets in the United States and because of evidence suggesting possible harm from routine ingestion of specially formulated high-protein supplements, the use of special protein powders or formulated high-protein beverages should be discouraged.

However, there is no contraindication to increased use of food sources of protein such as milk and flesh foods as part of a well-balanced diet, especially because these foods are also rich sources of vitamins and minerals.

Although some studies in nonpregnant populations suggest that caffeine intake may decrease the availability of certain nutrients such as calcium, zinc, and iron, there is only inconsistent and fragmentary evidence that the consumption of coffee or caffeine during pregnancy exerts adverse effects on the fetus. It nevertheless appears sensible to limit the consumption of caffeine-containing products during pregnancy, although data are insufficient for setting a specific limit on intake or for recommending nutrient supplementation for women who continue to consume caffeine during pregnancy.

Special recommendations on the basis of ethnic background alone do not seem to be warranted at present. There is no evidence of substantial differences in nutrient requirements among various ethnic groups, but ethnic differences in food choices and, consequently, in the mean intake of certain nutrients do exist. For example, because ethnic groups with a high prevalence of lactose intolerance customarily consume relatively low amounts of milk, their intakes of calcium and vitamin D deserve special attention.

The adequacy of calcium and vitamin D intake among pregnant women under age 25 also deserves special attention, since bone mineral density is still increasing during that period of life. For older women who become pregnant, there is no evidence that high calcium intake will protect against later bone loss caused by osteoporosis.

There is some evidence that periconceptional use of multivitamins or folate may provide some protection against the occurrence of neural tube defects. Data to support a recommendation to use periconceptional vitamins for this purpose are not conclusive at this time.

Because of accumulating data that excessive vitamin A consumption poses a teratogenic risk, supplementation with preformed vitamin A should be avoided during the first trimester unless there is specific evidence of a deficiency. Carotene intake need not be restricted.

Clinical Recommendations

Dietary Assessment

Routine assessment of dietary practices is recommended for all pregnant women in the United States to allow evaluation of the need for improved diet or vitamin or mineral supplements.

Iron

For the general population of pregnant women, supplements of 30 mg of ferrous iron are recommended daily during the second and third trimesters. This amount of ferrous iron is provided, for example, by approximately 150 mg of ferrous sulfate, 300 mg of ferrous gluconate, or 100 mg of ferrous fumarate. Administration between meals or at bedtime on an empty stomach will facilitate iron absorption, but taking ascorbic acid with supplements containing ferrous iron does not enhance iron absorption.

Folate

Although routine folate supplementation of pregnant women is not recommended, a supplement of 300 μg/day may be given when there are doubts about the adequacy of dietary folate. Women who ingest fruit, juices, whole-grain or fortified cereals, and green vegetables infrequently are likely to have low folate intake.

Multivitamin Mineral Supplements

For pregnant women who do not ordinarily consume an adequate diet and for those in high-risk categories, such as women carrying more than one fetus, heavy cigarette smokers, and alcohol and drug abusers, the subcommittee recommends a daily multivitamin-mineral preparation containing the following nutrients beginning in the second trimester:

Iron	30 mg	Vitamin B_6	2 mg
Zinc	15 mg	Folate	300 μg
Copper	2 mg	Vitamin C	50 mg
Calcium	250 mg	Vitamin D	5 μg

To promote absorption of these nutrients, the supplement should be taken between meals or at bedtime.

Nutrient Supplementation in Special Circumstances

As mentioned above, supplementation of other nutrients may be desirable for certain pregnant women in the United States. The following are the subcommittee's recommendations for those special circumstances.

Vitamin D: 10 μg (400 IU) daily for complete vegetarians (those who consume no animal products at all) and others with a low intake of vitamin D-fortified milk. Vitamin D status is a special concern for women at northern latitudes in winter and for others with minimal exposure to sunlight and thus reduced synthesis of vitamin D in the skin.

Calcium: 600 mg daily for women under age 25 whose daily dietary calcium intake is less than 600 mg. To enhance absorption and limit interaction with iron supplements, the calcium supplement should be taken at mealtime. There is no evidence that older pregnant women (i.e., those over age 35) have a special need for supplemental calcium.

Vitamin B_{12}: 2.0 μg daily for complete vegetarians.

Zinc and copper: When therapeutic levels of iron (>30 mg/day) are given to treat anemia, supplementation with approximately 15 mg of zinc and 2 mg of copper is recommended because the iron may interfere with the absorption and utilization of those trace elements.

Research Recommendations

Survey Needs

• Representative data should be collected on the nutrient status of pregnant women and their usual dietary and supplement intake, especially with regard to iron and folate. Pregnant women should be oversampled in national surveys (e.g., the National Health and Nutrition Examination Survey and the Continuing Survey of Food Intake of Individuals) to improve the data base regarding health and usual nutrient intake in relation to age, income, and ethnic background.

Nutritional Assessment

• Special purpose longitudinal studies should be conducted from before pregnancy to parturition to relate food and nutrient intake of individual women to maternal and fetal nutritional status and pregnancy outcome. Priority should be given to iron; zinc; copper; calcium; magnesium; and vitamins D, B_6, and folate.

• Better practical diagnostic tests should be developed for detecting deficiencies of the following in pregnancy: folate, zinc, copper, vitamin B_6, calcium, and magnesium.

• Further work is needed to determine the intakes of nutrients by pregnant teenagers in specific age and economic groups and by women of different ethnic backgrounds.

• In view of the increasing number of women who bear more than one fetus, it is important to acquire data on their food and nutrient intakes in order to develop appropriate nutritional interventions.

• Strategies are needed for investigating the nutritional consequences of nausea, vomiting, and food cravings and aversions to provide data that are useful for determining the appropriateness of nutritional interventions for these conditions.

• Trials should be conducted to assess the effects of nutrient-nutrient interactions on the absorption and utilization of specific nutrients when they are included in multinutrient supplements.

Iron Supplementation

• Studies are needed on the prevention of iron deficiency without the use of iron supplements. Such methods would include counseling in the selection of diets to enhance iron absorption. The effectiveness of iron-fortified foods in preventing iron deficiency requires further study, and the improvement of fortification methods should be given a high priority.

• Randomized, controlled trials are recommended to study the effects of iron in 15- to 60-mg doses in different formulations that include iron compounds alone, with folate, and in multinutrient preparations.

Periconceptional Supplements

Further studies should be conducted to investigate the effectiveness of routine periconceptional use of vitamins and minerals in the prevention of birth defects.

Supplementation for High-Risk Groups

Possible benefits of vitamin-mineral supplementation should be studied for substance abusers, adolescents, and other groups at high risk of nutritional deficiency.

REFERENCES

American Red Cross. 1984. Better Eating for Better Health: Participant's Guide. I'm Pregnant: What Should I Eat? American Red Cross, Washington, D.C. 10 pp.

Corruccini, C.G. 1977. Nutrition for Pregnancy and Breast Feeding: Eating Right for Your Baby. Maternal and Child Health Branch, Family Health Services Section, California Department of Health Services, Sacramento, Calif. 20 pp.

DHHS (Department of Health and Human Services). 1989. Caring for Our Future: the Content of Prenatal Care. A Report of the Public Health Service Expert Panel on the Content of Prenatal Care. Public Health Service, U.S. Department of Health and Human Services, Washington, D.C. 125 pp.

DHHS/USDA/March of Dimes Birth Defects Foundation (Department of Health and Human Services/U.S. Department of Agriculture/March of Dimes Birth Defects Foundation). 1982. Food For the Teenager: During and After Pregnancy. DHHS Publ. No. (HRSA) 82-5106. Public Health Service, U.S. Department of Health and Human Services, Rockville, Md. 31 pp.

Dimperio, D. 1988. Prenatal Nutrition: Clinical Guidelines for Nurses. March of Dimes Birth Defects Foundation, White Plains, N.Y. 134 pp.

IOM (Institute of Medicine). 1985. Preventing Low Birthweight. Report of the Committee to Study the Prevention of Low Birthweight, Division of Health Promotion and Disease Prevention. National Academy Press, Washington, D.C. 284 pp.

IOM (Institute of Medicine). 1988. Prenatal Care: Reaching Mothers, Reaching Infants. Report of the Committee to Study Outreach for Prenatal Care, Division of Health Promotion and Disease Prevention. National Academy Press, Washington, D.C. 254 pp.

Metropolitan Life Insurance Company. 1959. New weight standards for men and women. Stat. Bull. Metrop. Life Insur. Co. 40:1-4.

NRC (National Research Council). 1970. Maternal Nutrition and the Course of Pregnancy. Report of the Committee on Maternal Nutrition, Food and Nutrition Board. National Academy of Sciences, Washington, D.C. 241 pp.

USDA (U.S. Department of Agriculture). 1979. Food. Home and Garden Bulletin No. 228. Science and Education Administration, Food and Nutrition Service, U.S. Department of Agriculture, Alexandria, Va. 65 pp.

USDA (U.S. Department of Agriculture). 1989. Preparing Foods & Planning Menus Using the Dietary Guidelines. Home and Garden Bulletin No. 232-8. Human Nutrition Information Service, U.S. Department of Agriculture. U.S. Government Printing Office, Washington, D.C. 31 pp.

PART I

NUTRITIONAL STATUS
AND
WEIGHT GAIN

2

Introduction

Efforts to improve maternal and fetal nutrition during pregnancy have focused on achieving appropriate energy intake and ensuring that the intake of specific nutrients is adequate to meet maternal and fetal requirements. Although the need for appropriate weight gain during pregnancy has long been recognized, clinical and public health recommendations for weight gain have changed over the years as new data have become available.

In the 1940s and 1950s it was standard practice in the United States to restrict weight gain during pregnancy to less than 9 kg (20 lb), with the intent of reducing the risk of toxemia and of birth complications that were believed to occur more often with larger babies. In 1967, the Food and Nutrition Board's (FNB's) Committee on Maternal Nutrition referred to a 10.9-kg (24-lb) average weight gain for pregnant women in the United States in *Nutrition in Pregnancy and Lactation* (NRC, 1967), a report transmitted to the Children's Bureau of the Department of Health, Education, and Welfare. Following publication of results from the Collaborative Perinatal Project (Eastman and Jackson, 1968), there was increased awareness that mothers who gained less than 9 kg had smaller babies who had poorer chances for survival. Shortly thereafter, the FNB's Committee on Maternal Nutrition completed a more comprehensive report entitled *Maternal Nutrition During the Course of Pregnancy* (NRC, 1970a), which reviewed problems, practices, and research bearing on the relation between nutrition and the course and outcome of pregnancy and provided recommendations for weight gain and intake of certain nutrients. That volume, along with

27

its companion *Summary Report* (NRC, 1970b), had a major impact on the medical and nutrition community.

Since publication of the 1970 report, a number of studies have shown that desirable weight gain during pregnancy varies as a function of prepregnancy weight for height (Abrams and Laros, 1986; Miller and Merritt, 1979; Naeye, 1979, 1981; Peckham and Christianson, 1971; Winikoff and Debrovner, 1981). In particular, the evidence suggests that in order to achieve optimal fetal growth, women with inadequate prepregnancy weight for height may need to gain more weight during pregnancy and that women who are overweight prior to pregnancy may not need to gain as much (Borberg et al., 1980; Brown, 1988; Brown et al., 1981; Campbell, 1983; Edwards et al., 1978; Gormican et al., 1980; Harrison et al., 1980). In light of these new data, it has been suggested that recommendations for nutritional guidelines during pregnancy should be revised to take prepregnancy nutritional status into account (Koops et al., 1982; Rosso, 1985).

In considering the relationship between gestational weight gain and pregnancy outcome, attention has centered on birth weight. One reason for this is that birth weight is the pregnancy outcome most frequently examined in epidemiologic studies. But a more fundamental justification for the emphasis on birth weight is its widely recognized association with infant mortality and morbidity.

The United States has lagged behind a number of other developed countries in reducing infant mortality, despite recent advances in perinatal intensive care and marked improvements in birth weight-specific mortality rates (McCormick, 1985; Wegman, 1988). The lag appears to be related to an unfavorable birth weight distribution and, in particular, a high proportion of infants with low (<2,500 g) and very low (<1,500 g) birth weights, particularly among blacks (Kessel et al., 1984; Kleinman and Kessel, 1987). Although in the United States most neonatal deaths (which account for most deaths in the first year of life) are related to preterm birth (i.e., <37 weeks of gestation), and although the effects of gestational weight gain on fetal growth are better documented than those on length of gestation (see Chapter 8), a shift in the distribution of birth weight for gestational age would nonetheless lead to some reduction in perinatal deaths (Prentice et al., 1988; Sappenfield et al., 1987).

The specific task assigned to the Subcommittee on Nutritional Status and Weight Gain During Pregnancy was to "evaluate and document the current scientific evidence and formulate recommendations for desirable weight gain during pregnancy." The subcommittee was asked to consider several issues in its deliberations and report, including the effect of prepregnancy nutritional status on overall weight gain and the patterns of weight gain, the effect of dietary intake during pregnancy on overall weight gain and patterns of weight gain, and the relative advantages and disadvantages

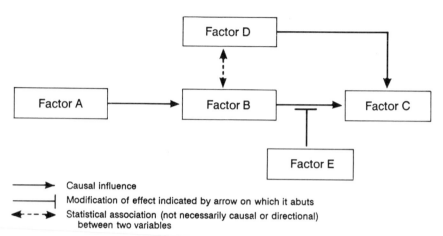

Causal influence
Modification of effect indicated by arrow on which it abuts
Statistical association (not necessarily causal or directional) between two variables

FIGURE 2-1   Schematic diagram of causal paths: determinants, consequences, confounders, and effect modifiers. Factor A is a *determinant* (cause) of Factor B, which, therefore, is a *consequence* (effect) of Factor A. Factor B is a determinant of Factor C. Therefore Factor A is also a determinant of Factor C. Factor B can be called a *mediating variable* by which Factor A causes Factor C. Alternatively, Factor A is sometimes referred to as an *indirect* determinant of Factor C, whereas Factor B is a *direct* determinant. Factor D is a *confounding variable* (confounder) in the relationship between Factors B and C, i.e., it biases (increases or decreases) the apparent effect of Factor B on Factor C. Because of this bias, the true effect of Factor B on Factor C is actually different from (less or more than) the apparent effect. Note that Factor B does *not* confound the relationship between Factors A and C, since it lies on the causal path between the two (see text). Factor E is an *effect modifier* in the relationship between Factors B and C, i.e., it modifies (increases or decreases) the true effect of Factor B on Factor C.

of various anthropometric methods for assessing nutritional status during pregnancy. In addition to the specific request to consider special recommendations for women with different prepregnancy nutritional statuses, the subcommittee was also asked to consider differential recommendations according to age and ethnic background, in particular the needs of pregnant adolescents; women over age 35; and women of black, Hispanic, and Southeast Asian origin.

The section that follows concerns the relationships among maternal factors, nutritional intervention, gestational weight gain, and maternal and child health in healthy women in a developed country (especially the United States). Standard epidemiologic terms and concepts are used to characterize these relationships (particularly as they relate to cause and effect) by making frequent reference to determinants, consequences, confounders, and effect modifiers. These concepts are illustrated in Figure 2-1.

Determinants are causal (etiologic) factors; *consequences* are the health outcomes caused by those determinants. The health outcomes considered in this report all have multifactorial etiologies; thus, no single factor is a sufficient cause of any of these outcomes. (The use of the word determinant, therefore, does not imply that a given factor automatically determines the outcome.) A given factor can be both a consequence of a factor that precedes it and a determinant of a factor that succeeds it (e.g., Factor B in Figure 2-1). Thus, gestational weight gain can be a consequence of energy intake during pregnancy and a determinant of fetal growth. The term *mediating variable* is sometimes used to indicate a factor that, like gestational weight gain, lies on the causal path between a preceding determinant (energy intake) and a subsequent consequence (fetal growth). Another way of expressing the same idea is to refer to a determinant (weight gain) immediately preceding a given consequence (fetal growth) as a *direct* determinant, and to an earlier factor on the causal path (energy intake) as an *indirect* determinant.

A *confounding variable* (confounder) distorts (biases up or down) the apparent relationship between an exposure (putative determinant) and outcome (putative consequence) under study; i.e., it makes the relationship appear stronger or weaker than it really is. This factor must fulfill three criteria:

• It must itself be a determinant of the outcome.
• It must be associated (without implying causality or directionality) with the exposure.
• It must not lie on the causal path between exposure and outcome.

As an example, energy intake is likely to confound the apparent relationship between maternal anemia and fetal growth. Women with low energy intake are also likely to have low iron intake. Energy intake is a likely determinant of fetal growth, but does not lie on the causal path between maternal anemia or iron status and fetal growth. Gestational weight gain does not confound the relationship between energy intake and fetal growth, even though it is associated with energy intake and is a determinant of fetal growth, because it lies on the causal path between the two.

An *effect modifier* is a factor that modifies (i.e., increases or decreases) the magnitude of the effect of a determinant on a particular consequence. Factor E in Figure 2-1 alters the degree to which Factor B affects Factor C. Thus, despite the apparent simplicity suggested by the causal arrow from Factor B to Factor C, the magnitude and perhaps even the existence of the causal effect depend on Factor E. Effect modifiers do not cause bias per se, but failure to consider effect modification by reporting only an overall effect can be extremely misleading. For example, if large weight gains were beneficial for thin women but deleterious for overweight women, there might not be a net effect in women examined overall. But this would hide the fact that there are important (and opposite) effects in the two subgroups. Unlike confounders, effect modifiers may have no association with either exposure (determinant) or outcome (consequence). The principal effect modifiers under consideration by the subcommittee are those that may alter the impact of gestational weight gain on pregnancy outcome: prepregnancy weight for height, age, and ethnic origin.

Figure 2-2 summarizes the potential determinants, consequences, and effect modifiers of gestational weight gain. Figure 2-3 presents the factors explicitly addressed in this report. It is essential to consider the determinants of gestational weight gain, because clinicians and public health policymakers cannot intervene directly to influence maternal weight gain during pregnancy. Nor do changing maternal attitudes have a direct impact on gestational weight gain, whether they arise from alterations in public awareness that filter into the community through media reports of research findings and expert opinions or from more formal health education efforts. Instead, interventions and attitude changes should be aimed at energy intake and expenditure. The resultant changes in energy balance would affect gestational weight gain. The consequences of physical activity and energy expenditure during pregnancy were reviewed by another FNB committee (IOM, 1989). The present report focuses on the intake component. The recommendations in Part I are intended to be used by clinicians in advising their patients on energy intake and gestational weight gain; by those involved in planning and implementing health education, counseling, and supplementation programs for pregnant women; and by those who deliver health messages to the general public, thereby increasing awareness and reshaping attitudes.

To gain an understanding of the consequences of different gestational weight gains for both mother and fetus, it is important to separate nutritional and nonnutritional contributions. As discussed in greater detail in subsequent chapters, many of the studies in this area have not distinguished changes in fat stores or lean body mass from weight increases as a result of increases in the size of the fetus, placenta, and amniotic fluid, on the one hand, or from increases in the size of the maternal breast and uterus and in plasma volume and extravascular body water, on the other. Ideally, in examining the maternal and child health consequences of different gestational weight gains, distinctions in components of weight gain should be considered.

As indicated above, the term *consequence* implies causality. Any association between gestational weight gain and subsequent maternal and child health outcomes will be most important to the extent that gestational weight gain is a cause of those outcomes. Any clinical or public health interventions to affect gestational weight gain will be ineffective in improving maternal and child health outcomes if the associations between weight

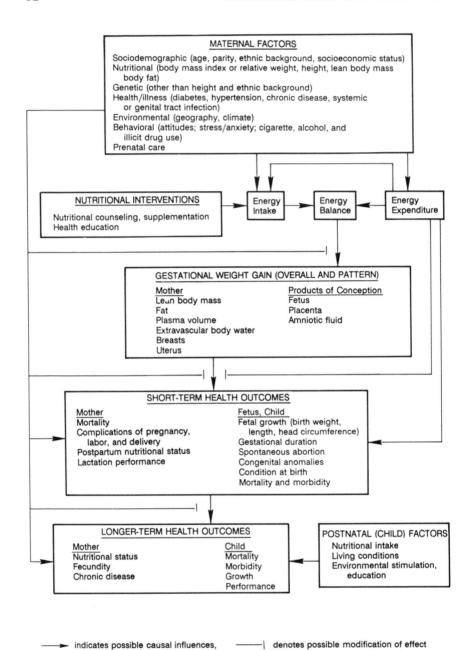

FIGURE 2-2 Schematic summary of potential determinants, consequences, and effect modifiers for gestational weight gain.

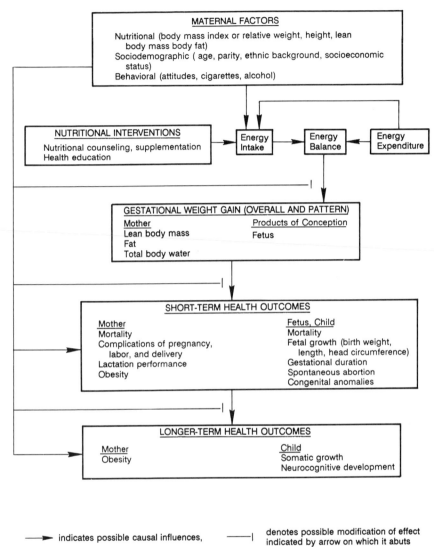

──▶ indicates possible causal influences, ────| denotes possible modification of effect indicated by arrow on which it abuts

FIGURE 2-3 Determinants, consequences, and effect modifiers discussed in this report.

gain and those outcomes are noncausal (or if the direction of causality is reversed). The elements used by the subcommittee to assess the epidemiologic evidence for causality are based on the report of the Surgeon General's Advisory Committee on Smoking and Health (DHEW, 1964), and on the work of Hill (1965) and Susser (1973, 1988). These elements include the strength, biologic gradient (dose-response effect), lack of bias, statistical significance, specificity, consistency, and biologic plausibility and coherence of the association.

In emphasizing gestational weight gain as a potential cause of maternal and fetal outcomes, the subcommittee in no way wishes to impugn its potential value as a *marker* of risk for adverse pregnancy outcome. For example, women with low gestational weight gain could be targeted for an intervention aimed at a modifiable causal determinant, e.g., cigarette smoking. Unfortunately, there are no data demonstrating the efficacy of this type of approach. Moreover, detailed consideration of interventions that do not have either a direct or indirect impact on gestational weight gain lies outside the mandate of the subcommittee.

The subcommittee has given considerable thought to the problem of reverse causality (discussed in greater detail in Chapter 10). A larger fetus and placenta and a greater volume of amniotic fluid will obviously lead to a larger maternal weight gain. It may even be that faster-growing fetuses provide a greater physiologic stimulus to increase maternal plasma and extracellular fluid volume. Another obvious, but surprisingly unappreciated, source of reverse causality is the effect of gestational age. Shorter pregnancies are, of course, associated with smaller total gestational weight gains. This does not necessarily indicate, however, that decreased total weight gain is a *cause* of shortened gestation. As discussed in Chapters 4 and 8, basing analyses on the rate of weight gain (e.g., grams of weight gained per week) is one way of adjusting for length of gestation.

It is important to distinguish short-term maternal and child outcomes from longer-term outcomes. Both may be worthy of consideration, but such short-term outcomes as early postpartum maternal nutritional status and birth weight are potentially less serious than longer-term maternal nutritional status and child morbidity, growth, and performance. Despite the importance the subcommittee attaches to these longer-term outcomes, however, the majority of the epidemiologic evidence concerning the effects of gestational weight gain bears on birth weight and fetal growth. The following nine chapters are based on the concepts summarized above. Chapter 3 provides a historical background, including secular trends in gestational weight gain, prepregnancy nutritional status, age at menarche, parity, cigarette smoking, birth weight, gestational age, and utilization of prenatal care and supplementation programs. Chapter 3 also contains a history of recommendations regarding weight gain and energy intake. Chapter 4 focuses on definitions and methodologic issues in the assessment of maternal weight gain and body composition in the clinical, research, and surveillance settings.

In Chapter 5, the subcommittee describes total weight gain and the pattern of weight gain over the course of pregnancy. It also examines physiologic and maternal determinants of gestational weight gain, including prepregnancy nutritional status, age, ethnic origin, cigarette smoking, parity, alcohol consumption, marital status, and work and physical activity. Chapter 6 summarizes knowledge about changes in body composition during pregnancy, including alterations in body fat, lean tissue, and body water. Energy requirements during pregnancy and the relationship between energy intake and gestational weight gain are considered in Chapter 7. In Chapter 8, the subcommittee reviews the evidence concerning the maternal and child health consequences of variations in gestational weight gain, including fetal/infant mortality, fetal growth, gestational duration, spontaneous abortion, congenital anomalies, maternal mortality, complications of pregnancy, lactation performance, and maternal obesity. Chapter 9 is a summary of the literature bearing on weight gain in twin gestations, including its description, determinants, and consequences.

Chapter 10 relates the material covered in Chapters 3 through 9 to the causal links in the overall conceptualization shown in Figure 2-3, with an emphasis on feasible interventions and their likely impact on short- and long-term maternal and child health. Chapter 1 presents the conclusions and recommendations reached by the subcommittee as a result of its research and deliberation.

REFERENCES

Abrams, B.F., and R.K. Laros, Jr. 1986. Prepregnancy weight, weight gain, and birth weight. Am. J. Obstet. Gynecol. 154:503-509.

Borberg, C., M.D.G. Gillmer, E.J. Brunner, P.J. Gunn, N.W. Oakley, and R.W. Beard. 1980. Obesity in pregnancy: the effect of dietary advice. Diabetes Care 3:476-481.

Brown, J.E. 1988. Weight gain during pregnancy: what is "optimal"? Clin. Nutr. 7:181-190.

Brown, J.E., H.N. Jacobson, L.H. Askue, and M.G. Peick. 1981. Influence of pregnancy weight gain on the size of infants born to underweight women. Obstet. Gynecol. 57:13-17.

Campbell, D.M. 1983. Dietary restriction in obesity and its effect on neonatal outcome. Pp. 243-250 in Nutrition in Pregnancy: Proceedings of the Tenth Study Group in the Royal College of Obstetricians and Gynaecologists, September, 1982. The Royal College of Obstetricians and Gynaecologists, London.

DHEW (Department of Health, Education, and Welfare). 1964. Smoking and Health: Report of the Advisory Committee to the Surgeon General of the Public Health Service. PHS Publ. No. 1103. Public Health Service, U.S. Department of Health, Education, and Welfare. U.S. Government Printing Office, Washington, D.C. 387 pp.

Eastman, N.J., and E. Jackson. 1968. Weight relationships in pregnancy: I. The bearing of maternal weight gain and pre-pregnancy weight on birth weight in full term pregnancies. Obstet. Gynecol. Surv. 23:1003-1025.

Edwards, L.E., W.F. Dickes, I.R. Alton, and E.Y. Hakanson. 1978. Pregnancy in the massively obese: course, outcome, and obesity prognosis of the infant. Am. J. Obstet. Gynecol. 131:479-483.

Gormican, A., J. Valentine, and E. Satter. 1980. Relationships of maternal weight gain, prepregnancy weight, and infant birthweight. Interaction of weight factors in pregnancy. J. Am. Diet. Assoc. 77:662-667.

Harrison, G.G., J.N. Udall, and G. Morrow III. 1980. Maternal obesity, weight gain in pregnancy, and infant birth weight. Am. J. Obstet. Gynecol. 136:411-412.

Hill, A.B. 1965. The environment and disease: association or causation? Proc. R. Soc. Med. 58:295-300.

IOM (Institute of Medicine). 1989. The Impact of Diet and Physical Activity on Pregnancy and Lactation: Women's Work in the Developing World. Report of the Subcommittee on Diet, Physical Activity, and Pregnancy Outcome, Committee on International Nutrition Programs, Food and Nutrition Board. Report transmitted to the Office of Nutrition, Bureau for Science and Technology, U.S. Agency for International Development, Washington, D.C. 129 pp.

Kessel, S.S., J. Villar, H.W. Berendes, and R.P. Nugent. 1984. The changing pattern of low birth weight in the United States: 1970 to 1980. J. Am. Med. Assoc. 251:1978-1982.

Kleinman, J.C., and S.S. Kessel. 1987. Racial differences in low birth weight: trends and risk factors. N. Engl. J. Med. 317:749-753.

Koops, B.L., L.J. Morgan, and F.C. Battaglia. 1982. Neonatal mortality risk in relation to birth weight and gestational age: update. J. Pediatr. 101:969-977.

McCormick, M.C. 1985. The contribution of low birth weight to infant mortality and childhood morbidity. N. Engl. J. Med. 312:82-90.

Miller, H.C., and T.A. Merritt. 1979. Fetal Growth in Humans. Year Book Medical Publishers, Chicago. 180 pp.

Naeye, R.L. 1979. Weight gain and the outcome of pregnancy. Am. J. Obstet. Gynecol. 135:3-9.

Naeye, R.L. 1981. Maternal nutrition and pregnancy outcome. Pp. 89-111 in J. Dobbing, ed. Maternal Nutrition in Pregnancy: Eating for Two? Academic Press, London.

NRC (National Research Council). 1967. Nutrition in Pregnancy and Lactation. Report of the Committee on Maternal Nutrition, Food and Nutrition Board. National Academy of Sciences, Washington, D.C. 67 pp.

NRC (National Research Council). 1970a. Maternal Nutrition and the Course of Pregnancy. Report of the Committee on Maternal Nutrition, Food and Nutrition Board. National Academy of Sciences, Washington, D.C. 241 pp.

NRC (National Research Council). 1970b. Maternal Nutrition and the Course of Pregnancy: Summary Report. Report of the Committee on Maternal Nutrition, Food and Nutrition Board. National Academy of Sciences, Washington, D.C. 23 pp.

Peckham, C.H., and R.E. Christianson. 1971. The relationship between prepregnancy weight and certain obstetric factors. Am. J. Obstet. Gynecol. 111:1-7.

Prentice, A.M., T.J. Cole, and R.G. Whitehead. 1988. Food supplementation in pregnant women. Eur. J. Clin. Nutr. 42:87-91.

Rosso, P. 1985. A new chart to monitor weight gain during pregnancy. Am. J. Clin. Nutr. 41:644-652.

Sappenfield, W.M., J.W. Buehler, N.J. Binkin, C.J.R. Hogue, L.T. Strauss, and J.C. Smith. 1987. Differences in neonatal and postneonatal mortality by race, birth weight, and gestational age. Public Health Rep. 102:182-192.

Susser, M. 1973. Causal Thinking in the Health Sciences: Concepts and Strategies of Epidemiology. Oxford University Press, New York. 181 pp.

Susser, M. 1988. Falsification, verification and causal inference in epidemiology: reconsiderations in the light of Sir Karl Popper's philosophy. Pp. 33-57 in K.J. Rothman, ed. Causal Inference. Epidemiology Resources, Chestnut Hill, Mass.

Wegman, M.E. 1988. Annual summary of vital statistics—1987. Pediatrics 82:817-827.

Winikoff, B., and C.H. Debrovner. 1981. Anthropometric determinants of birth weight. Obstet. Gynecol. 58:678-684.

3
Historical Trends in Clinical Practice, Maternal Nutritional Status, and the Course and Outcome of Pregnancy

Improvement of maternal and fetal health and nutrition has been a public health goal since the beginning of organized medicine. As knowledge has accumulated over time, standard clinical practices, attitudes, and beliefs regarding prenatal care and nutrition have changed. Furthermore, the socioeconomic status of the U.S. population has improved along with technological advancements. Changes in clinical practice and socioeconomic status undoubtedly have influenced the nutrition and health of women entering and during their pregnancies, as well as both maternal and fetal outcomes. The following review of historical trends provides a foundation for evaluating current standards of practice and relationships between those standards and gestational weight gain and pregnancy outcome.

TRENDS IN RECOMMENDATIONS

Over the past century, there have been substantial changes in recommendations made to women about weight gain during pregnancy. In the sixteenth, seventeenth, and eighteenth centuries, much emphasis was placed on the maternal diet since the mother was known to be the only source of nutrients for the fetus (Rosso and Cramoy, 1979). In the nineteenth century, the idea that pregnant women should not overeat became a recurrent theme. Overeating was believed to be a cause of large babies and, as a consequence, more difficult labors. In a period when maternal mortality was extremely high and cesarean deliveries were a desperate alternative, limitation of fetal size by restricting maternal food intakes was an

37

understandable goal. This formed the basis for the first published study of diet and pregnancy (Prochownick, 1901). This report showed that restricted food intake throughout pregnancy reduced the birth weights of males by approximately 400 g and those of females by 500 g.

In the 1920s in the United States, Davis (1923) reported that maternal weight gain could be used as an indicator of maternal nutritional status and that, in turn, maternal nutritional status influenced fetal growth. Mean birth weight increased with increasing gestational weight gain from approximately 3,100 g with a 7-kg (15-lb) gain to about 3,600 g with a 13.6-kg (30-lb) gain.

Following publication of these and successive studies, documentation of gestational weight gain became an increasingly common clinical practice. Emphasis was first placed on identification of excessive weight gains rather than insufficient gains. An excessive weight gain was regarded as a clinical sign of edema and impending toxemia. Controlling weight gain during pregnancy was encouraged as a means of preventing toxemia. Salt-free diets were advocated to control tissue fluid retention (McIlroy and Rodway, 1937), and women were commonly told to restrict their food intake to limit their total gestational weight gain to no more than 6.8 kg (15 lb) (Bingham, 1932; McIlroy and Rodway, 1937). Up to World War II, most published studies of gestational weight gains reported average gains that were low; several were less than 9.1 kg (20 lb) (Hytten, 1980).

Hytten and Leitch (1971) analyzed several large studies of gestational weight gain that were conducted during the 1950s and 1960s (Eastman and Jackson, 1968; Humphreys, 1954; Singer et al., 1968; Thomson and Billewicz, 1957) and concluded that an average gain of 12.5 kg (27.5 lb) is the "physiological normality" in apparently healthy, young, primigravid women. These data show that weight gain before and during pregnancy had independent, but additive, effects on birth weight; e.g., a high prepregnancy weight and a high gestational weight gain resulted in a higher birth weight than did a low prepregnancy weight with a high gestational weight gain. In 1970 the Food and Nutrition Board's (FNB's) Committee on Maternal Nutrition stated that "the desirable average gain is 24 pounds within a range of 20 to 25 pounds" (NRC, 1970, p. 190). Two years later, the adhoc Committee on Nutrition of the American College of Obstetricians and Gynecologists (ACOG) published the same recommendation (Pitkin et al., 1972), and in 1974, the ACOG Committee on Nutrition repeated the recommendation in the booklet *Nutrition and Maternal Health Care* (Committee on Nutrition, 1974). The ACOG booklet emphasized that the pattern of weight gain is equally important, if not more so, than the total amount of gain and recommended a linear gain from week 13 of gestation through term. These recommendations were supported in the 1978 booklet *Assessment of Maternal Nutrition* published jointly by ACOG and the American Dietetic Association (Task Force on Nutrition,

TABLE 3-1 Weight Gain Recommendations in a Sample of Medical Textbooks

Reference	Recommendation
Clinical Obstetrics Lull and Kimbrough, 1953	A total gain of 10.9 kg (24 lb), based on the authors' own research in which they recorded a 9.5-kg (21-lb) average linear gain after the first trimester. Weight gain was related to prematurity and toxemia. The importance of prepregnancy weight was emphasized, and a protein intake of 1.5 g/kg of body weight was recommended.
Williams Obstetrics 12th edition Eastman and Hellman, 1961	A limitation on weight gain to 11.4 kg (25 lb), at most, or to 9.1 kg (20 lb), which was considered better. Restriction of weight gain to 8.2 kg (18 lb) with an 1,800-kcal diet was emphasized. The 1943 RDA of 2,500 kcal/day was suggested.
14th edition Hellman and Pritchard, 1971	A gain of 9.1 to 11.4 kg (20 to 25 lb), because it was associated with the most favorable outcome. Eastman and Jackson (1968) was cited. The recommendations of the ACOG Committee on Maternal Nutrition were summarized, and the 1968 RDAs were listed.
15th edition Pritchard and MacDonald, 1976	A weight gain of at least 9.1 kg (20 lb) in most cases, and women should be encouraged to eat as much as they wish. The 1974 RDAs were listed.
16th edition Pritchard and MacDonald, 1980	The 1978 ACOG Task Force on Nutritional Status criteria were reviewed, and the 1980 RDAs were presented.
Beck's Obstetrical Practice 9th edition Taylor, 1971	A total gain of 9.1 to 11.4 kg (20 to 25 lb), and instructions were given to gain no more than 0.9 to 1.8 kg (2 to 4 lb) per month. An increase above this amount was recommended for underweight women, and obese women were allowed to diet and lose weight.

1978). Further emphasis on the weight gain recommendation appeared in *Guidelines for Perinatal Care* (AAP/ACOG, 1983) and in *Standards for Obstetric,Gynecologic Services* (ACOG, 1985). In 1981, the FNB's *Nutrition Services in Perinatal Care*(NRC, 1981) presented the following guidelines for evaluation of weight gain, which were published initially by Pitkin (1977):

Inadequate gain: Gain of 1 kg or less per month during the second or third trimesters.
Excessive gain: Gain of 3 kg or more per month (NRC, 1981, p. 12).

Frequently, but not always, these authoritative recommendations were incorporated into textbooks, usually at least 1 year after they first appeared (Table 3-1). *Williams Obstetrics* (e.g., Eastman and Hellman, 1961)

a primary reference used in many medical schools, is an example. Editions published between 1961 and 1980 in general recommended a total gain of 9.1 to 11.4 kg (20 to 25 lb). The earlier editions recommended some restriction of gain; the later ones advised a more liberal approach. The suggestion that weight gain should not be limited and that women should be allowed to eat as much as they want did not appear until 1976 (Pritchard and MacDonald, 1976). The FNB's Recommended Dietary Allowances (RDAs) were used as standards for dietary intakes throughout these editions. *Beck's Obstetrical Practice* (Taylor, 1971) and *Clinical Obstetrics* (Lull and Kimbrough, 1953) were widely used sources on obstetric care. The recommendations in these books differed from those in *Williams Obstetrics*. Lull and Kimbrough (1953) recommended a total gain of 10.9 kg (24 lb). They also emphasized that prepregnancy weight as well as gestational weight gain influenced pregnancy outcome. *Beck's Obstetrical Practice* (Taylor, 1971) emphasized the existence of a relationship between prepregnancy weight and gestational weight gain. They suggested that underweight women should be allowed to gain more weight than women of normal weight and that obese women should be allowed to diet and lose weight.

The FNB has prepared 10 editions of the RDAs between 1943 and 1989. During that time, energy recommendations for pregnant women have ranged from 2,200 kcal/day in 1968 to 2,700 kcal/day in 1953 (Table 3-2). Ironically, the highest energy intakes were recommended during the 1950s, when women were also advised to restrict their weight gain. In the 1960s, the total energy recommendation for pregnant women decreased to a range of 2,200 to 2,300 kcal/day. In 1974, 2,400 kcal was recommended for pregnant women. In 1989, the nonpregnant RDA for energy rose another 100 kcal, bringing the total recommended energy intake during pregnancy to 2,500 kcal.

Recommended gestational weight gains have nearly doubled during the past 50 years—from 6.8 kg (15 lb) in the 1930s to a range of 11.4 to 15.9 kg (25 to 35 lb) in the 1980s. Concurrently, standard clinical practice changed from restricting to encouraging weight gain during gestation. In dietetic practice, changes were made from a limited to an unlimited food intake. The most recent RDAs for energy are consistent with these changes in clinical practice, but the total amount recommended still falls below that recommended in the 1950s (NRC, 1953, 1958).

TABLE 3-2 Recommended Energy Intakes for Pregnant Women Made by the Food and Nutrition Board (FNB) from 1943 to 1989

Reference	Recommended Energy Intake for Nonpregnant Women, kcal/day (activity level or age group)	Recommended Energy Intake for Pregnant Women	
		Increment, kcal	Total kcal/day
NRC, 1943, 1945	2,100 (sedentary) 2,500 (moderately active) 3,000 (very active)	NR[a]	2,500
NRC, 1948	2,000 (sedentary) 2,400 (moderately active) 3,000 (very active)	NR[a]	2,400 (sedentary)[b]
NRC, 1953	2,300	+400	2,700
NRC, 1958	2,300	+300	2,600
NRC, 1964	2,100	+200	2,300
NRC, 1968	2,000	+200	2,200
NRC, 1974	2,100	+300	2,400
NRC, 1980	2,100 (19–22 yr) 2,000 (23–50 yr)	+300	2,400 2,300
NRC, 1989	2,200	+300	2,500

[a] NR = Not reported.
[b] Recommendations for women in the other two activity groups are calculated by adding 20% to the recommendation for nonpregnant women.

TRENDS IN MATERNAL NUTRITIONAL STATUS AND CHARACTERISTICS ASSOCIATED WITH OUTCOME

Not only have standards for clinical practice changed in the past 50 years, but there also have been substantial changes in the health status and the health habits of women who are entering pregnancy.

Maternal Body Size

Maternal weight, height, and weight-for-height ratios are used frequently as indirect measures of nutritional status. The ability to establish a trend in body size requires serial data from representative subjects from the same population over time. Changes in maternal body size have not been studied systematically, but national surveys of representative samples of U.S. women of reproductive age can be used to identify trends in body weight, height, and weight-for-height ratios. The weight-for-height ratio used most frequently in the analysis of these data is the body mass index (BMI), which is calculated from weight and height (see Chapter 4). BMI measurements generally correlate well with more accurate measurements of body fat content such as body density or total body water (Garrow, 1983).

Three large national health surveys have been conducted in the United

TABLE 3-3   Trends in the Heights of U.S. Women Aged 18 to 24 Years
from 1960 to 1980

Years of Study and Reference	Height, cm (in.)		Percentage of Population by Height	
	Mean	Median	<157 cm (<62 in.)	<160 cm (<63 in.)
1960–1962 NCHS, 1965	162 (63.8)	162 (63.9)	24.6	40.1
1971–1974 Abraham et al., 1979	163 (64.3)	163 (64.3)	16.6	29.8
1976–1980 Najjar and Rowland, 1987	163 (64.3)	164 (64.5)	17.8	29.1

States since 1960: the National Health Examination Survey, Cycle I (HES)
(1960-1962); the first National Health and Nutrition Examination Survey
(NHANES I) (1971-1974); and the second National Health and Nutrition
Examination Survey (NHANES II) (1976-1980). These data show that the
mean height of women between 18 and 24 years of age increased 1.8 cm
(0.7 in.) between the 1960-1962 (NCHS, 1965) and 1971-1974 (Abraham
et al., 1979) surveys; the median height increased 1 cm (0.4 in.) during
the same period (Table 3-3). Changes in the percentage of women who
were less than 160 cm (63 in.) in height are much more dramatic. In the
1960-1962 survey, 40% of the women surveyed were less than 160 cm tall;
this dropped to 30% in the 1971-1974 survey. During the 1970s, there was
little change in the mean heights of women or in the proportion of short
women.

Using data from these three national surveys, Flegal et al. (1988)
calculated the trends in BMI. The skinfold thicknesses of the women in
these three surveys were also summarized. Data were provided for women
in two age groups (18 to 24 and 25 to 34 years), for blacks and whites, and
for level of education and income. Between the 1960-1962 and 1976-1980
surveys, an increase in body weight of 2.5 to 3.0 kg (5.5 to 6.6 lb) resulted in
a statistically significant increase in BMI for women of both races and for
women under and over age 25. Increases in triceps and subscapular skinfold
thicknesses paralleled the trends in BMI and body weight, suggesting that
much of the change in BMI was due to an increase in body fat.

Using the same data base, Harlan et al. (1988) searched for evidence
of an increase in the prevalence of obesity. They found that the proportion
of white women with BMIs above the 75th percentile for age and sex,
based on the 1959 Metropolitan Life Insurance Standards (Metropolitan
Life Insurance Company, 1959), increased from approximately 22 to 30%
between the 1960-1962 and 1976-1980 surveys, and that the proportion of
black women above the 75th percentile increased from about 43 to 49%.

Thus, during the past two decades, women in the United States have become taller and heavier. But the increase in body weight was greater than the increase in height, resulting in an increase in BMI and, therefore, the prevalence of overweight women of reproductive age. These changes in maternal body size may influence pregnancy outcomes: infant birth weight has been correlated with maternal height, weight, and weight-for-height ratios (Kramer, 1987).

Age of Menarche

The onset of menstruation is believed to be related to body size (Frisch, 1980); i.e., a particular ratio of fat to lean mass and total body weight is necessary for puberty. Since adult female body size has increased during the past two decades, the possibility of a lowered age of menarche was investigated. Earlier menarche could be accompanied by an increased prevalence of young mothers, which in turn might influence the course and outcome of pregnancy.

There are some data on the average age at onset from the first half of the nineteenth century in studies from Scandinavia, Great Britain, and Germany (Tanner, 1981). These data suggest that there has been a 3-year decrease in the average age of menarche from the early 1800s to the mid-twentieth century. If the decrease is linear, this is equivalent to a decrease of 3 to 4 months per decade (Frisch, 1984). However, in four individual studies published between 1948 and 1976, the average age at menarche remained at 12.9 years in the United States (Zacharias et al., 1976).

Maternal Age and Parity

Maternal age and parity are reported to influence the size of the baby at birth (Kramer, 1987). In general, primiparous women give birth to infants who are smaller than those of multiparous women. In some studies, very young mothers tend to have smaller babies than do older women. National vital statistics data provide information on the distribution of births among women of different ages and parities. For this report, data on the birth weights of singleton infants born in 1960, 1971, 1980, and 1985 were tabulated by race of infant, maternal age, and live birth order. Maternal age was categorized into four groups: under 18, 18 to 19, 20 to 29, and 30 and over. Parity was based on live birth order and categorized into three groups: primiparas, low-parity multiparas, and high-parity multiparas. High parity was defined as third- or higher-order births to mothers under age 20 and fourth- or higher-order births to mothers age 20 and over.

There have been changes in the distribution of live births according to the age of the mother (Figure 3-1), but the 1985 distribution is quite similar

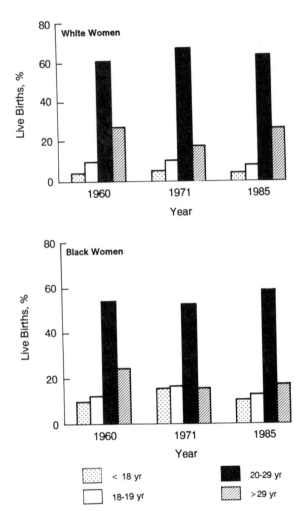

FIGURE 3-1 Distribution of live births according to maternal age, by race. Based on unpublished data from the National Vital Statistics System, computed by the Division of Analysis from data compiled by the Division of Vital Statistics, National Center for Health Statistics.

to the 1960 distribution for both whites and blacks. The distribution of births according to maternal parity changed much more markedly over the same period. In 1960, approximately 25% of the white births and almost 50% of the black births were to high-parity mothers (Figure 3-2). By 1985, high-parity births accounted for only 9% of white and 15% of black births. This reduction in the prevalence of high-parity births was accompanied by a sharp increase in the proportion of first births. Between 1960 and 1985, the percentage of births that were first births increased by 55% among white women and by 80% among black women. There was a relatively large change in the proportion of first births to mothers aged 30 and over—from 2 to 6% of total births among whites and from 1 to 3% of total births among blacks. However, the proportion of total births to women in this age group was lower than that in 1960.

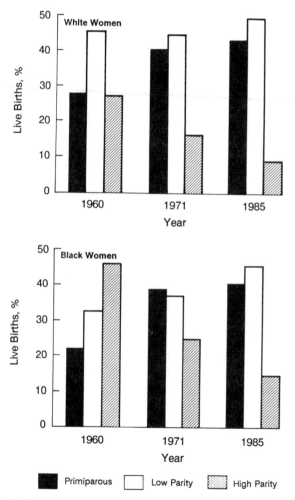

FIGURE 3-2 Distribution of live births according to maternal parity, by race. Based on unpublished data from the National Vital Statistics System, computed by the Division of Analysis from data compiled by the Division of Vital Statistics, National Center for Health Statistics.

TABLE 3-4   Ethnic Origin of Infants Born in the
United States in 1960[a] and 1987[b]

Ethnic Origin	Percentage of Births		Number of Births (in thousands)	
	1960	1987	1960	1987
White[c]	84.6	78.6	3,600	2,992
Black	14.1	16.9	602	642
American Indian	0.5	1.2	6	44
Chinese	0.1	0.5	6	19
Japanese	0.3	0.3	12	10
All others	0.3	2.5	15	112

[a] From NCHS, 1962.
[b] From NCHS, 1989a.
[c] Hispanics were not coded separately prior to 1980. Data from 22
reporting states indicate that there were 289,000 births of Hispanic
origin in 1980 (Ventura, 1983) compared to 405,000 in 1987 (NCHS,
1989a).

Ethnic Origin of Mothers

Maternal ethnic origin has been linked with infant birth weight. In
general, black and Asian mothers give birth to smaller infants than do white
mothers (Kramer, 1987). Thus, a substantial shift in the ethnic origin of
mothers having babies could influence national data on infant birth weights.
    Although the total number of births in the United States decreased
by about 10% between 1960 and 1987, the number of births to nonwhites
other than blacks grew substantially (Table 3-4). The number of Hispanic
births increased by 40% between 1980 and 1987. (The Hispanic designation
was not on the birth certificate until 1978.)

Smoking Habits of Women of Reproductive Age

Smoking during pregnancy has a detrimental effect on fetal growth
(see the review by Kramer [1987]). Thus, any changes in birth weight
should be compared with changes in maternal smoking habits during the
same period of time.
    Between 1965 and 1987, the prevalence of smoking among women
of childbearing age (20 to 44 years of age) decreased from approximately
40 to 30%. Among men in the same age group, the decline was much
greater—from 60 to 30% (NCHS, 1989b). Smoking among girls aged 12
to 17 years also decreased from 24% in 1974 to 15% in 1985 (NCHS,
1989b). Between 1974 and 1985, education replaced gender as the major sociodemographic predictor of smoking status. Smoking prevalence
has declined across all educational groups, but the decline has occurred
five times faster among the more educated groups compared with those who

are less educated (Pierce et al., 1989). In 1985, the prevalence of smoking among people with less than a high school education (34%) was almost twice that of people with 4 or more years of college education (18%).

Smoking during pregnancy also decreased during the late 1960s and the 1970s. Kleinman and Kopstein (1987) analyzed data from two national samples of live births to married mothers, the 1967 and the 1980 National Natality Surveys, and showed that the proportion of white married mothers age 20 and over who smoked decreased from 40 to 25%; the proportion of pregnant black smokers decreased from 33 to 23% (Figure 3-3). Unfortunately, this decline in smoking was only seen in women over age 20. The prevalence of smoking among mothers less than age 20 did not change during this period; approximately 40% of whites and 30% of blacks under age 20 smoked during their pregnancies in 1967 and 1980.

The higher prevalence of smoking among those with lower levels of education (Figure 3-4) may account in part for the substantial portion of the excess incidence of low-birth-weight infants among these mothers. Kleinman and Madans (1985) estimated that elimination of smoking would reduce the incidence of low birth weight by 11% for those with more than 12 years of education and by 35% for those with less than 12 years of education. In the future, public health programs designed to help women stop smoking during pregnancy should be directed toward teenagers and women with less than a high school education.

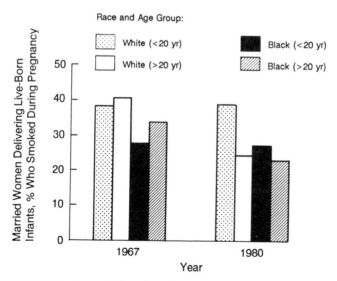

FIGURE 3-3 Smoking characteristics of married pregnant women, by race and age. Based on data from Kleinman and Kopstein (1987).

Use of Selected Substances

Information on the use of alcohol, marijuana, and cocaine during the previous month were collected in national surveys conducted between 1972 and 1988 (NCHS, 1990). Data are not available for all age and sex groups in each year. In 1976, 58% of the women aged 18 to 25 reported using alcohol in the past month. This increased to 68% in 1979 and declined slightly to 57% in 1988. Data on the use of marijuana by women aged 18 to 25 have been tabulated for the period from 1976 to 1988. In 1976, 19% reported using marijuana in the past month. This increased to 26% in 1979 and fell to 11% in 1988. Data on cocaine use among women between the ages of 18 and 25 years are only available for the years from 1982 to 1988. During this period, the number of women who reported using cocaine in the past month increased by one-third—from 4.7 to 6.3%—but then declined to 3.0% in 1988. It should be noted, however, that emergency room admissions with mention of cocaine for women aged 18 to 25 quadrupled between 1984 and 1988 (A. Kopstein, National Institute on Drug Abuse, personal communication, 1989). If we assume that the lifestyles of women who became pregnant in 1985 were similar to those of the women in the survey, we can also assume that the prevalence of substance use would be the same, i.e., alcohol, 64%; marijuana, 17%; and cocaine, >6%. There are no specific data on alcohol, marijuana, and cocaine use among pregnant women in the United States. However, studies of selected populations show cocaine use during pregnancy up to 25% (Chasnoff, 1989).

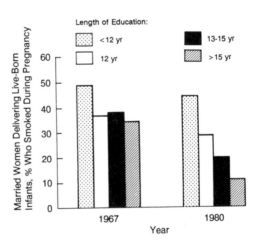

FIGURE 3-4 Smoking habits of white married women over age 20, by level of education. Based on data from Kleinman and Kopstein, (1987).

TRENDS IN USE OF PRENATAL CARE AND FOOD SUPPLEMENTATION PROGRAMS

Changes in the availability of prenatal care and food supplementation programs can have a great impact on the general and nutritional health of pregnant women. Poor prenatal care and insufficient food intake both have been associated with poor pregnancy outcomes. Trends in the use of prenatal care since 1969 were recently summarized in the Institute of Medicine report *Prenatal Care: Reaching Mothers, Reaching Infants* (IOM, 1988). Steady increases in the percentage of births to mothers who received prenatal care in the first trimester of pregnancy occurred for both whites and blacks between 1969 and 1980. In 1980, about 76% of the babies were born to women who had begun receiving prenatal care in the first trimester. This proportion has remained essentially constant between 1980 and 1987. Among black women, 8.8% of the new mothers had received late or no prenatal care in 1980. By 1987, the prevalence had increased to 11%. Of the white women giving birth, 4.3% and 5.0% received little or no prenatal care in 1980 and 1987, respectively (NCHS, 1990). Social, economic, and other changes in the 1980s have been offered as explanations for this disturbing trend. These include the increase in unemployment in the early 1980s and the resulting loss of employer-based health insurance and personal income; the increasing proportion of women of childbearing age living in poverty; and the increasing number of employed people with inadequate or no health insurance, along with the continuing erosion of maternity benefits under private health insurance plans. The increasing proportion of births to unmarried women and the growth in the number of households headed by single women may also have contributed to this trend.

The Special Supplemental Food Program for Women, Infants, and Children (WIC), administered by the U.S. Department of Agriculture (USDA), has had an increasing impact on the provision of food to disadvantaged pregnant women in the United States since 1974 (Rush et al., 1988). Before then, there was distribution of supplemental food to a relatively small number of pregnant women through USDA's Supplemental Food Program. This program provided allotments of canned meat or poultry, peanut butter or dried beans, egg mix, nonfat dry milk powder, canned fruits or vegetables, canned juice, evaporated milk, and hot or cold cereal. The primary objective of the Supplemental Food Program was distribution of surplus commodity foods to low-income people in general; there was no special attempt to supply foods to pregnant women. In contrast, the WIC program provides nutrition education, counseling, and referrals, in addition to food or vouchers, for a carefully tailored, nutritious food pack-

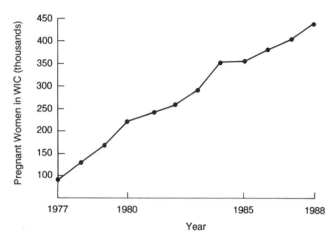

FIGURE 3-5 Estimated WIC participation, 1977 through 1988. "Pregnant" includes women up to 6 weeks post partum. The percentage of all women participants who are pregnant is assumed to be constant at the level of 53.7% as found in the 1984 *Study of WIC Participant and Program Characteristics* (Richman et al., 1986). Based on data from USDA (1988).

age to pregnant, low-income women who meet state criteria for nutritional risk. Other priority groups targeted by the WIC program include lactating women and children from infancy up to age 5. The WIC program has reached increasing numbers of pregnant women each year (Figure 3-5). Estimated average participation per year grew from 9,000 pregnant women in 1974 to approximately 440,000 in 1988 (J. Hirschman, Food and Nutrition Service, USDA, personal communication, 1989), but it still does not serve all those who are eligible. In 1987, 78.1% of pregnant women who were certified to receive food or food instruments (vouchers) took advantage of the program; only the actual participants are included in Figure 3-5.

Each month, an average WIC package provides the equivalent of 20.5 quarts of milk, 1.9 pounds of cheese, 2.1 dozen eggs, 259.6 ounces of juice, 33.3 ounces of cereal, and 12 ounces of dried beans, dried peas, or peanut butter. If this food is consumed evenly over a month, this package would provide about 900 to 1,000 kcal/day and 40 to 50 g of protein per day. The effects of the WIC program on maternal weight gain and birth weight are briefly reviewed in Chapter 7.

TRENDS IN PREGNANCY OUTCOME

The changes in maternal health habits and characteristics noted above could have both a positive and negative impact on infant mortality and birth weight. The increase in maternal body size, decrease in smoking prevalence, and improved accessibility to supplemental foods would be expected to be associated with an improved outcome, whereas the increased prevalence of late or no prenatal care would be expected to cause poorer outcomes. Given these divergent changes in maternal health characteristics and habits, it is not possible to predict trends in infant mortality rates or birth weights based on these data alone.

Infant Mortality

Infant mortality is used frequently as an indicator of infant health. Neonatal mortality (deaths occurring during the first 28 days of life) is considered to be related to the course of pregnancy. Between 1950 and 1987, infant mortality rates for all races declined from 29.2 to 10.1 deaths per 1,000 live births (Figure 3-6) (NCHS, 1990). Infant mortality among black infants was about twice that observed among white infants. After a plateau during the 1950s and early 1960s, infant mortality declined rapidly from 1965 to 1980 for both whites and blacks. The rate of decline slowed during the 1980s, especially among blacks. Most of the improvement in infant mortality was due to reductions in birth weight-specific mortality; relatively little was due to improvement in the birth weight distribution (Buehler et al., 1987). In other words, through improved neonatal intensive care, deaths among high risk births were reduced.

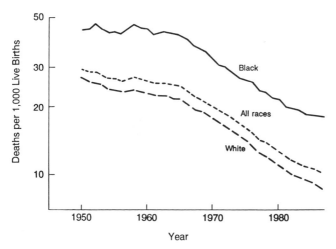

FIGURE 3-6 Infant mortality rates in the United States, 1950 through 1987, by race. From NCHS (1990).

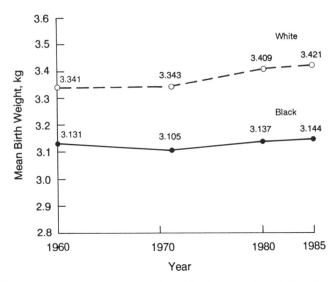

FIGURE 3-7 Trends in mean birth weight of live-born singleton infants in the United States from 1960 through 1985, by race. Based on unpublished data from the National Vital Statistics System, computed by the Division of Analysis from data compiled by the Division of Vital Statistics, National Center for Health Statistics.

Birth Weight

U.S. national vital statistics data for 1960 through 1985 provide information on the trends in mean birth weight as well as the incidence of low-birth-weight (LBW; <2,500 g), very-low-birth-weight (VLBW; <1,500 g), and high-birth-weight (>4,000 g) infants. For use in this report, data on the birth weight of singleton, live infants in 1960, 1971, 1980, and 1985 were tabulated. Between 1960 and 1971, the mean birth weight was constant for both white and black infants (Figure 3-7), but between 1971 and 1980 it increased by 60 g for white infants and 30 g for black infants. Between 1980 and 1985, the rate of increase slowed for both whites and blacks. Adjustment of these trends for the changing maternal age and parity distribution had little effect on the mean birth weights. In 1985, the mean birth weight of white infants born in the United States averaged 3,421 g and that of black infants averaged 3,144 g.

Estimates of trends in the mean birth weight of Canadian infants are based on Statistics Canada data (Arbuckle and Sherman, 1989). Arbuckle and Sherman reported that the mean birth weight of Canadian singleton male infants increased 132 g—from 3,325 to 3,457 g—between 1972 and 1986; the mean birth weight of female infants increased 135 g—from 3,199 to 3,334 g. (Data from vital statistics consistently demonstrate that mean birth weight of males is higher than that of females.) This net change in the mean birth weight of Canadian infants is nearly double that seen for white infants in the United States over a similar period.

Changes in mean birth weight are of some interest, but the extremes of the birth weight distribution are most important. Figure 3-8 shows the trends in LBW (<2,500 g) for white and black infants, both full term and preterm, based on national vital statistics data. From 1960 to 1985, the incidence of LBW infants declined to 4.7% of white births and to 11% of black births. The values shown for LBW in 1960 may be lower than the actual values because of underreporting of LBW during that period (Kleinman, 1986).

Adjustment for the changing age-birth order distribution of births had essentially no effect on these trends. However, there was a large decline in the percentage of LBW infants born to white women age 30 and over, especially primiparas. This is probably due in part to the changing mix of women in this group: during the 1960s, first live births to older mothers probably included a large proportion of women who had prior fetal losses. By 1985, a much larger proportion of the women in this group had intentionally postponed childbirth. The socioeconomic status of women over age 30 having babies in 1985 probably was higher than that of women of the same age delivering in 1960. In addition, the medical

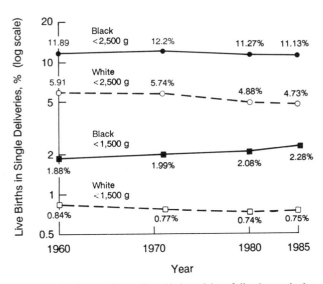

FIGURE 3-8 Trends in low and very low birth weight of live-born singleton infants in the United States from 1960 through 1985, by race. Based on unpublished data from the National Vital Statistics System, computed by the Division of Analysis from data compiled by the Division of Vital Statistics, National Center for Health Statistics.

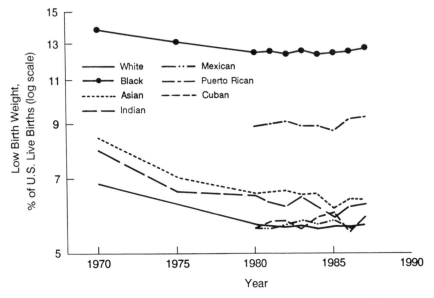

FIGURE 3-9 Trends in low birth weight of live-born singleton infants in the United States from 1970 through 1987, by race and ethnic background. From NCHS (1990).

management of pregnancies among older women with chronic illness, such as hypertension or diabetes, has improved.

Trends in the incidence of VLBW show a sharper divergence by race (Figure 3-8). Between 1960 and 1985, the incidence of VLBW white infants dropped from 0.84 to 0.75% of all births, while the incidence of VLBW among black infants increased from 1.9 to 2.3%.

The incidence of VLBW among blacks is triple the rate among whites and the incidence of LBW is double. In an analysis of trends in racial differences in low birth weight in the United States between 1973 and 1983, Kleinman and Kessel (1987) report that the rate of LBW dropped by 14% among white women but only 3% among black women. Kleinman and Kessel (1987) attributed 15% of the decline among the white women to favorable changes in maternal characteristics, primarily an increase in educational level. They reported no change in incidence of VLBW infants among white women, but an increase among black women; 35% of this increase was attributed to an increase in births to unmarried women.

Published data show national trends in LBW for white, black, American Indian, and Asian births since 1970 and Hispanic births since 1980 (NCHS, 1990). These data, which include both single and multiple births, are shown in Figure 3-9. There was a flattening of the downward trend in LBW for all ethnic groups during the 1980s. In 1987, LBW infants accounted for about

5 to 7% of the births in all groups except Puerto Ricans (9.3%) and blacks (12.7%).

An infant may be born small because it was born too early (i.e., preterm) or because it experienced growth retardation in utero. Between 1970 and 1980, the incidence of preterm LBW infants declined to the same degree for both white and black women—7.1% (Kessel et al., 1984). The incidence of full-term LBW infants decreased almost three times as much—20.9%. Consequently, the incidence of preterm LBW infants among all LBW infants has risen from 51% in 1970 to 56% in 1980. Thus, the overall decline in LBW has occurred primarily as a result of declines in full-term LBW infants. Decreased cigarette smoking, improved diets, and improved utilization of early prenatal care during the 1970s may have contributed to improved intrauterine growth and, therefore, a reduced rate of full-term LBW infants.

At the other end of the birth-weight scale, changes in the incidence of high birth weights for white and black women have been observed (Figure 3-10). Among whites, the proportion of infants who weighed 4,000 g or more at birth remained constant during the 1960s but increased by 31% between 1971 and 1985. For blacks, however, there was a sharp decline between 1960 and 1971, followed by a 17% increase between 1971 and 1985. In 1985, 12.7% of the white infants and 5.5% of the black infants weighed 4,000 g or more at birth. An increase in prepregnancy weight

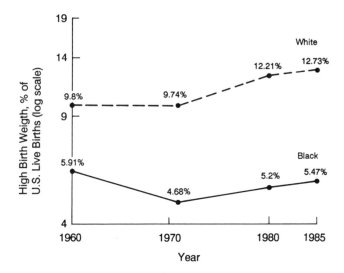

FIGURE 3-10 Trends in high birth weight (4 kg or more) of live-born singleton infants in the United States from 1960 through 1985, by race. Based on unpublished data from the National Vital Statistics System, computed by the Division of Analysis from data compiled by the Division of Vital Statistics, National Center for Health Statistics.

and the prevalence of obesity may contribute to the increase in high-birth-weight infants. It may also be related to the fact that pregnant women are now encouraged to let their appetite guide the amount they eat, whereas in the 1960s, women were advised to restrict their weight gain by limiting food intake.

TRENDS IN GESTATIONAL WEIGHT GAIN

Trends in gestational weight gain are difficult to determine, because it has not been monitored in representative samples of the U.S. population over time. A comparison of mean reported weight gains from studies with large sample sizes completed during the past 45 years provides some information on weight gain trends. Data from 11 studies of maternal weight gain and birth weight completed between 1946 and 1983 are summarized in Table 3-5. Of the women studied in the 1940s, 1950s, and 1960s, the reported mean weight gain was 10 kg (22 lb) or less. An exception is the study by Peckham and Christianson (1971) in which weight gain data were collected from 1963 to 1965 and the average gain was 11.8 kg (26 lb). This was a study of white, primiparous women who were attending Kaiser prenatal clinics in northern California. There was a smaller group of women in this study than in the other studies, and the socioeconomic status of the women was relatively high, as is characteristic of a health maintenance organization. Women studied in Boston during World War II (Beilly and Kurland, 1945) gained as much weight, on average, as did women from another urban area, Baltimore, about 15 years later (Eastman and Jackson, 1968).

After 1970, there appears to be an incremental increase in reported mean gestational weight gains. All studies conducted after 1970 show a mean gain of more than 12.5 kg (27 lb). These data were collected after the 1970 FNB report *Maternal Nutrition and the Course of Pregnancy*, (NRC, 1970), in which it was recommended that women gain an average of 11 kg (24 lb) during pregnancy. Thus, the upward shift may be related to a more liberal attitude regarding weight gain and, therefore, food intake in the 1970s. Gormican et al. (1980) reported that the mean gain of women attending their clinics in Madison, Wisconsin, during the last two trimesters averaged 7.2 kg (16 lb) before 1971 and 11 kg (24 lb) afterward, when clinic philosophy regarding weight gain was liberalized. In that study the higher gain after 1971 was associated with a 2-kg (4.4-lb) net increase in maternal body weight at 4 to 8 weeks postpartum, whereas a small average weight loss occurred in the women who were given advice to restrict their energy intake prior to 1971, suggesting that the increased gestational weight gains were associated with a gain of maternal fat.

In the early 1980s, mean gains of as much as 15 kg (33 lb) were

TABLE 3-5 Gestational Weight Gain and Birth Weights of Full-Term Deliveries, 1942 through 1983

Reference	Period of Data Collection	Number of Subjects	Mean Weight Gain, kg (lb)		Mean Birth Weight, g
Prior to 1970					
Beilly and Kurland, 1945	1942–1943	979	10.1	(22.3)	3,263
Simpson et al., 1975[a]	1946–1966	26,468	8.9	(19.6)	3,237
Eastman and Jackson, 1968[a]	1954–1961	11,911	9.4	(20.7)	3,314
Niswander and Jackson, 1974[a]	1959–1966	16,894	9.8	(21.6)	3,202
Peckham and Christianson, 1971	1963–1965	352[b]	11.8	(25.9)	3,389
Nyirjesy et al., 1968	1964–1966	12,569	9.9[c]	(21.9)	NR[d]
Meyer, 1978	1960–1961	51,490	10.2	(22.6)	NR[d]
After 1970					
Brown et al., 1981	1969–1976	247	12.6	(27.7)	3,234
Taffel, 1986	1980	2,930,000	13.2	(29.1)	3,387
Shepard et al., 1986	1980–1982	4,186	14.9	(32.8)	3,442
Abrams and Laros, 1986	1980–1983	1,535[e]	15.2	(33.4)	3,414

[a] Data for blacks and whites were originally reported separately but are combined for this table.
[b] Includes only white, primiparous women in medium weight group.
[c] Median (not mean) weight gain.
[d] NR = Not reported.
[e] Includes only women of ideal weight for height.

observed in two studies (Abrams and Laros, 1986; Shepard et al., 1986). Early returns from the 1988 National Maternal and Infant Health Survey suggest that there has been a continuing increase in maternal weight gain in the 1980s. Final results will not be available until 1991 (K. Keppel, National Center for Health Statistics, personal communication, 1989). Between the 1960s and the 1980s, there was an approximately 50% increase in gestational weight gain, from about 10 to 15 kg (22 to 33 lb). The change in average birth weight increased 100 to 150 g. Although the increase in weight gain was contemporaneous with an increase in birth weight, the change in birth weight was small, about a 20- to 30-g increase in birth weight for every 1-kg increase in total weight gain.

SUMMARY

On average, in the early 1980s women gained approximately 3.6 to 4.5 kg (8 to 10 lb) more weight than was reported during studies between 1940 and 1970. Since 1970, there has been a shift away from limiting weight gain, a decline in the percentage of women who are short, an increase in the percentage of women who began prenatal care in the first trimester, and initiation and growth of the WIC program, which provides

58   NUTRITIONAL STATUS AND WEIGHT GAIN

food supplements or vouchers to eligible low-income, pregnant women. Each of these changes may have contributed to the increase in average gestational weight gain.

This upward shift in gestational weight gain occurred simultaneously with lower infant mortality rates, increased average birth weights, a decreased incidence of LBW infants but an increased incidence of VLBW infants among blacks and little change in the incidence of VLBW white infants. Most impressive is the increase in high birth weight (>4,000 g) infants during the 1970s—from 9.7 to 12.2% among whites and 4.7 to 5.2% among blacks.

Several sociodemographic changes occurring in the 1980s suggest that a decline in gestational weight gain may occur. In the early 1980s, for example, enrollment for early prenatal care declined, and alcohol and cocaine use became more prevalent among women of reproductive age. Potential deterioration of maternal health habits should be kept in mind as future standards for prenatal care are established. If socioeconomic barriers make it more difficult for pregnant women to achieve good health and nutrition, it is even more important that care providers continue to encourage weight gain and good nutrition.

REFERENCES

AAP/ACOG (American Academy of Pediatrics/American College of Obstetricians and Gynecologists). 1983. Guidelines for Perinatal Care. American Academy of Pediatrics, Elk Grove, Ill. 288 pp.

Abraham, S., C.L. Johnson, and M.F. Najjar. 1979. Weight and Height of Adults 18-74 Years of Age, United States, 1971-74. Vital and Health Statistics, Series 11, No. 211. DHEW Publ. No. (PHS) 79-1659. National Center for Health Statistics, Public Health Service, U.S. Department of Health, Education, and Welfare, Hyattsville, Md. 49 pp.

Abrams, B.F., and R.K. Laros, Jr. 1986. Prepregnancy weight, weight gain, and birth weight. Am. J. Obstet. Gynecol. 154:503-509.

ACOG (American College of Obstetricians and Gynecologists). 1985. Standards for Obstetric-Gynecologic Services, 6th ed. The American College of Obstetricians and Gynecologists, Washington, D.C. 109 pp.

Arbuckle, T.E., and G.J. Sherman. 1989. An analysis of birth weight by gestational age in Canada. Can. Med. Assoc. J. 140:157-165.

Beilly, J.S., and I.I. Kurland. 1945. Relationship of maternal weight gain and weight of newborn infant. Am. J. Obstet. Gynecol. 50:202-206.

Bingham, A.W. 1932. The prevention of obstetric complications by diet and exercise. Am. J. Obstet. Gynecol. 23:38-44.

Brown, J.E., H.N. Jacobson, L.H. Askue, and M.G. Peick. 1981. Influence of pregnancy weight gain on the size of infants born to underweight women. Obstet. Gynecol. 57:13-17.

Buehler, J.W., J.C. Kleinman, C.J. Hogue, L.T. Strauss, and J.C. Smith. 1987. Birth weight-specific infant mortality, United States, 1960 and 1980. Public Health Rep. 102:151-161.

Chasnoff, I.J. 1989. Drug use and women: establishing a standard of care. Ann. N.Y. Acad. Sci. 562:208-210.

Committee on Nutrition. 1974. Nutrition in Maternal Health Care. American College of Obstetricians and Gynecologists, Washington, D.C. 13 pp.

Davis, C.H. 1923. Weight in pregnancy; its value as a routine test. Am. J. Obstet. Gynecol. 6:575-581.

Eastman, N.J., and L.M. Hellman. 1961. Williams Obstetrics, 12th ed. Appleton-Century-Crofts, New York. 1230 pp.

Eastman, N.J., and E. Jackson. 1968. Weight relationships in pregnancy: I. The bearing of maternal weight gain and pre-pregnancy weight on birth weight in full term pregnancies. Obstet. Gynecol. Surv. 23:1003-1025.

Flegal, K.M., W.R. Harlan, and J.R. Landis. 1988. Secular trends in body mass index and skinfold thickness with socioeconomic factors in young adult women. Am. J. Clin. Nutr. 48:535-543.

Frisch, R.E. 1980. Pubertal adipose tissue: is it necessary for normal sexual maturation? Evidence from the rat and human female. Fed. Proc., Fed. Am. Soc. Exp. Biol. 39:2395-2400.

Frisch, R.E. 1984. Body fat, puberty and fertility. Biol. Rev. 59:161-188.

Garrow, J.S. 1983. Indices of adiposity. Nutr. Abstr. Rev. 53:697-708.

Gormican, A., J. Valentine, and E. Satter. 1980. Relationships of maternal weight gain, prepregnancy weight, and infant birthweight. Interaction of weight factors in pregnancy. J. Am. Diet. Assoc. 77:662-667.

Harlan, W.R., J.R. Landis, K.M. Flegal, C.S. Davis, and M.E. Miller. 1988. Secular trends in body mass in the United States, 1960-1980. Am. J. Epidemiol. 128:1065-1074.

Hellman, L.M., and J.A. Pritchard. 1971. Williams Obstetrics, 14th ed. Appleton-Century-Crofts, New York. 1242 pp.

Humphreys, R.C. 1954. An analysis of the maternal and foetal weight factors in normal pregnancy. J. Obstet. Gynaecol. Br. Commonw. 61:764-771.

Hytten, F.E., and I. Leitch. 1971. The Physiology of Human Pregnancy, 2nd ed. Blackwell Scientific Publications, Oxford. 599 pp.

Hytten, F.E. 1980. Weight gain in pregnancy. Pp 193-233 in F. Hytten and G. Chamberlain, eds. Clinical Physiology in Obstetrics, Blackwell Scientific Publications, Oxford.

IOM (Institute of Medicine). 1988. Prenatal Care: Reaching Mothers, Reaching Infants. Report of the Committee to Study Outreach for Prenatal Care, Division of Health Promotion and Disease Prevention. National Academy Press, Washington, D.C. 254 pp.

Kessel, S.S., J. Villar, H.W. Berendes, and R.P. Nugent. 1984. The changing pattern of low birth weight in the United States: 1970 to 1980. J. Am. Med. Assoc. 251:1978-1982.

Kleinman, J.C. 1986. Underreporting of infant deaths: then and now. Am. J. Public Health 76:365-366.

Kleinman, J.C., and S.S. Kessel. 1987. Racial differences in low birth weight: trends and risk factors. N. Engl. J. Med. 317:749-753.

Kleinman, J.C., and A. Kopstein. 1987. Smoking during pregnancy, 1967-80. Am. J. Public Health 77:823-825.

Kleinman, J.C., and J.H. Madans. 1985. The effects of maternal smoking, physical stature, and educational attainment on the incidence of low birth weight. Am. J. Epidemiol. 121:843-855.

Kramer, M.S. 1987. Determinants of low birth weight: methodological assessment and meta-analysis. Bull. W.H.O. 65:663-737.

Lull, C.B., and R.A. Kimbrough, eds. 1953. Clinical Obstetrics. Lippincott, Philadelphia. 732 pp.

McIlroy, A.L., and H.E. Rodway. 1937. Weight-changes during and after pregnancy with special reference to early diagnosis of toxaemia. J. Obstet. Gynaecol. Br. Empire 44:221-244.

Metropolitan Life Insurance Company. 1959. New weight standards for men and women. Stat. Bull. Metrop. Life Insur. Co. 40:1-4.

Meyer, M.B. 1978. How does maternal smoking affect birth weight and maternal weight gain? Evidence from the Ontario Perinatal Mortality Study. Am. J. Obstet. Gynecol. 131:888-893.

Najjar, M.F., and M. Rowland. 1987. Anthropometric Reference Data and Prevalence of Overweight, United States, 1976-80. Vital and Health Statistics, Series 11, No. 238. DHHS Publ. No. (PHS) 87-1688. National Center for Health Statistics, Public Health Service, U.S. Department of Health and Human Services, Hyattsville, Md. 73 pp.

NCHS (National Center for Health Statistics). 1962. Vital Statistics of the United States, 1960. Vol. I—Natality. National Center for Health Statistics, Public Health Service, U.S. Department of Health, Education, and Welfare, Washington, D.C. (various pagings).

NCHS (National Center for Health Statistics). 1965. Weight, Height, and Selected Body Dimensions of Adults, United States 1960-1962. Vital and Health Statistics, Series 11, No. 8. (PHS) Publ. No. 1000. National Center for Health Statistics, Public Health Service, U.S. Department of Health and Human Services. Hyattsville, Md. 44 pp.

NCHS (National Center for Health Statistics). 1989a. Advance report of final natality statistics, 1987. Mon. Vital Stat. Rep. 38:1-48.

NCHS (National Center for Health Statistics). 1989b. Health United States 1988. DHHS Publ. No. (PHS) 89-1232. National Center for Health Statistics, Public Health Service, U.S. Department of Health and Human Services. Hyattsville, Md. 208 pp.

NCHS (National Center for Health Statistics). 1990. Health United States 1989. DHHS Publ. No. (PHS) 90-1232. National Center for Health Statistics, Public Health Service, U.S. Department of Health and Human Services, Hyattsville, Md. 291 pp.

Niswander, K., and E.C. Jackson. 1974. Physical characteristics of the gravida and their association with birth weight and perinatal death. Am. J. Obstet. Gynecol. 119:306-313.

NRC (National Research Council). 1943. Recommended Dietary Allowances. Report of the Food and Nutrition Board. Reprint and Circular Series No. 115. National Academy of Sciences, Washington, D.C. 6 pp.

NRC (National Research Council). 1945. Recommended Dietary Allowances, revised 1945. Report of the Food and Nutrition Board. Reprint and Circular Series No. 122. National Academy of Sciences, Washington, D.C. 18 pp.

NRC (National Research Council). 1948. Recommended Dietary Allowances, revised 1948. Report of the Food and Nutrition Board. Reprint and Circular Series No. 129. National Academy of Sciences, Washington, D.C. 31 pp.

NRC (National Research Council). 1953. Recommended Dietary Allowances, revised 1953. Report of the Food and Nutrition Board. Publication 302. National Academy of Sciences, Washington, D.C. 36 pp.

NRC (National Research Council). 1958. Recommended Dietary Allowances, revised 1958. Report of the Food and Nutrition Board. Publication 589. National Academy of Sciences, Washington, D.C. 36 pp.

NRC (National Research Council). 1964. Recommended Dietary Allowances, 6th revised ed. Report of the Food and Nutrition Board. Publication 1146. National Academy of Sciences, Washington, D.C. 59 pp.

NRC (National Research Council). 1968. Recommended Dietary Allowances, 7th revised ed. Report of the Food and Nutrition Board. Publication 1694. National Academy of Sciences, Washington, D.C. 101 pp.

NRC (National Research Council). 1970. Maternal Nutrition and the Course of Pregnancy. Report of the Committee on Maternal Nutrition, Food and Nutrition Board. National Academy of Sciences, Washington, D.C. 241 pp.

NRC (National Research Council). 1974. Recommended Dietary Allowances, 8th ed. Report of the Committee on Dietary Allowances, Committee on Interpretation of the Recommended Dietary Allowances, Food and Nutrition Board. National Academy of Sciences, Washington, D.C. 128 pp.

NRC (National Research Council). 1980. Recommended Dietary Allowances, 9th ed. Report of the Committee on Dietary Allowances, Food and Nutrition Board, Division of Biological Sciences, Assembly of Life Sciences. National Academy Press, Washington, D.C. 185 pp.

NRC (National Research Council). 1981. Nutrition Services in Perinatal Care. Report of the Committee on Nutrition of the Mother and Preschool Child, Food and Nutrition Board, Assembly of Life Sciences. National Academy Press, Washington, D.C. 72 pp.

NRC (National Research Council). 1989. Recommended Dietary Allowances, 10th ed. Report of the Subcommittee on the Tenth Edition of the RDAs, Food and Nutrition Board, Commission on Life Sciences. National Academy Press, Washington, D.C. 284 pp.

Nyirjesy, I., W.M. Lonergan, and J.J. Kane. 1968. Clinical significance of total weight gain in pregnancy. I. Primipara. Obstet. Gynecol. 32:391-396.

Peckham, C.H., and R.E. Christianson. 1971. The relationship between prepregnancy weight and certain obstetric factors. Am. J. Obstet. Gynecol. 111:1-7.

Pierce, J.P., M.C. Fiore, T.E. Novotny, E.J. Hatziandreu, and R.M. Davis. 1989. Trends in cigarette smoking in the United States: educational differences are increasing. J. Am. Med. Assoc. 261:56-60.

Pitkin, R.M. 1977. Obstetrics and gynecology. Pp. 407-421 in H.A. Schneider, C.E. Anderson, and D.B. Coursin, eds. Nutritional Support of Medical Practice. Harper & Row, New York.

Pitkin, R.M., H.A. Kaminetzky, M. Newton, and J.A. Pritchard. 1972. Maternal nutrition: a selective review of clinical topics. J. Obstet. Gynecol. 40:773-785.

Pritchard, J.A., and P.C. MacDonald. 1976. Williams Obstetrics, 15th ed. Appleton-Century-Crofts, New York. 1003 pp.

Pritchard, J.A., and P.C. MacDonald. 1980. Williams Obstetrics, 16th ed. Appleton-Century-Crofts, New York. 1179 pp.

Prochownick, L. 1901. Ueber Ernährungscuren in der Schwangerschaft. Ther. Monatsh. 15:446-463.

Richman, L., T. Hildlebaugh, L. Ku, N. McMahon-Cox, C.M. Dayton, and N. Goodrich. 1986. Study of WIC Participant and Program Characteristics. Office of Analysis and evaluation, Food and Nutrition Service, U.S. Department of Agriculture, Alexandria, Va. 179 pp.

Rosso, P., and C. Cramoy. 1979. Nutrition and pregnancy. Pp. 133-228 in M. Winick, ed. Human Nutrition: A Comprehensive Treatise, Vol. 1. Nutrition: Pre- and Postnatal Development. Plenum Press, New York.

Rush, D., D.G. Horvitz, W.B. Seaver, J.M. Alvir, G.C. Garbowski, J. Leighton, N.L. Sloan, S.S. Johnson, R.A. Kulka, and D.S. Shanklin. 1988. The National WIC Evaluation: evaluation of the Special Supplemental Food Program for Women, Infants, and Children. I. Background and Introduction. Am. J. Clin. Nutr. 48:389-393.

Shepard, M.J., K.G. Hellenbrand, and M.B. Bracken. 1986. Proportional weight gain and complications of pregnancy, labor, and delivery in healthy women of normal prepregnant stature. Am. J. Obstet. Gynecol. 155:947-954.

Simpson, J.W., R.W. Lawless, and A.C. Mitchell. 1975. Responsibility of the obstetrician to the fetus. II. Influence of prepregnancy weight and pregnancy weight gain on birthweight. Obstet. Gynecol. 45:481-487.

Singer, J.E., M. Westphal, and K. Niswander. 1968. Relationship of weight gain during pregnancy to birth weight and infant growth and development in the first year of life: a report from the Collaborative Study of Cerebral Palsy. Obstet. Gynecol. 31:417-423.

Taffel, S.M. 1986. Maternal Weight Gain and the Outcome of Pregnancy: United States, 1980. Vital and Health Statistics, Series 21, No. 44. DHHS Publ. No. (PHS) 86-1922. National Center for Health Statistics, Public Health Service, U.S. Department of Health and Human Services, Hyattsville, Md. 25 pp.

Tanner, J.M. 1981. Growth and maturation during adolescence. Nutr. Rev. 39:43-55.

Task Force on Nutrition. 1978. Assessment of Maternal Nutrition. The American Dietetic Association and The American College of Obstetricians and Gynecologists, Washington, D.C. 25 pp.

Taylor, E.S. 1971. Beck's Obstetrical Practice, 9th ed. Williams & Wilkins, Baltimore, Md. 665 pp.

Thomson, A.M., and W.Z. Billewicz. 1957. Clinical significance of weight trends during pregnancy. Br. Med. J. 1:243-247.

USDA (U.S. Department of Agriculture). 1988. Annual Historical Review of FNS Programs: Fiscal Year 1988. Food and Nutrition Service, U.S. Department of Agriculture, Alexandria, Va. 32 pp.

Ventura, S.J. 1983. Births of Hispanic parentage, 1980. Mon. Vital Stat. Rep. 32:1-18.

Zacharias, L., W.M. Rand, and R.J. Wurtman. 1976. A prospective study of sexual development and growth in American girls: the statistics of menarche. Obstet. Gynecol. Surv. 31:325-337.

4

Assessment of Gestational Weight Gain

In this chapter, methods and issues related to the assessment of maternal weight gain during pregnancy are discussed. The types of data essential to assessment of gestational weight gain in the clinical setting are identified, and desirable methods of collecting, using, and interpreting these data are described. The subcommittee then discusses various definitions of gestational weight gain and other factors that have complicated interpretation of the research on health implications of gestational weight gain.

METHODOLOGICAL ISSUES RELATED TO DATA COLLECTION IN THE CLINIC

When weight and weight gain are used to screen individual women for special treatment or to monitor the progress of a pregnancy, the consequences of misdiagnosis resulting from poor data quality may be substantial. Therefore, major emphasis should be placed on establishing and implementing data collection techniques that provide the most reliable and accurate data possible for the particular clinical setting.

Clinical data relevant to gestational weight gain include weight, height, and gestational age. Other measures, such as skinfold thickness and indicators of frame size, are also occasionally recommended but are not included in this critique. For reasons discussed in Chapter 6, the measurement of skinfold thickness to assess composition of weight gain and nutritional status during pregnancy has not been thoroughly studied or validated. Similarly, there have been no studies on pregnant women to validate the functional meaning of frame size indicators (e.g., elbow breadth and wrist circumference or diameter—measurements suggested as a basis for improving weight-for-height classification schemes). Therefore, the subcommittee believes it is premature to recommend specific techniques for making these measurements. Before making any of the measurements described below, one should consult a reliable source such as Lohman et al. (1988) for a thorough review of methods and techniques.

Weight

Weights measured in the clinic are preferable to self-reported or recalled weights. However, measurement alone does not ensure accuracy. Factors that can affect measurements of a woman's weight include the type of scale used (e.g., spring or beam balance scale), the accuracy of its calibration, the clothing worn by the woman, the time of day the measurement is made, and the contents of the bowel and bladder at that time. When considering efforts to improve the reliability of measurements, it is useful to keep in mind their purpose. Control of errors is most crucial when weights are collected over a short period (e.g., 1 to 2 weeks). For example, normal weight gain during the second trimester is approximately 0.4 to 0.5 kg (~1 lb) per week, or 1.6 kg (3.5 lb) per month, but it is not unusual for the accumulated errors in weekly or monthly weighings to total 0.4 to 0.7 kg (1 to 1.5 lb) in many clinics. Since a subnormal gain is often defined as less than 1 kg (2 lb) per month, with this degree of error, it might be very difficult to distinguish abnormal weight gains from measurement error over relatively short intervals.

Subjects should be weighed on a platform beam balance scale with movable weights or on a high-quality electronic scale. The scale should be graduated to the nearest 100 g (0.25 lb) and calibrated periodically against a known weight or series of weights approximating the range of weights encountered in clinic patients. For example, barbell weights or boxes of books with known (recorded) weights can be stacked to cover the range of calibration weights. Subjects need not be weighed while they are nude, but procedures should be followed to promote consistency in the amount of clothing worn by all patients. The fewer clothes the better, as long as the weight of the clothing can be kept relatively constant for all women and all seasons of the year. This requires weighing women without purses, shoes, boots, coats, jackets, or any accompanying young children. All personnel responsible for taking weights and other measurements should be trained in the standard procedures chosen by the clinic. It should not be assumed that everyone knows how to obtain weight measurements properly. For clinical management of the patient, it is most important to have accurate measurements taken sequentially throughout the pregnancy.

Prepregnancy weights are determined primarily to establish whether the patient's weight is high, low, or normal and to provide a basis for identifying extreme first-trimester weight changes. Prepregnancy weight is best determined from objective data from the patient's chart reflecting a recent preconceptional visit. Self-reported prepregnancy weights must be evaluated for plausibility and discarded if they are suspect.

Height

Knowledge of standing height (stature) is indispensable when careful classification by prepregnancy weight status is desired. Such classifications are based on body mass index (BMI; see the section Assessing Prepregnancy Weight for Height below) or on a percentage of a standard reference weight for a given height, e.g., the Metropolitan Life Insurance (MLI) Company standards for ideal body weight (1959, 1983). Height can be measured with reasonable precision in a clinical setting if standard procedures are followed. A low-cost stadiometer can be constructed from a metal measuring tape and a headboard. The tape is attached to a vertical wall against which the patient can stand erect with the back, buttocks, and heels against the tape. The headboard can be constructed from two pieces of wood joined to form a right angle. The vertical board is pushed flat against the wall and lowered along the tape measure until the horizontal board makes contact with the patient's head. The measurement is taken at the point where the horizontal board touches the patient's scalp. Commercially available stadiometers can also be used, but the ones built into weighing scales are unsuitable for research purposes. The stadiometer should be inspected periodically to ensure that its position has not changed with use. Height should be measured as early in the pregnancy as possible to avoid errors caused by body posture changes, which may affect measurements beginning approximately 20 weeks into gestation. Postural change may reduce measured height by approximately 1 cm (0.4 in.).

Gestational Duration

The adequacy of accumulated weight gain or achieved weight status at any given stage of pregnancy can be determined only when the length of gestation is known. An accurate estimate of length of gestation is also essential for research on gestational weight gain and fetal growth. By far the most common method of estimating length of gestation is calculation of the time since the last menstrual period (LMP) based on dates provided by the woman at her first prenatal visit. There is an established literature (e.g., Oates and Forrest, 1984; Wilcox and Horney, 1984) dealing with the accuracy of recall of this date. Recall becomes increasingly problematic as the LMP becomes more distant in time and memory becomes less reliable. Also, a small percentage of conceptions in the United States occur during amenorrheic cycles. In some pregnancies, vaginal bleeding occurs within the first 4 to 6 weeks after conception and is falsely reported as a menstrual flow. Moreover, the date of the LMP does not denote the beginning of the pregnancy but only the presumed beginning of the cycle that produced the ovum that was fertilized 10 to 14 days later. *Actual* gestational length, or time from conception, is rarely known and is even less likely to be accurately self-reported several months after conception. *Actual* length of gestation is generally calculated from the estimated date of conception up to the date of the prenatal exam or delivery, whichever is applicable.

In the clinic, a gestational age calculator or table, special computer program, or programmed hand calculator should be used to estimate the length of time since last menstruation, rather than calculations made in the head or on paper. Early (prior to 20 weeks) ultrasound measurement of the fetal biparietal diameter represents an alternative for estimating gestational duration.

Although errors in estimating gestational duration may pose problems of interpretation when one uses incremental weight gain from conception to a point later in gestation, they do not do so when estimating the rate of weight gain between two or more prenatal visits after the first trimester. A shift of several weeks in the gestational age estimate does not affect the interpretation of the rate of gain, since it is generally linear over a broad range of pregnancy from 13 to 35 weeks of gestation.

Assessing Prepregnancy Weight for Height

To assess prepregnancy weight for height, it is necessary either to calculate BMI or to compare the weight for height to a weight-for-height reference standard (e.g., MLI ideal weight tables). To minimize the chance of calculation errors, it is advisable to use the units of measure used in the clinic (i.e., metric or English system).

BMI is the most common expression of body weight corrected for height in use today. It is computed as follows:

$$BMI = \frac{wt}{ht^2} = \frac{kg}{m^2} \times 100, \text{ or } \frac{lb}{in.^2} \times 100.$$

BMI can be easily determined from the table in Appendix C. A similar weight-for-height index is achieved by expressing body weight as a percentage of desirable body weight adjusted for height in the following form:

$$\text{Percentage of reference weight} = \frac{\text{observed weight}}{\substack{\text{expected or desirable weight} \\ \text{given the patient's height}}} \times 100.$$

The most widely used values for bracketing normal weight seem to be 90 and 120% of the 1959 MLI (Metropolitan Life Insurance Company, 1959) reference weights. This, in turn, corresponds to a metric BMI of approximately 19.8 to 26.0. However, some clinicians use 80% of the 1959 MLI reference as the cutoff point for distinguishing those who are underweight, while others may use 95% as the cutoff point. The cutoff point for overweight may be as low as 110% to as high as 130% of MLI reference weights. Moreover, an increasing number of clinics are using the 1983 version of the MLI reference weights (Metropolitan Life Insurance Company, 1983).

There is no statistical or scientific basis for prescribing one set of cutoff values or reference standards over another when assessing prepregnancy weight. The relationship between prepregnancy weight and various fetal or maternal outcomes is generally considered to be linear, with no well-defined threshold at either end of the prepregnancy weight distribution, but this view has not been verified by research. Pending further research, the subcommittee recommends using a metric BMI of 19.8 to 26.0 as the definition of normal (moderate) prepregnancy weight for height. This BMI range (see Appendix C) encompasses the 25th to 75th percentiles of prepregnancy weight for height of women in the 1980 National Natality Survey (Kleinman, 1990).

BMI is a preferred indicator of nutritional status because it depends on two commonly measured aspects of body morphology—weight and height. BMI is often viewed as a proxy for more accurate indicators of body composition such as body fat content or lean body mass, but it is not simply an obesity index. Women with BMIs greater than 26.0 do not necessarily have excess body fat deposition; in some, the extra weight may be attributable predominantly to muscle tissue or skeletal mass. Studies relating BMI or its equivalent to estimates of body fat obtained from more complex methods, such as those described in Chapter 6, have indicated a good correlation between percentage of body fat and BMI (e.g., $R = .7$; Jackson et al., 1988), but there will be considerable misclassification of undernutrition or obesity.

Using Weight Gain Data in the Clinic

It is desirable to plot cumulated weight gain (weight gain to date) sequentially on a weight gain chart that has a reference curve that reflects normal weight gain. This allows visual inspection of the overall trajectory or slope of the patient's weight gain and comparison with the standard. It thus provides the clinician with a visual impression of whether or not weight gain is progressing normally for the mother. Toward the end of gestation, cumulated weight gain becomes increasingly predictive of birth weight because the weight contributed by the fetus becomes relatively greater.

Gestational weight gain can be monitored in a manner similar to methods recommended for monitoring child growth (see Griffiths, 1985). For example, at the third prenatal visit it is useful to compare the rate of gain between the second and third visits to the rate of gain between the first and second visits. A rapid weight gain is more acceptable if the starting weight was unusually low for the woman's height or if the weight gain between the first and second visits was unusually low. In both cases, one might interpret the rapid weight gain as catching up to or compensating for poor earlier weight status. In contrast, if a woman were obese before pregnancy and she gained weight rapidly between each successive measurement, there is cause for concern. Unusually high or low gains should be checked for possible measurement or recording error.

To determine numerically whether the rate of weight gain is close to that recommended, the following equation can be used:

$$\text{weight gain} = \frac{\text{wt}_t - \text{wt}_{t-1}}{\text{GA}_t - \text{GA}_{t-1}},$$

where wt is weight, GA is gestational age in weeks, t is time of most recent measurement, and $t - 1$ = time of previous measurement. As an example, if body weight is 135 lb at week 20 of the pregnancy and 139 lb at week 25, then

$$\text{weight gain (lb/wk)} = \frac{139 \text{ lb} - 135 \text{ lb}}{25 \text{ wk} - 20 \text{ wk}} = \frac{4 \text{ lb}}{5 \text{ wk}} = 0.8 \text{ lb/wk}.$$

It is less useful to calculate rate of gain for periods including part or all of the first trimester, when the rate of gain is normally low, than for periods within the second and third trimesters.

Weight Gain Charts

Many different weight gain charts and tables are available for use in the clinical assessment of gestational weight gain; Table 4-1 presents selected examples representing a wide range of applications. An evaluation of the characteristics of these various charts is useful in considering their application in the clinical setting. Weight gain charts evolved over the past

40 years in four basic stages: (1) early, normative charts constructed from a homogeneous sample (usually a very small sample) of healthy women who delivered normal infants, (2) modification of the early normative charts to account for maternal prepregnancy weight, (3) elaboration of the charts that incorporate prepregnancy weight status by inclusion of more recent normative data on gestational weight gain, and (4) elaboration of prepregnancy weight classification to establish target weights based on some percentage of the ideal or reference prepregnancy weight. However, there is still a need for a validated chart, with the characteristics outlined in Appendix A.

In Table 4-1, the large number of charts from the 1980s reflects an increased interest by the scientific community and a growing awareness of the inadequacy of early weight gain charts among practitioners. Also, the expansion of prenatal services in the Supplemental Food Program for Women, Infants, and Children (WIC) created a demand for gestational weight gain charts. The subcommittee had access to weight gain charts used by WIC in 21 states. They represent a broad range of different types of charts, based on different sources of information on normal weight gain. As described in Table 4-1, most of the charts developed for WIC at the state level include the normative curve originally reported by Tompkins and Wiehl (1951) (Figure 4-1) and make some allowance for prepregnancy weight for height. The mean total gestational weight gain for the 60 women in Tompkins and Wiehl's sample was 10.9 kg (24 lb), but no ranges, standard deviations, or percentiles were reported.

The curve developed by Tompkins and Wiehl has been used differently in different charts. Some states (e.g., Ohio, Georgia, Oregon, Massachusetts, New Hampshire, and Rhode Island) use the curve to represent the average or target weight gain for women with normal prepregnancy weight. In the chart used by Oregon WIC (Oregon WIC Staff, 1981) (Figure 4-2), upper and lower limits have been added to the original Tompkins and Wiehl curve, but their derivation is not given. Other states use different curves for women who are overweight or underweight before pregnancy (e.g., Figure 4-3). Some states (e.g., Wisconsin, Florida, New Jersey, Idaho, Washington, Wyoming, and New York) use the Tompkins and Wiehl curve to depict the lower limits of normal. Some use separate charts for normal weight, overweight, and underweight women, and also include upper and lower limits, such as those in Figure 4-4A through D. The limits have not been based on systematic studies of the consequence of misclassification resulting from the use of specific cutoff points or limits—such studies have not yet been conducted.

Dimperio (1988) has developed a weight gain chart which includes an 11.4-kg (25-lb) total gain marking the lower limit and a procedure for adjusting the single curve for different prepregnancy weights for height

TABLE 4-1 Characteristics of Gestational Weight Gain Charts and Tables

Reference and Description	Basis	Characteristics of Reference Population	Target Gestational Weight Gain, kg (lb)[a]	Comments
Early normative, average only				
Tompkins and Wiehl, 1951 (most widely published chart)	Average gain for 60 healthy women with favorable pregnancy outcomes	Within 10% of ideal body weight, other characteristics not reported	11 (24)	Often credited to other sources such as Lull and Kimbrough (1953), Pritchard et al. (1985). No adjustments made for prepregnancy weight for height.
Hytten and Leitch, 1971	Average gain for a healthy group of 2,870 women with favorable pregnancy outcomes	White, British, normotensive, primiparous women between ages 20 and 29	12.5 (27.5)	No adjustments made for prepregnancy weight for height.
Early normative, modified for WIC				
Oregon WIC Staff, 1981 Chart used in Oregon WIC	Curve drawn by Tompkins and Wiehl (1951) used as average curve; upper and lower limits added	NA	11 (24); range, 7 to 14.5 (15 to 32)	Methods not described for setting limits for insufficient (<15 lb) or excessive (>32 lb) gain.
Butman, 1982 Chart used in Massachusetts WIC	Curve drawn by Tompkins and Wiehl (1951) used to set lower limits for women of normal weight; curve drawn by Hytten and Leitch (1971) used as average	NA	Underweight: 13.5 (30) Normal weight: 11 to 13.5 (24 to 30) Overweight: 8 to 10 (18 to 22)	Adjustments made for prepregnancy weight for height below 95% or above 105% of 1959 MLI standards. Reasons for lower limit of gain of 22 lb not specified; no upper limit set.

Idaho WIC Program, 1988 Chart used in Idaho WIC	Same as for Massachusetts WIC	NA	Underweight: 12.5 to 16.5 (28 to 36) Normal weight: 11 to 13.5 (24 to 30) Overweight: 8 to 10 (18 to 22)	Combines recommendations from many sources. Adjustments made for prepregnancy weight for height below 85% or above 120% of 1959 MLI standard. Provides separate recommendations for teens and women carrying multiple fetuses.

Recent normative curves by prepregnancy weight for height

Brown et al., 1986 Four separate curves for undersized, normal-weight, overweight, and obese women	Average gain for 459 healthy women delivering infants weighing between 3,000 and 4,500 g	Mixed ethnic background, age, and parity; low income; Cleveland and Minneapolis Maternal-Infant Care clinics	Underweight: 12.5 to 16.5 (28 to 36) Normal weight: 11 to 14.5 (24 to 32) Overweight: 9 to 11 (20 to 24) Obese: 9 (20)	No limits specified on graphs. Adjustments made for prepregnancy weight for height below 95% or above 115% of 1959 MLI standard.
Dimperio, 1988 Single set of curves for lower and upper limits of gain that is adjusted depending on four levels of prepregnancy weight for height	Appears to use modified version of Tompkins and Wiehl (1951) as lower limit; upper limit is 4.5 kg (10 lb) higher than lower limit after 13 weeks	NA	Underweight: 15.5 to >13.5 (25 to >30) Normal weight: 11.5 to 13.5 (25 to 30) Moderately obese: 7 to 11.5 kg (15 to 25) Massively obese: 7 to 9 (15 to 20)	Adjustments made for prepregnancy weight for height below 90%, above 120%, or above 150% of 1959 MLI standard. Recommends that underweight women gain as much weight as normal-weight women plus enough to make up their weight deficit. Not clear how to interpret overweight on grid.

Table 4-1 continues

TABLE 4-1—Continued

Reference and Description	Basis	Characteristics of Reference Population	Target Gestational Weight Gain, kg (lb)[a]	Comments
Single grids or tables, to provide targets for proportional weight gain based on prepregnancy weight for height				
Gueri et al., 1982 One table of recommended weights to achieve for specific week of gestation and maternal height	Average gain of 12 kg (26 lb) over 40 weeks and average weight for height of women aged 18 to 24 years in NHANES I	NA	120% of ideal body weight	Validity of ideal body weight was not tested; chart appears to recommend weight loss for obese women.
Rosso, 1985 One chart with many weight gain curves depending on prepregnancy weight for height	Target gains based on weight gains of women delivering an infant weighing 3,500 g	Black and Hispanic women, 20 to 25 years of age, of mixed parity	Underweight and normal weight gain to 120% of ideal weight for height; overweight gain to 115% of prepregnancy weight	Standard weight is based on 1959 MLI table. Recommends very large weight gains for underweight women and potentially high gains for massively obese women.
Husaini et al., 1986 One chart with many weight gain curves depending on maternal height	Target weight gains based on weight gains of women delivering infants weighing more than 2,500 g	1,332 Indonesian women of mixed parity aged 14 to 44	10 (22)	Reference population is very short in stature.

NOTE: WIC = Supplemental Food Program for Women, Infants, and Children. NA = Not available given that various charts are generally combined or modified. MLI = Metropolitan Life Insurance Company's tables of ideal weight for height (Metropolitan Life Insurance Company, 1959). NHANES I = First National Health and Nutrition Examination Survey.
[a] Rounded to the nearest half pound or kilogram.

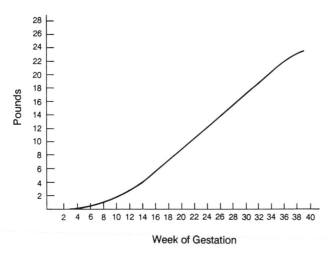

FIGURE 4-1 Weight gain grid from Tompkins and Wiehl (1951).

(Figure 4-5). Several states (e.g., Indiana, Kansas, Mississippi, and Colorado) use weight gain charts based on normative data for a group of low-income pregnant women from Cleveland and Minneapolis (Brown et al., 1986) (Figure 4-6). For these charts, the total target weight gain for women with a normal prepregnancy weight is 14.3 kg (31.5 lb), which is approximately 2.9 kg (6.5 lb) higher than specified on most of the charts mentioned above. Several authors (e.g., Gueri et al., 1982; Husaini et al., 1986; and Rosso, 1985) have developed single charts or tables to be applied across a range of prepregnancy weights, heights, or weights for height. A table of reference weights for height developed by Gueri et al. (1982) is intended to be used at any stage of pregnancy. Figure 4-7 is based on data from that table to illustrate the weight gain patterns suggested by Gueri et al. The basis for and limitations of this table are discussed later in this chapter.

In order to accommodate inconsistency in the application of proportionate weight gain recommendations across the range of prepregnancy weight for height, Rosso (1985) developed a weight gain grid that applies different assumptions of weight gain patterns for underweight and overweight women (Figure 4-8). Rosso's grid suggests that normal-weight women should be advised to achieve 120% of their prepregnancy reference weight for height but that overweight women (e.g., those weighing up to 140% of reference weight for height) should gain up to 115% of their prepregnancy reference weight. Rosso's chart, like that of Gueri et al. (1982), suggests that underweight women gain all their weight deficit up to their prepregnancy reference weight as well as the additional weight

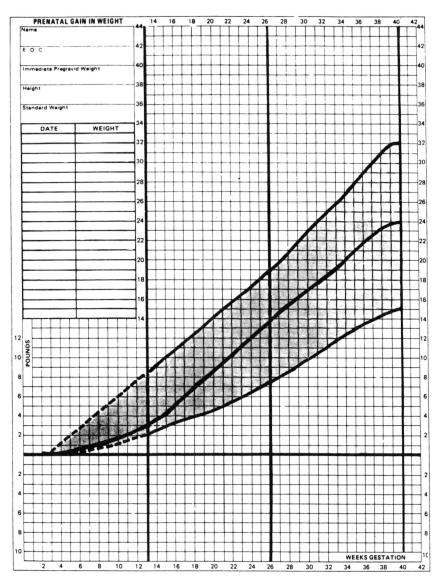

FIGURE 4-2 Weight gain grid from Oregon WIC (Oregon WIC Staff, 1981). Lower and upper lines represent extremes of achieved weight gain.

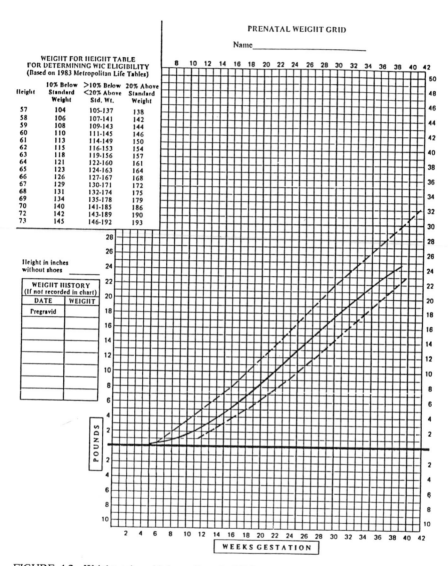

FIGURE 4-3 Weight gain grid from Georgia WIC (Georgia Dietetic Association, 1987). Lower dashed line is recommended gain for overweight women; upper dashed line is recommended gain for underweight women.

76

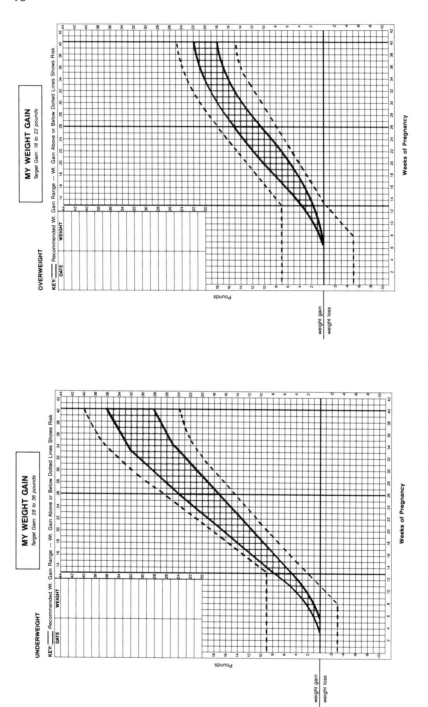

FIGURE 4-4 Weight gain grids from Idaho WIC Program (1988) for underweight (A), overweight (B), teenage (C), and normal (standard) weight (D) women.

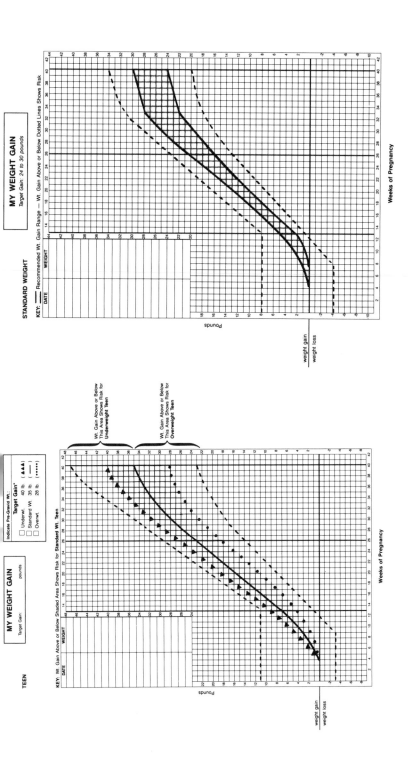

Instructions on Use of Weight Grid. The weight grid shown in [this figure] was developed to facilitate [use of] the guidelines given in [the accompanying] manual [i.e., in Dimperio, 1988], particularly for underweight women. It shows a weight gain range between 25 and 35 pounds over baseline weight. Baseline weight (zero) is standard weight or actual prepregnancy weight, whichever is greater. Women who are at standard weight at conception and obese women have their prepregnancy weight plotted at zero. The woman who is at standard weight, with a singleton pregnancy, should gain somewhere in the normal range shown. The grid does not show the recommended weight gain for obese women. These lines will need to be drawn by hand. The prepregnancy weight of the underweight woman should be plotted below the line showing the number of pounds she is underweight. [Following is an example given by Dimperio (1988) for a normal weight woman.]

Step 1: Assess PPW [prepregnancy weight]: [in this example, it is in] the normal range of standard weight.

Step 2: Plot standard weight of 126 at zero.

Step 3: Calibrate [vertical] scale based on patient's weight.

Step 4: Plot today's weight of 136 lb at her current gestational age of 20 weeks.

Step 5: Continue to plot weight at each visit and encourage a total gain of 25-30 lb.

WOMEN AT STANDARD WEIGHT

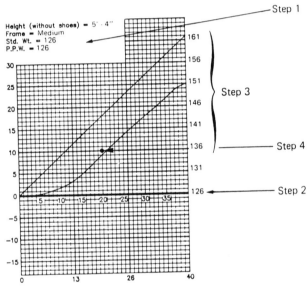

FIGURE 4-5   Weight gain grid from Dimperio (1988).

needed to achieve 120% of that reference weight during gestation. The theoretical assumptions on which proportionate weight gain recommendations are made clearly need to be evaluated through careful research. Special attention should be directed toward women at the extremes of prepregnant weight. Assumptions based on *average* women with *average* gains, delivering *average* infants may not apply to women at the extremes.

Interpretation of charts and tables is confounded by the unresolved differences concerning the optimal reference standards and cutoff points to be used in classifying women as underweight, normal weight, overweight,

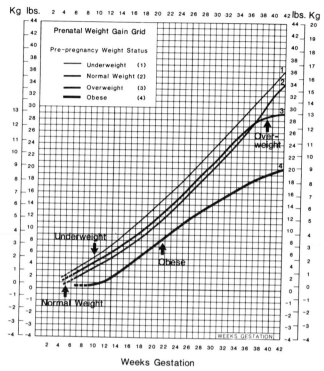

Weeks Gestation

FIGURE 4-6   Weight gain grid from J. Brown, University of Minnesota, 1987, unpublished; used with permission.

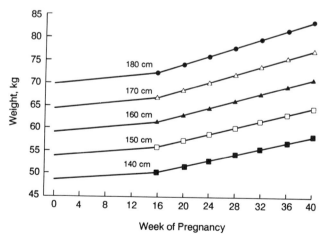

Week of Pregnancy

FIGURE 4-7   Weight gain chart based on tabular data reported by Gueri et al. (1982).

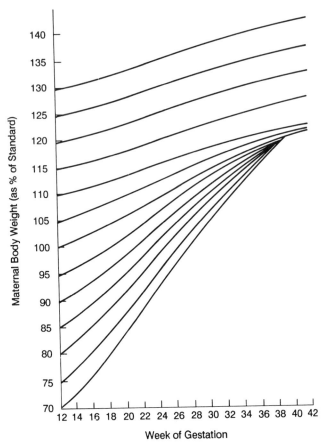

FIGURE 4-8   Chart designed for use in monitoring weight gain during pregnancy considering prepregnancy weight for height as a percentage of a standard. From Rosso (1985).

and obese. Normative data from the First National Health and Nutrition Examination Survey (NHANES I) for women aged 18 to 24 give mean values of weight for a given height that are 2.5 to 6 kg (5 to 13 lb) heavier than the 1959 MLI ideal weights [used by Rosso (1985) and in many WIC programs], but they are only about 1 kg (2.2 lb) heavier than the 1983 MLI values (Metropolitan Life Insurance Company, 1983) used, for example, with the chart depicted in Figure 4-3.

Another problem related to the choice of reference values for BMI arises when classifying young adolescent mothers. No widely accepted standards of weight for height exist for adolescents. The National Center for Health Statistics has developed weight and height standards for children from birth through 18 years of age (Hamill et al., 1977), but weight-for-height charts only up to 137 cm (54 in.)—the median height of 10-year-old girls in the United States. The large variation in weight and height at adolescence and the dependence of weight for height on age in late adolescence have presented major barriers to the establishment of weight-for-height standards in that age group. Except for very young girls or those who conceive within two years of menarche, adult BMI recommendations may be used provisionally to classify girls as underweight, moderate weight, overweight, and obese. However, new research should be directed toward the construction of appropriate adolescent standards for BMI that consider variation in maturational status and subsequent pregnancy outcome.

Although the data from such national probability surveys as NHANES I are normative, they were not intended to be used as target or recommended weights. The MLI tables of desirable weights for height give weights that are based on actuarial analyses of the mortality risks associated with body weight for height in a large sample of insurance policy holders over the previous five decades (Society of Actuaries, 1959, 1960; Society of Actuaries/Association of Life Insurance Medical Directors of America, 1980). BMI values associated with the lowest mortality in the 1959 MLI desirable weight tables are nearly identical to the normative values reported by Flegal et al. (1988) for 18- to 24-year-old white women in 1960. Compared with the 1959 MLI tables, the recommended weights in the 1983 MLI revision are higher, equaling the increase in average body weight observed in the U.S. population over the same period. Burton et al. (1985) raise questions about the advisability of using the 1983 MLI tables because of their higher recommended weights.

The actuarial analysis on which the MLI tables are based may not be relevant in categorizing the prepregnancy weight for height of U.S. women because it is based on mortality data that are unrelated to pregnancy outcomes. There is no evidence that the desirable weights for height in either of the MLI tables, which are associated with the lowest mortality later in life, are also associated with favorable reproductive outcome earlier in life. Thus, the subcommittee has no scientific basis on which to accept or reject any of the existing reference standards for evaluating prepregnancy weight-for-height status, but it has adopted the BMI ranges shown in Table 4-2 to define four weight-for-height categories. The BMI ranges in Table 4-2 approximate 1959 MLI cutoff values for 90, 120, and 135% of ideal body weight for height. Since there is no empirical basis for establishing specific cutoff values for pregnant women, further refinement of the BMI cutoff values would be inappropriate at this time. The 1959 MLI cutoff values seem to be as appropriate as any others (such as 1983 MLI cutoff values) because most weight gain charts in current use refer to the 1959 MLI classification criteria. Also, the 19.8 and 26.0 cutoff

TABLE 4-2   Classifying Maternal Prepregnancy
Weight-for-Height Status: BMI[a] Compared with 1959
MLI[b] Standards

Weight-for-Height Status	BMI	1959 MLI, %
Very low	<16.5	<80
Low	16.5 to 19.7	80 to 90
Normal	19.8 to 26.0	91 to 120
High	>26.0 to 29.0	121 to 135
Very high	>29	>135

[a] BMI expressed in metric units.
[b] From Metropolitan Life Insurance Company (1959).

values for BMI approximate the 25th and 85th percentiles, respectively, of
the distribution of prepregnancy weight for height from the 1980 National
Natality Survey, which is the basis for much of the discussion of the
effect that prepregnancy weight and weight gain have on fetal growth (see
Chapter 8). Within programs such as WIC, there would be advantages to
the consistent use of a single reference standard and common cutoff values.
    Given the considerable differences across various weight gain charts
and tables in current use and the large differences between these charts
and the normative values from the 1980 National Natality Survey (see
Chapter 8), the subcommittee does not recommend one of these charts
above another. None of the charts reviewed contains all the elements the
subcommittee considers important in constructing a scientifically valid chart
(Appendix A). Based on data reviewed in Chapter 8, the subcommittee
presents provisional charts in Appendix B.

INTERPRETATION OF RESEARCH INVOLVING GESTATIONAL
WEIGHT GAIN

    In interpreting studies bearing on the health implications of gestational
weight gain, it is necessary to pay careful attention to definitions, which
suffer from uncertainties in three areas: (1) the method of designating
prepregnancy weight, (2) the length of the period during which weight
changes are recorded, and (3) the inclusion of fetal weight as part of
maternal weight gain. In addition, regardless of the ways weight gain is
measured and expressed, it should be assessed in light of such factors
as prepregnancy weight, maternal height, pattern of weight changes by
trimester of the pregnancy, and comparison with an appropriate reference
standard. Table 4-3 summarizes five ways in which gestational weight gain
is commonly defined and presents criteria for evaluating their utility.

TABLE 4-3 Definitions of Gestational Weight Gain and Comments on Their Applications

Method of Expressing Gestational Weight	Availability of Measurements	Characteristics	Disadvantages[a]
1. *Total Weight Gain* (final weight minus initial weight)		Used in research and surveillance	Does not identify important patterns, not useful for monitoring during pregnancy, and is influenced by length of gestation
Initial weight is prepregnancy weight	Difficult to obtain in some population subgroups	Includes early gain but is subject to biased recall of prepregnancy weight	
Initial weight is weight at first prenatal visit	Commonly available	Does not rely on prepregnancy weight, but may seriously affect calculated weight change in late registrants	
Final weight is weight at delivery	Not routinely collected	Gives total weight gain and is important for research	
Final weight is weight at last prenatal visit	Commonly available	Practical, but may be obtained several weeks before delivery	
2. *Net Maternal Weight Gain*		Used in research and surveillance	
Total weight gain minus birth weight	Commonly available	Removes part-whole correlation with birth weight and provides estimate of maternal gain	Not particularly useful for clinical applications since fetal weight cannot be determined in utero and corrections cannot be made during gestation
Total weight gain minus weight of products of conception	Birth weight available, but not weight of placenta and amniotic fluid	Removes part-whole correlation as above; also subtracts weight of placenta and amniotic fluid, thus providing a better estimate of maternal tissue gain	

Table 4-3 continues

TABLE 4-3—Continued

Method of Expressing Gestational Weight	Availability of Measurements	Characteristics	Disadvantages[a]
Postpartum weight minus prepregnancy weight	Easy to measure, but not often available	Removes part-whole correlation as above; influenced by time since delivery (diuresis)	Usually assumes a linear pattern, which may not be the case if first trimester is included
		Used in the clinic, and in research and surveillance	
3. *Incremental Weight Gain* (weight gain between two or more specified dates)			
Weight gain by trimester or other long periods or intervals	Easy to measure, but not commonly available	Does not necessarily require prepregnancy weight but may need an accurate estimate of gestational age	
Cumulative gain to a specific point in gestation	Routinely available in the clinic but not commonly available for research	Partially removes time dependence but may be biased by poor prepregnancy weight and gestational age	
Weekly or monthly rate of gain	Routinely available in the clinic but not commonly available for research	Removes time dependence, but may be nonlinear and therefore affected by frequency of measurements	

Method			
4. Weight Gain as a Percentage of Body Weight (Pregnant weight/actual prepregnancy weight) $\times$ 100	Requires knowledge of prepregnancy weight	Potentially useful in the clinic and in research Expresses gain relative to initial weight, but does not consider differential responses of extremes of prepregnancy weight	Assumes that total weight gain should be proportional to initial or desirable weight. Does not distinguish patterns of gain. Suffers from same biases as total weight gain
(Pregnant weight/desirable prepregnancy body weight) $\times$ 100	Weight commonly available and prepregnancy weight not required	Standardizes gain for maternal height, but standards have not been validated	
5. As a Percentage of Recommended Gain (Total gain/recommended gain) $\times$ 100	No validated standards for recommended gain	Potentially useful in the clinic and in research Removes time dependence, but does not assume a specific pattern of gain; subject to same definitional problems as total weight gain	Assumes that percentages of gain at different points of gestation are comparable; the selection of standards is arbitrary
(Incremental gain/recommended incremental gain for the same period) $\times$ 100	No validated standards for recommended gain	Removes time dependence, but does not assume a specific pattern of gain; subject to same definitional problems as total weight gain	

[a] Pertains to the entire category of gestational weight gain, not to each item within the method.

Estimation of Gestational Weight Gain in Research

Information on gestational weight gain is commonly used in biomedical research, public health, and nutritional surveillance as well as in clinical care. Each application has its own requirements for the method of expressing weight gain, but each benefits from rigorous attention to collecting high-quality data. The following discussion deals primarily with uses of gestational weight gain in research, which has stringent requirements for data quality and completeness.

By far the most common expression of gestational weight gain in research is total weight gain based on the difference between an initial weight and a final weight taken in the last few weeks prior to delivery (Method 1 in Table 4-3). Rarely is it corrected for the weight of the fetus, placenta, and amniotic fluid in an effort to assess net weight gain or maternal tissue change (Method 2). Occasionally, total weight gain is corrected for gestational length to yield a rate of gain (Method 3). Increasingly, both researchers and clinicians are expressing gestational weight gain relative to either the observed or desirable prepregnancy weight (Method 4) or some recommended weight gain (Method 5), in which case the reference body weight (actual or desirable) should be expressed relative to maternal stature.

All the methods of expressing gestational weight gain shown in Table 4-3 have been used in research. A premium is placed on reliable weight measurements, accurate estimates of gestational age, and valid reference standards. Total weight gain based on recalled prepregnancy weight without correction for length of gestation has severe limitations. This is particularly true in the study of mechanisms by which weight gain and, more specifically, changes in maternal tissue and nutritional status affect maternal and fetal well-being. Measures of rate of weight gain, especially for specific phases of gestation, provide insight into the timing of intrauterine insults and, perhaps, into the mechanisms of fetal growth retardation and pregnancy and postpartum complications. However, the data needed to compute weight gain by stages of gestation are difficult to collect with adequate quality in all but the best-controlled prospective studies.

Prepregnancy Weight Estimates

Recalled prepregnancy weights may be acceptable for research under many circumstances (Stevens-Simon et al., 1986); however, U.S. women of reproductive age tend to report current weights approximately 1.4 kg (3 lb) lower than their actual weights. Moreover, U.S. women who perceive themselves as overweight or who have less than a high school education underestimate their weight to a greater extent than do those who believe their weights are normal or who have more formal education (Stewart, 1982).

Unlike weight, height tends to be overreported by an average of 1.1 cm (0.42 in.), especially among short women with limited formal education (Stewart, 1982). Considering the negative bias in recalled weight and the positive bias in self-reported height, BMIs based on self-reported rather than measured prepregnancy weights and heights tend to be underestimated to a greater degree than is weight alone.

Weights determined at the first prenatal visit during the first trimester of pregnancy have been used to estimate total weight gain and early-gestation weight gain, but they do not necessarily reflect prepregnancy weights. Although average weight gain in the first trimester is small relative to that in later periods of pregnancy, individual variation may be considerable. Total gestational weight gains may be overestimated by self-reporting or underestimated if based on late first trimester weight.

Gestational Duration Estimates

The use of reported LMP to estimate gestational duration has been shown (Kramer et al., 1988) to result in substantial misclassification of preterm and postterm ($\geq$42 weeks of gestation) births and thus, possibly, incorrect diagnosis of intrauterine growth retardation. This error in gestational age could cause an overestimate of the rate of weight gain in women delivering at full-term but whose LMP dates suggest a preterm birth. Kramer et al. suggest an even greater error in overestimating gestational age among women with postterm LMP dates. Women who deliver their infants at full-term rather than postterm (as estimated from their LMP) may have an underestimate of their true rate of gain when that rate is calculated based on the LMP gestational age.

To improve upon estimates of gestational length based on LMP dates, several methods have been used during pregnancy (sonography, symphysis-uterine fundal height) and at delivery (newborn maturity indicators). All these methods are based on measurements that are dependent upon length of gestation. In all cases, the estimates of gestational age were validated against gestational duration based on LMP, which is itself an imperfect measure. Moreover, all these techniques are based on measurements of fetal development that are also influenced by intrauterine environmental factors. Therefore, a 20-week-old fetus (whose age was estimated by sonography) who is determined to be growth retarded to the size of a 16-week-old fetus will be given a gestational age of 16 weeks, and the gestational weight gain of the mother may be charted at 16, not 20, weeks from conception. If there is an association between gestational weight gain and fetal growth, this relationship might be obscured by the fact that both the dependent variable (fetal weight or birth weight for gestational age) and the independent variable (weight gain) are biased in the same direction by errors in estimating gestational age.

Determining Final Weight and Rates of Weight Gain

Rarely is the final maternal weight measured at admission to the hospital just before delivery, but rather, it is measured at the last prenatal visit. Moreover, weights taken at the hospital vary according to the status of the membranes, i.e., whether or not they have ruptured, the content of the bladder and bowel, and the amount of clothing worn during the weighing, which is likely to have been done in a hurry.

An alternative to using total weight gain is to compute a rate of weight gain up to the date of the last prenatal visit. Of course, any estimate of a rate of weight gain based only on initial and final weights assumes a linear pattern, which is not likely to be the case. Most evidence suggests that the lowest rates of weight gain occur during the earliest and latest weeks of a term pregnancy (see Chapter 5), when the frequency of the weighings may be most variable. A nonlinear pattern of weight gain plus the irregular time between weighings could result in more error in estimating the rate of weight gain as opposed to total weight gain. For example, a woman who gains a total of 11 kg (25 lb) between 12 and 37 weeks of gestation would have gained weight at a linear rate of 0.5 kg/week (1 lb/week). But if (as sometimes occurs) this initial weight is used as the prepregnancy weight (i.e., weight at week zero of gestation) and the weight at the last prenatal visit (e.g., at 37 weeks of gestation) is used as the delivery weight (e.g., at 39 weeks of gestation), then the computed rate is 0.3 kg/week (0.64 lb/week). More frequent weighings enable investigators to make more precise estimates of weight gain patterns according to the trimester of pregnancy, and would facilitate identification of the occurrence of fetal or maternal health problems by period of gestation.

Including the Fetus in Total Weight Gain

Total gestational weight gain includes the products of conception as well as maternal tissue (Method 1 in Table 4-3). The definition may lead to problems of misinterpretation of studies relating maternal weight gain to birth weight. When the weight of the newborn is included in both the dependent and independent variables, a statistical situation known as part-whole correlation occurs. This is of considerable concern in research on maternal factors relating to variation in fetal growth when causal mechanisms are being investigated (see Chapter 8). In clinical settings, however, where total weight gain is used as a screening tool to assess fetal well-being, it is advantageous that maternal weight gain reflects fetal size, especially if the screening takes place at a stage of pregnancy that allows intervention. To estimate maternal tissue mass more closely, researchers generally subtract the infant's birth weight from the total weight gain. At times, this procedure is refined by subtracting placental weight and an estimate of amniotic fluid weight. Or, when the data are available, net weight gain may be estimated by subtracting prepregnancy weight from postpartum weight obtained after delivery.

Comparison of Gestational Weight Gain with Reference Standards

The expression of maternal weight or weight gain relative to a reference standard is especially useful if initial weights were taken after the first trimester of pregnancy and total or cumulative weight gain could not be calculated. One approach is to express weight at a given gestational age relative to prepregnancy body weight or desirable body weight (Method 4 in Table 4-3). This is based on the assumption that weight gain should be proportional to either initial or desirable body weight. These two ways of expressing the reference prepregnancy weight can yield very different results at the extremes of the observed body weight distribution in a population. An overweight woman who is 165-cm (65-in.) tall and whose prepregnancy weight was 80 kg (176 lb) serves as an example. If she gains 15 kg (33 lb) during a pregnancy, she achieves 119% of her actual prepregnancy weight (95 kg/80 kg) but 161% of her "ideal" prepregnancy weight (i.e., 59 kg, according to 1959 MLI tables). On the other hand, a woman of the same height who weighs 45 kg (99 lb) and gains 15 kg (33 lb) during pregnancy would achieve 133% of her observed prepregnancy weight and 102% of her ideal weight.

One advantage to the use of ideal prepregnancy weight as a reference weight is that it does not require knowledge of actual prepregnancy weight. Also, any analysis that includes weight gain expressed as a percentage of observed prepregnancy weight will be confounded by prepregnancy weight, the very factor that is independently related to pregnancy outcome and that may modify the effect of weight gain on the outcome.

Using ideal body weight as the reference weight from which total pre-scribed weight gain is estimated, Gueri et al. (1982) presented a rationale for recommending a total gestational weight gain equal to 20% of the mother's ideal weight for height. They based their weight gain recommendations on four assumptions: (1) the desirable prepregnancy weights for height used are the average weights for U.S. women of different heights, as obtained for women between 18 and 24 years of age in the NHANES I survey, (2) the average total gestational weight gain should be 12 kg (26.4 lb), (3) the average increment of gestational weight gain should be 20% of the ideal prepregnancy weight, and (4) the average gestational weight gain of 1 kg (2.2 lb) in the first trimester and the gain of 11 kg (24.2 lb) in the next two trimesters follow a linear pattern.

As illustrated in Figure 4-7, the target maternal weight at any gestational age differs according to maternal height. A total gain of 12 kg (26.5 lb) equals 20% of the average weight of U.S. women of average height (163 cm, or 64 in.) in the reference population. Taller women have a higher desirable body weight and would be expected to gain proportionately more than 12 kg. Similarly, shorter women would be expected to gain proportionately less weight. The adjustments for weight gain by trimester made by Gueri and colleagues were based on the assumption that regardless of the total prescribed weight gain, one-twelfth (8.3%) of the total gain should occur in the first trimester, and the remaining eleven-twelfths of the total gain should be divided equally between the remaining two trimesters (i.e., 45.8% of the total gain in each trimester).

The application of this recommendation to women at the extremes of the weight-for-height spectrum poses a problem. Underweight women would be expected not only to compensate for their entire deficit in prepregnancy body weight but also to add the tissues of pregnancy during a 9-month period. For a 160-cm (63-in.) tall woman whose prepregnancy weight was 47.5 kg (104 lb), this would amount to a gain of 23.5 kg (52 lb)—50% of her prepregnancy weight—during the course of the pregnancy. The subcommittee found no evidence that such a large weight gain would be desirable for underweight women. Another serious problem with the table of Gueri et al. occurs at the upper end of the range of prepregnancy weight for height. Women at 120% of the reference weight would be advised to gain no weight during pregnancy, and those over 120% of the reference weight would be advised to lose weight during pregnancy.

Husaini et al. (1986) developed a weight gain grid for Indonesian women based on the same principles used by Gueri and colleagues, but they used observed weight gain among women who delivered infants weighing more than 2,500 g (5.5 lb) at birth. Overweight was not a factor in this poor, rural Javanese population, so their patterns of weight gain for different heights appear to follow those presented by Gueri et al. However, the achieved weights at any given height and at any given week of gestation are considerably lower than those suggested by Gueri and associates. Furthermore, the weight gain chart for Indonesian women does not assume a proportionate weight gain; short women of any prepregnancy weight would gain the same absolute amount of weight during gestation as taller women of the same relative weight for height.

Another modification of this approach is to express weight gain as a percentage of recommended gain, either over the entire pregnancy or over specified periods (Method 5 in Table 4-3). This requires the same measurements as in Methods 1 and 3 but expresses the resulting gains relative to a standard. This is similar to the way one expresses weight or height in children relative to a postnatal growth standard. The advantage of this method is that it allows weights collected at different frequencies during different stages of pregnancy to be compared on a similar scale (as percentages of reference weight gain) and thus removes the time dependence of weight changes described above. This is also the preferred way of expressing gestational weight gain when studying its effect on length of gestation or risk of premature delivery. Since premature delivery will shorten the time over which weight gain occurs, there is a need to express weight gain in a way that is independent of the length of gestation. Many researchers choose to express weight gain as a rate. However, this approach usually does not account for the nonlinear nature of weight gain throughout gestation, which will result in a bias toward underestimating the true rate of weight gain if the pregnancy is terminated early. This bias could lead to an observed negative relationship between rate of weight gain and risk of preterm delivery that may not actually exist. One solution to this problem is to express weight gain as a percentage of a reference weight for a given week of gestation. Of course, the method is valid only if the correct standard is used and if the percentage deviation from the reference curve is interpreted similarly at different weeks of gestation.

Given current knowledge of the use of this approach to evaluate early postnatal growth, it is likely that a given percentage of reference maternal weight for gestational age at 20 weeks of gestation implies a different degree of risk than the same percentage of reference weight at 35 weeks of gestation (Haas and Habicht, 1990). At the very least, the method requires knowing if the coefficient of variation (standard deviation/mean) of weight gain in normal pregnancies with favorable outcomes is constant over all gestational ages. If it is not constant, then a given percent deviation from a mean weight at a given week of gestation will not have the same percentile standing as it would at another week of gestation.

USES OF GESTATIONAL WEIGHT GAIN IN NUTRITIONAL SURVEILLANCE

In recent years, a system of nutritional surveillance has been under development in the United States. The major objective of such a system is to provide accurate information to decision makers who are responsible for policy, program development, and management in areas that affect nutrition and public health (DHHS/USDA, 1986; Mason et al., 1984). The information derived from nutritional surveillance can also be of use in clinical practice (Wong and Trowbridge, 1984). The Centers for Disease Control have been charged with the coordination of nutrition surveillance activities, which include identifying data sources, standardizing data collection instruments, training people in data collection, conducting data analysis, and disseminating information to appropriate users. Two components of nutritional surveillance related to the work of this subcommittee are the Pregnancy Risk Assessment Monitoring System and the Pregnancy Nutrition Surveillance System. The goal of these two systems is to contribute to the reduction of pregnancy-related health risk factors and adverse pregnancy outcomes in both the general population and the low-income population of the United States.

In these surveillance systems, gestational weight gain is included as a maternal measure associated with health risk and pregnancy outcome. The extensive standardized data collection instrument developed for these two systems includes questions on prepregnancy weight and height as well as total gestational weight gain and length of gestation (from LMP). There appears to be no information on patterns of weight gain or a specific identification code for the sources of data on weight and height (measured versus recalled). Since these systems are still in the development stage, it has not been possible to evaluate how these data are to be analyzed and whether some of the concerns raised elsewhere in this chapter have been addressed.

The analytical depth and sophistication often required of scientific research cannot be applied to nutritional surveillance data. Reports must be generated in a timely fashion if they are to be of use to decision makers, and a sophisticated statistical analysis may not be understood by many of the potential users. However, most of the concerns regarding data quality and interpretation raised under research applications also apply to use of gestational weight gain data in nutritional surveillance.

Operation of the two relevant surveillance systems may produce benefits in addition to those previously stated. Because of increased efforts to standardize data collection methods among the many state programs, there is likely to be an increase in the amount and quality of data available on gestational weight gain, its antecedents, and its consequences, so that important research can progress. Also, this standardization process may extend to clinical uses of gestational weight gain charts such as those found in individual state WIC programs.

SUMMARY

Clinical practice, research, and surveillance activities benefit from the implementation of proper measurement techniques. Interpretation of results from studies of gestational weight gain requires careful attention to definitions of gestational weight gain and gestational duration.

CLINICAL IMPLICATIONS

• Prepregnancy weight is an important factor. Objective data, such as those obtained from a medical record, are preferred. Information provided by the patient should be evaluated for its accuracy.

• Height without shoes should be determined at the first prenatal visit, preferably with a wall stadiometer whose accuracy has been verified.

• Gestational age should be estimated from the date of onset of the woman's last menstruation, preferably supplemented by estimates based on the obstetric clinical examination and perhaps by early ultrasound.

• A weight-for-height category is derived from the patient's height and prepregnancy weight. The resulting BMI can be compared to the recommended classification in Appendix C.

• This comparison will provide a foundation for specific nutrition counseling and the creation of a plan for overall and incremental weight gain.

• The patient's weight should be obtained at the beginning of each prenatal visit. Consistently, the patient should be weighed without her purse and outdoor clothing. If weight cannot be obtained routinely without shoes, a marked variation in the type of footwear should be noted.

• The immediate recording of measurements directly on an appropriate form is encouraged.

• Recording data on a chart that depicts weight gain by gestational age provides a visual impression of sequential changes. Abrupt or inconsistent changes should be scrutinized to determine whether they reflect errors or accurate data.

• Members of the clinical staff should be trained in proper measurement techniques. Their performance should be monitored periodically.

• Equipment for taking measurements should be calibrated periodically.

• Only the patient's *approximate* weight is obtained at the time of measurement. An exact measurement is not possible because of clothing, contents of bladder and bowel, time of day, time of last meal, and other such factors. Therefore, interpretation of weight change should focus on sequential data or trends.

• The patient's weight should be compared with the target weights and rates of gains depicted in Chapter 1, Table 1-1, and Appendix B. Investigation to determine the cause of inappropriate patterns will permit specific remedial action to be taken.

REFERENCES

Brown, J.E., K.W. Berdan, P. Splett, M. Robinson, and L.J. Harris. 1986. Prenatal weight gains related to the birth of healthy-sized infants to low-income women. J. Am. Diet. Assoc. 86:1679-1683.

Burton, B.T., W.R. Foster, J. Hirsch, and T.B. Van Itallie. 1985. Health implications of
    obesity: an NIH Concensus Development Conference. Int. J. Obesity 9:155-170.
Butman, M., ed. 1982. Prenatal Nutrition: A Clinical Manual. WIC Program, Massachusetts
    Department of Public Health, Boston, Mass. 158 pp.
DHHS/USDA (Department of Health and Human Services/U.S. Department of Agriculture).
    1986. Nutrition Monitoring in the United States: A Progress Report from the Joint
    Nutrition Monitoring Evaluation Committee. DHHS Publ. No. (PHS) 86-1255. Public
    Health Service. U.S. Government Printing Office, Washington, D.C. 356 pp.
Dimperio, D. 1988. Prenatal Nutrition: Clinical Guidelines for Nurses. March of Dimes
    Birth Defects Foundation, White Plains, N.Y. 134 pp.
Flegal, K.M., W.R. Harlan, and J.R. Landis. 1988. Secular trends in body mass index and
    skinfold thickness with socioeconomic factors in young adult women. Am. J. Clin.
    Nutr. 48:535-543.
Georgia Dietetic Association. 1987. Diet Manual of the Georgia Dietetic Association, 3rd
    ed. Georgia Dietetic Association, Duluth, Ga. 441 pp.
Griffiths, M. 1985. Growth Monitoring of Preschool Children: Practical Considerations
    for Primary Health Care Projects. World Federation of Public Health Associations,
    Washington, D.C. 79 pp.
Gueri, M., P. Jutsum, and B. Sorhaindo. 1982. Anthropometric assessment of nutritional
    status in pregnant women: a reference table of weight-for-height by week of pregnancy.
    Am. J. Clin. Nutr. 35:609-616.
Haas, J.D., and J.P. Habicht. 1990. Growth and growth charts in the assessment of
    preschool nutritional status. Pp. 160-183 in G.A. Harrison and J.C. Waterlow, eds.
    Diet and Disease in Traditional and Developing Societies. Cambridge University Press,
    Cambridge.
Hamill, P.V.V., T.A. Drizd, C.L. Johnson, R.B. Reed, and A.F. Roche. 1977. NCHS Growth
    Curves for Children from Birth to 18 Years: United States. Vital and Health Statistics,
    Series 11, No. 165. DHHS Publ. No. (PHS) 78-1650. National Center for Health
    Statistics, Public Health Service, U.S. Department of Health, Education, and Welfare,
    Hyattsville, Md. 74 pp.
Husaini, Y.K., M.A. Husaini, Z. Sulaiman, A.B. Jahari, Barizi, S.T. Hudono, and D. Karyadi.
    1986. Maternal malnutrition, outcome of pregnancy, and a simple tool to identify
    women at risk. Food Nutr. Bull. 8:71-76.
Hytten, F.E., and I. Leitch. 1971. The Physiology of Human Pregnancy, 2nd ed. Blackwell
    Scientific Publications, Oxford. 599 pp.
Idaho WIC Program. 1988. Idaho WIC Program Procedure Manual: Special Supplemental
    Food Program for Women, Infants, & Children. Bureau of Maternal and Child
    Health, Division of Health, Department of Health and Welfare, State of Idaho, Boise,
    Idaho. (various pagings).
Jackson, A.S., M.L. Pollock, J.E. Graves, and M.T. Makar. 1988. Reliability and validity of
    bioelectrical impedance in determining body composition. J. Appl. Physiol. 64:529-534.
Kleinman, J.C. 1990. Maternal Weight Gain During Pregnancy: Determinants and Conse-
    quences. NCHS Working Paper Series No. 33. National Center for Health Statistics,
    Public Health Service, U.S. Department of Health and Human Services, Hyattsville,
    Md. 24 pp.
Kramer, M.S., F.H. McLean, M.E. Boyd, and R.H. Usher. 1988. The validity of gestational
    age estimation by menstrual dating in term, preterm, and postterm gestations. J. Am.
    Med. Assoc. 260:3306-3308.
Lohman, T.G., A.F. Roche, and R. Martorell, eds. 1988. Anthropometric Standardization
    Reference Manual. Human Kinetics Books, Champaign, Ill. 177 pp.
Lull, C.B., and R.A. Kimbrough, eds. 1953. Clinical Obstetrics. Lippincott, Philadelphia.
    732 pp.
Mason, J.B., J.P. Habicht, H. Tabatabai, and V. Valverde. 1984. Nutritional Surveillance.
    World Health Organization, Geneva. 194 pp.
Metropolitan Life Insurance Company. 1959. New weight standards for men and women.
    Stat. Bull. Metrop. Life Insur. Co. 40:1-4.
Metropolitan Life Insurance Company. 1983. 1983 Metropolitan height and weight tables.
    Stat. Bull. Metrop. Life Found. 64:3-9.

Oates, R.K., and D. Forrest. 1984. Reliability of mothers' reports of birth data. Aust. Paediatr. J. 20:185-186.

Oregon WIC Staff. 1981. WIC Program Manual. WIC Program, Oregon Health Division, Department of Human Resources, State of Oregon, Portland, Oreg. (various pagings).

Pritchard, J.A., P.C. MacDonald, and N.F. Gant. 1985. Williams Obstetrics, 17th ed. Appleton-Century-Crofts, Norwalk, Conn. 976 pp.

Rosso, P. 1985. A new chart to monitor weight gain during pregnancy. Am. J. Clin. Nutr. 41:644-652.

Society of Actuaries. 1959. Build and Blood Pressure Study 1959, Vol. I. Society of Actuaries, Chicago. 268 pp.

Society of Actuaries. 1960. Build and Blood Pressure Study 1959, Vol. II. Society of Actuaries, Chicago. 240 pp.

Society of Actuaries/Association of Life Insurance Medical Directors of America. 1980. Build Study 1979. Society of Actuaries/Association of Life Insurance Medical Directors of America, Chicago. 255 pp.

Stevens-Simon, C., E.R. McAnarney, and M.P. Coulter. 1986. How accurately do pregnant adolescents estimate their weight prior to pregnancy? J. Adol. Health Care 7:250-254.

Stewart, A.L. 1982. The reliability and validity of self-reported weight and height. J. Chronic Dis. 35:295-309.

Tompkins, W.T., and D.G. Wiehl. 1951. Nutritional deficiencies as a causal factor in toxemia and premature labor. Am. J. Obstet. Gynecol. 62:898-919.

Wilcox, A.J., and L.F. Horney. 1984. Accuracy of spontaneous abortion recall. Am. J. Epidemiol. 120:727-733.

Wong, F.L., and F.L. Trowbridge. 1984. Nutrition surveys and surveillance: their application to clinical practice. Clin. Nutr. 3:94-99.

5
Total Amount and
Pattern of Weight Gain:
Physiologic and Maternal Determinants

Total weight change during pregnancy can vary from a weight loss to a gain of more than 30 kg (66 lb). This wide variation in gain among healthy pregnant women appears to be attributable to several physiologic and environmental factors. For example, changes in the secretion of maternal hormones and other physiologic adjustments associated with pregnancy undoubtedly affect the utilization of energy sources and thus the amount of weight gained. Certain maternal characteristics and health habits may also exert an influence. In this chapter, the subcommittee reviews these physiologic factors and evaluates the relationship between selected maternal characteristics and the amount and pattern of gain. A discussion of relationships between dietary- and supplemental energy intake and weight gain is found in Chapter 7.

NORMS FOR TOTAL GAIN, RATE OF GAIN, AND
COMPOSITION OF GAIN

Pattern and Amount of Gain

In 1971, Hytten and Leitch established physiologic norms for total weight gain, the rate of gain in the last half of pregnancy, and the rate of gain associated with the best reproductive performance. Using data from two British studies (Humphreys, 1954; Thomson and Billewicz, 1957) of more than 3,800 women, they concluded that the physiologic average total gain of "healthy primigravidae women eating without restriction" is 12.5

96

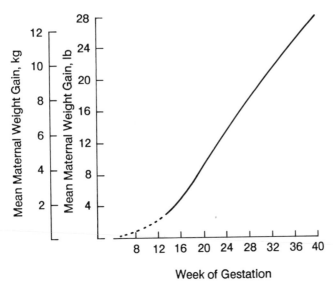

Week of Gestation

FIGURE 5-1   Mean rate of weight gain during pregnancy of 2,868 normotensive, primigravid women, from Thomson and Billewicz (1957) by permission of Blackwell Scientific Publications, Inc.

kg (27.5 lb)—approximately 1 kg (2.2 lb) in the first trimester and the remainder during the last two trimesters. For multigravid women, they made no specific estimates but suggested that a slightly lower gain could be expected.

To determine a physiologic norm for rate of gain during the last half of pregnancy, Hytten and Leitch (1971) extracted weight gain data from records maintained by the Aberdeen Maternity Hospital for 486 healthy women aged 20 to 29 and at least 160 cm (63 in.) tall, who delivered their infants between weeks 39 and 41 of pregnancy (between 1950 and 1955). No attempt was made to control weight gain by food restriction in this population. The most common value for the rate of gain during the last half of pregnancy was between 0.41 and 0.45 kg (~1 lb) per week, but the range of gain was very wide—from less than 0.1 to 0.9 kg (0.2 to 2 lb) per week. The data from this study are shown in Figure 5-1, which has been used widely to evaluate the rate and total amount of weight gained by pregnant woman. Hytten and Leitch emphasized, however, that considerable variation of this pattern is consistent with good pregnancy outcomes. The lowest incidence of preeclampsia, low birth weight, and perinatal death was associated with gaining 0.45 kg/week during the last 20 weeks of pregnancy. The following rates were established for each quarter of pregnancy among primigravid women:

0 to 10 weeks, 0.065 kg/week
10 to 20 weeks, 0.335 kg/week
20 to 30 weeks, 0.450 kg/week
30 to 40 weeks, 0.335 kg/week

Components of Gain

The components of gain can be divided into two parts—the products of conception and maternal tissue accretion. The products of conception comprise the fetus, placenta, and amniotic fluid. On the average, the fetus represents approximately 25% of the total gain, the placenta about 5%, and the amniotic fluid about 6% (Hytten, 1980b). Cross-sectional data indicate that fetal growth follows a sigmoid curve, with growth slowing in the final week of gestation. The rate of placental growth declines toward the end of pregnancy.

Expansion of maternal tissues accounts for approximately two-thirds of the total gain. In addition to increases in uterine and mammary tissue mass, there is an expansion of maternal blood volume, extracellular fluid, fat stores, and possibly other tissues. In laboratory animals, an increase in liver and intestinal mucosal mass during gestation is evident, but there is no evidence that these tissues increase in pregnant women.

Expansion of the blood volume accounts for 10% of the total gain. The increase in plasma volume (approximately 50%) is greater than that of the red blood cell mass increase, but expansion of both is related to fetal size (Hytten, 1980b). Most of the increase in plasma volume occurs before week 34 of gestation; the increase in red blood cell mass is believed to be linear from the end of the first trimester to term. Iron supplementation increases the expansion of the red blood cell mass (see Chapter 14).

In women without generalized edema or with only leg edema, an expansion of the extracellular, extravascular fluid volume accounts for approximately 13% of the total gain. The retention of extracellular fluid can be highly variable; some women accumulate more than 5 liters (5 kg, or 11 lb). The physiologic basis for extracellular fluid retention is uncertain. Placental estrogens may increase the affinity for water of muco- or glycopolysaccharides in connective tissue (Hytten, 1980b), resulting in an expanded, softer tissue.

Women normally accumulate fat during pregnancy. Hytten (1980b) estimated that pregnant women who gain 12.5 kg (27.5 lb) without edema acquire about 3.5 kg (7.5 lb) of fat. (See Chapter 6 for other, more recent estimates.) The purpose of the fat store is uncertain: it may be a maternal energy reserve for use when the food supply is limited during either pregnancy or lactation.

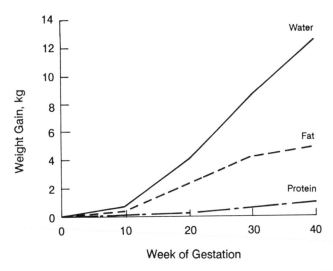

FIGURE 5-2   Composition of weight gain during pregnancy. From Hytten (1980b).

Proximate Composition of Gain

Hytten (1980b) estimated that, on average, water contributes approximately 62% of the total gain at term, fat contributes 30%, and protein contributes 8%; but there is considerable variation in these values. Of the total fat gain, 90% is deposited as maternal stores. About 60% of the total protein accretion is located in the products of conception; the remainder is accounted for by the gain of maternal uterine, mammary, and blood tissues. In early nitrogen balance studies, reported protein retentions were higher than could be accounted for by those fetal and maternal tissues. However, recent studies conducted in metabolic wards have reported protein retentions comparable to the estimated need for pregnancy.

Weight gain attributable to body water is the most variable of the components. A reported positive relationship between the increased total body water and infant birth weight (Hytten, 1980b) suggests that water accumulation is beneficial. An estimate of the pattern of weight composition for each quarter of pregnancy is depicted in Figure 5-2. Variation in the composition of gain is discussed in Chapter 6.

TOTAL WEIGHT GAIN AND PATTERN OF GAIN

The most representative data for total weight gain in the U.S. population are from the 1980 National Natality Survey (NNS) (Taffel, 1986), which is a probability sample of all live births to U.S. women in 1980. Because of the limited amount of information available from published reports, the subcommittee relied heavily on the data from the 1980 NNS to determine the independent effects of maternal characteristics on total weight gain (Kleinman, 1990; Taffel, 1986). The distribution of gains among white, non-Hispanic, married mothers by body mass index (BMI) (Kleinman, 1990) is shown in Figure 5-3 and Table 5-1.

Data from 12 other studies on gestational weight gain are shown in Table 5-2. These studies were selected because they provided data on cumulative increase in maternal weight at various times during pregnancy, thus permitting weight gain patterns to be estimated. These data were obtained from six countries and cover a span from 1925 to 1982. Three of the studies (Brown et al., 1986; Husaini et al., 1986; Kawakami et al., 1977) were reported after release of the Food and Nutrition Board's report, *Maternal Nutrition and the Course of Pregnancy* (NRC, 1970). The study by Brown et al. (1986) provides the most recent data regarding women living in the United States. Reported average total gains ranged from 10.1 to 14.9 kg (22 to 33 lb) across samples in these studies. From the published data, it is extremely difficult to identify a physiologic norm for total weight gain during pregnancy.

In the studies summarized in Table 5-2, women were weighed when they entered prenatal care (at 13 or 16 weeks of gestation), then usually once per month until about week 30 of gestation, and more frequently after that. Weight change at specific weeks of gestation was observed or interpolated from these data. In most studies, weight change was based on measured weight at the first visit; in others, it was based on recalled prepregnancy weight. Few studies collected data on weight gain during the first trimester. Most of them excluded women with obvious pregnancy complications, but some studies provided few descriptive data about their samples. Problematic characteristics of some studies include prescribed weight restriction, limitations of samples to poor women, and a complete lack of information about sample selection. Infant birth weight, an important criterion for healthy pregnancy outcome, was rarely considered.

Not only did total weight gain differ among studies, as mentioned above, but there were also differences in the amount of weight gained at specific points during gestation (Table 5-2). In the study by Brown et al. (1986), mean weight gains were higher at each gestational period. Patterns of gain are illustrated in Figure 5-4, which shows the cumulative gain reported in the 12 studies, and in Figure 5-5, which provides data from selected studies of well-nourished women with uncomplicated pregnancies in the United States and the United Kingdom.

Although the study designs and populations differed among these studies, the slopes of the lines representing cumulative weight gains were quite similar. As mentioned above, Hytten and Leitch (1971) suggested a gain of 0.41 to 0.45 kg (~1 lb) per week as a reference for the last half of

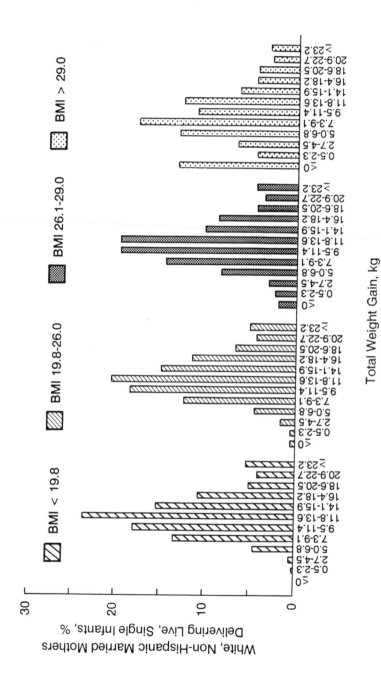

FIGURE 5-3 Distribution of maternal weight gain by prepregnancy weight-for-height category. Includes all white, non-Hispanic married mothers delivering live, singleton infants, regardless of infant birth weight or length of gestation in 1980. From Kleinman (1990).

TABLE 5-1   Mean Total Weight Gain and Coefficient of Variation for
White, non-Hispanic, Married Mothers Delivering Live Infants[a]

BMI Group	Number in Sample	Mean Weight Gain, kg	Coefficient of Variation, %	Weight Gain, kg, by Percentile	
				15th	85th
Low (<19.8)	1,027	13.8	37	8.6	18.2
Moderate (19.8–26.0)	2,393	13.8	38	7.7	18.6
High (26.1–29.0)	246	12.4	48	6.4	17.3
Very high (>29.0)	280	8.7	97	0.5	16.4
Total	3,946	13.3	45	8.2	17.7

[a] Based on unpublished data from 1980 National Natality Survey.

pregnancy. Similarly, Thomson and Billewicz (1957) concluded from their study of 2,868 normotensive Scottish primigravid women that an average gain of about 0.45 kg (1 lb) per week during the second half of pregnancy was a "sound and realistic average to aim at" (p. 247). Rates of gain observed by Thomson and Billewicz (1957) were 0.467 kg/week (standard deviation [SD] = 0.161) between 20 and 30 weeks of gestation and 0.395 kg/week (SD = 0.213) during weeks 30 to 36. Reported rates of gain of U.S. women during the same time period were lower than those observed in the United Kingdom (Robinson et al., 1943; Tompkins and Wiehl, 1951). Robinson and coworkers stressed that normal and overweight patients were told to limit their intake of carbohydrates and fat. The highest rate of gain occurred during the seventh lunar month of gestation (Robinson et al., 1943); between 20 and 28 weeks of gestation, the rate of gain averaged approximately 0.455 kg (1 lb) per week.

Only four reports of the *rate* of gain have appeared since 1971. In a 1977 study of weekly weights of 2,000 pregnant Japanese women, the mean rate of gain was 0.45 kg (1.0 lb) per week between 16 and 24 weeks and 0.48 kg/week between 24 and 32 weeks of gestation (Kawakami et al., 1977). Meserole and colleagues (1984) constructed a graph of the weight gain pattern of 80 pregnant girls aged 19 or less. The slope of the rate of gain for the adolescents was described as steeper than that for adult pregnant women. In a study of 1,000 pregnant women in Indonesia (Husaini et al., 1986), the rate of gain and total gain were lower than those reported in the other studies. The mean prepregnancy weight for the Indonesian women was 44.5 kg (98 lb), substantially less than that of women in the United

TABLE 5-2 Cumulative Increase in Maternal Weight

Country and Time of Data Collection	Selection Criteria	Number of Subjects	Gain, kg, by Period of Pregnancy, wks				Total Gain, kg	Reference
			13–16	13–20	13–32	13–Term		
United States 1925–1932	Private patients, uncomplicated pregnancy	1,000	1.45	3.45	9.31	10.31	10.94	Cummings, 1934
United States 1925–1932	Uncomplicated pregnancy	2,502[a]	1.57	3.87	10.1	13.46	13.96	Stander and Pastore, 1940
China 1934–1940	Uncomplicated pregnancy	200	1.09	2.91	7.81	10.44	10.59	Kuo, 1941
United States 1943	Private patients, live births within ±30 days of expected date of confinement (diet restriction in normal-weight and overweight women)	484	0.64	2.0	7.08	10.07	11.04	Robinson et al., 1943
United Kingdom 1941–1944	First prenatal care ≤16 weeks, extra dietary rations	360	NR[b]	1.92[c]	7.40	10.09	10.10[c]	Scott and Benjamin, 1948
United States 1947–1949	Uncomplicated pregnancy, ±10% of ideal prepregnancy weight for height, full-term living infant	60	1.18	2.86	7.27	9.76	10.90	Tompkins and Wiehl, 1951

Table 5-2 continues

TABLE 5-2—Continued

Country and Time of Data Collection	Selection Criteria	Number of Subjects	Gain, kg, by Period of Pregnancy, wks				Total Gain, kg	Reference
			13–16	13–20	13–32	13–Term		
Scotland 1949–1954	Primiparous, normotensive	2,868	1.41	3.27	8.80	11.84	12.50	Thomson and Billewicz, 1957
Scotland 1950–1955	Primiparous, age 20 to 29, ≥160 cm (63 in.) tall, live births at 39 to 41 weeks of gestation	486	2.01[b]	4.0	8.50	NR	12.50	Hytten and Leitch, 1971
India (dates not reported)	Poor women	130	0.88	3.43	5.25	6.36	NR	Venkatachalam et al., 1960
Japan (dates not reported)	Not described	2,000	1.9[d]	4.5	9.4	NR	11.7	Kawakami et al., 1977
United States 1979–1982	Low income, uncomplicated pregnancy, birth weight >3,000 g	384	4.40[d]	6.47	12.01	12.00	14.85	Brown et al., 1986
Indonesia (dates not reported)	Uncomplicated pregnancy; low to mid-socioeconomic status; live birth at 36 to 40 weeks of gestation	1,332	3.8[d]	5.2	8.6	9.4	NR	Husaini et al., 1986

[a] Interpolated from data reported for other weeks. All values based on change in weight from prepregnancy weight.
[b] NR = Not reported.
[c] Values based on change in weight from week 16 of gestation.
[d] Values based on change in weight from prepregnancy weights.

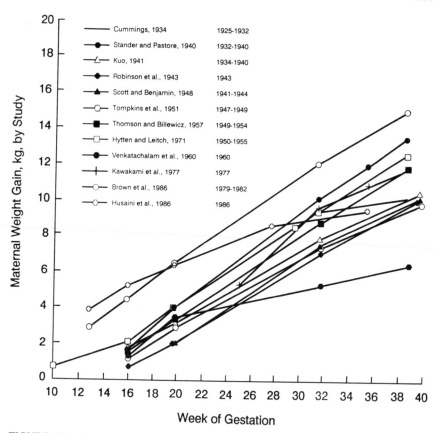

FIGURE 5-4 Pattern of maternal weight gain shown by data from 12 studies.

States. Brown and coworkers (1986) studied the pattern of gain of 459 low-income women who delivered infants weighing between 3,000 and 4,500 g. The weekly rates of maternal weight gain by this group were higher during the first two trimesters than has been reported in other studies (Table 5-2), namely, 0.22 kg (0.5 lb) per week during the first trimester and 0.52 kg (1.1 lb) per week during the second trimester, but they were comparable (0.40 kg, or 0.9 lb, per week) during the third trimester. A slowing of weight gain or a slight weight loss has been consistently reported as women approached term (Cummings, 1934; Kuo, 1941; Robinson et al., 1943; Scott and Benjamin, 1948).

Few investigators have evaluated weight gain during the first trimester in detail. Clapp et al. (1988) weighed 20 physically active, well-nourished women serially from before conception to week 15 of gestation and showed

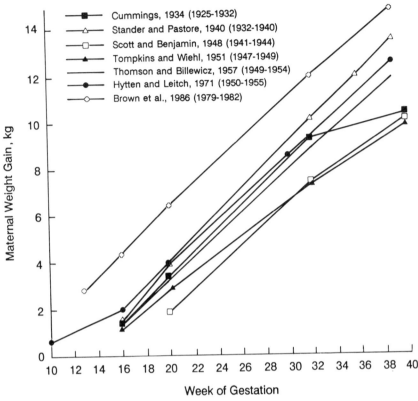

FIGURE 5-5 Pattern of maternal weight gain shown by the six studies in Figure 5-4 that focused on well-nourished women in Europe and the United States who had uncomplicated pregnancies.

that maternal gain averaged 2 kg (4.5 lb) at 7 weeks and 4.3 kg (9.5 lb) at 15 weeks; the average rate of gain from 0 to 15 weeks of gestation was 0.29 kg, or 0.6 lb, per week. Weights beyond this period were not given.

Thomson and Billewicz (1957) reported that 40% of their population gained their suggested amount of 3.6 to 5.4 kg (8 to 12 lb) during the second trimester, whereas almost 25% gained less. The investigators did not relate the pattern of gain to pregnancy outcome. However, only 14% of their sample gained amounts within the ranges the investigators considered to be ideal for both the second and third trimesters. Thus, the individual experience of many pregnant women is unlikely to fit the pattern depicted in Figure 5-1.

Estimated Normal Rates of Gain

There are no data on rates of weight gain by trimester that are representative of the U.S. population. However, given the remarkable similarity in the rates that can be interpreted from Figure 5-5, it is likely that a representative sample of the U.S. population would have rates similar to those represented by most other population groups. Studies suggest an average gain of approximately 0.45 kg (1 lb) per week during the second trimester and a slightly lower gain of about 0.40 kg (0.9 lb) per week during the third trimester.

Standard errors for the rates of weekly gain were given in only one published study that included a large sample size (Thomson and Billewicz, 1957). From these data, the subcommittee estimated the weight gain at the 15th and 85th percentiles of gain for Scottish primigravid women at different stages of pregnancy, as follows:

13 to 20 weeks = 0.15 to 0.69 kg (0.3 to 1.5 lb) per week
20 to 30 weeks = 0.31 to 0.65 kg (0.7 to 1.4 lb) per week
30 to 36 weeks = 0.18 to 0.61 kg (0.4 to 1.3 lb) per week

These ranges pertain to normal pregnancies of women with various maternal ages, heights, and prepregnancy weights for height.

ADJUSTMENTS IN INTAKE AND UTILIZATION OF ENERGY SOURCES DURING PREGNANCY

To estimate the energy cost for weight gain during pregnancy, the *theoretical* energy need (approximately 85,000 kcal) (Hytten, 1980a) was divided by the usual weight gain (12,500 g), yielding an energy cost of 6.4 kcal for every gram of weight gain. However, the *measured* energy requirement for pregnancy and weight gain in the recent Five Nation Study totaled 55,000 kcal for a 11,800-g gain (Durnin, 1987), or 4.7 kcal/g of weight gain. Both estimates of the energy cost of gain during pregnancy are lower than the 8.0 kcal/g required for weight gain by nonpregnant women (Forbes, 1988). The lower energy need for weight gain in pregnancy probably reflects the higher water content of the lean tissue that is gained.

It is uncertain whether a change in food intake is essential for a gain of maternal and fetal tissue. A positive energy balance and, therefore, a supply of energy for weight gain may be achieved by an increase in energy intake, a decrease in energy expenditure, an increase in the efficiency with which energy is used to synthesize new tissue, or some combination of these factors. (For a more detailed discussion of energy balance during pregnancy, see Chapter 7.) It is difficult to measure food intake precisely, but longitudinal studies of well-nourished pregnant women on unrestricted diets show a small, but not always significant or universal, increase in energy intake.

The hormonal adjustments of pregnancy may alter utilization of energy sources, resulting in a reduced energy cost for the synthesis of fat or protein. The energy cost of tissue synthesis has not been measured in pregnant women. The fetus requires an uninterrupted source of glucose and amino acids for growth. The placenta produces hormones, e.g., human placental lactogen, whose major metabolic effects are to promote greater use of lipids as an energy source by the mother. This may increase the availability of glucose and amino acids for fetal use. Following a meal, maternal glucose uptake is reduced, despite increased plasma concentrations of insulin (Kitzmiller, 1980). Human chorionic somatomammotropin, progesterone, and cortisol levels increase during pregnancy and contribute to a rise in maternal peripheral insulin resistance. This insulin resistance seems to be specific for maternal glucose uptake; amino acid uptake and the rate of hepatic conversion of glucose to triglycerides are not impaired. Following a meal, plasma amino acid concentrations are lower in pregnant women than they are in nonpregnant women, probably because of placental uptake and insulin-mediated increases in protein synthesis. The hepatic conversion of glucose to triglycerides also is increased in pregnant women after a meal. This increased tendency to synthesize triglycerides promotes energy storage. With fasting, these fat reserves are mobilized. At the same time, mobilization of maternal muscle mass remains low because of the higher insulin-to-glucagon ratio, and maternal lean tissue is conserved.

In summary, the net effects of the hormonal changes during pregnancy are increased tendencies to store excess energy as maternal fat after meals and to mobilize these energy-dense stores in the fasted state. Amino acid uptake is increased after meals, but amino acid release is reduced during fasting, causing a net conservation of maternal lean tissue. Adjustments in fat utilization occur between meals to provide for maternal energy needs while conserving glucose and amino acids for fetal fuel and synthesis of maternal and fetal lean tissue.

MATERNAL DETERMINANTS OF THE PATTERN AND AMOUNT OF WEIGHT GAIN

As mentioned earlier, gestational weight gain differs widely among healthy women delivering single, full-term infants, partly because of differences in maternal characteristics such as prepregnancy weight-for-height status, age, parity, ethnic origin, socioeconomic status, substance abuse, and physical activity level. The influence of these characteristics on gestational weight gain is discussed below.

Prepregnancy Weight-for-Height Status

The weight-for-height status of the mother before conception is frequently used as a marker for the mother's nutritional state before a pregnancy. A low weight-for-height is assumed to reflect marginal tissue reserves, whereas a high value is believed to be indicative of excessive reserves. Methods of expressing weight-for-height status are discussed in Chapter 4. Kleinman (1990) presented the distribution of total weight gains according to four BMI groups: <19.8, 19.8 to 26.0, 26.1 to 29.0 and >29.0, i.e., low, moderate, high, and very high weight for height. The subcommittee located 10 reports published between 1970 and 1989 on the relationship between maternal prepregnancy weight-for-height status and weight gain (see Table 5-3). The sample sizes ranged from 20 to approximately 1,500 women. Most studies included only women who were registered for prenatal care in the first trimester. Prepregnancy weight-for-height status usually was based on recalled prepregnancy weight and on height measured at the first prenatal visit. In a few cases, weight at the first visit was used. In some studies, the patients were classified by the 1959 Metropolitan Life Insurance Company's (MLI) standards (Metropolitan Life Insurance Company, 1959). Otherwise, the subcommittee calculated BMI from the reported data, and the women were assigned to one of the five groups identified in Table 5-3. All the studies excluded women with multiple births, preterm deliveries (<37 weeks of gestation), and women with obvious pregnancy complications. In several studies with fewer than 100 women per group, data collection was prospective. In the larger studies, the data were abstracted from clinic charts. Women from both public health clinics and private practices are included in the data presented in Table 5-3.

Table 5-3 shows that the amount gained by women in the five groups differed among the studies. For example, women in the low and normal weight-for-height groups studied by Mitchell and Lerner (1989) gained the least (9.3 and 8.4 kg, or 20.5 and 17.5 lb), whereas those studied by Haiek and Lederman (1989) gained the most (15.5 and 15.8 kg, or 34 and 35 lb). This discrepancy suggests that other differences in these two samples of women influenced total weight gain more than did their prepregnancy weight-for-height status. Divergent socioeconomic status may account for some of the differences: Haiek and Lederman (1989) studied women from public health clinics, including a high proportion of teenagers, whereas Mitchell and Lerner (1989) studied women from a private practice.

Given the disparate characteristics of the study samples, comparison of the influence of prepregnancy weight-for-height status can be made only within single studies. Only three of the studies (Abrams and Laros, 1986; Brown et al., 1981; Mitchell and Lerner, 1989) provide data from women in more than two of these five weight-for-height groups. Mitchell

TABLE 5-3   Gestational Weight Gain Reported by Maternal
Prepregnancy Weight-for-Height Status in Different Studies of U.S.
Women

Prepregnancy Weight for Height	Number in Sample	Total Mean Gain, kg	Coefficient of Variation, %	Reference
Very low (<80% of	155	12.6	29	Brown et al., 1981
standard,[a] or	79	9.3	34	Mitchell and Lerner, 1989
BMI[b] < 16.5)				
Low (80–90% of	243	12.9	36	Brown et al., 1981
standard or BMI	105	11.2	37	Winikoff and Debrovner, 1981
16.5–19.8)	62	11.7	71	Rosso, 1985
	268	14.3	31	Abrams and Laros, 1986
	80	14.3	NR[c]	Brown et al., 1986
	21	15.5	NR	Haiek and Lederman, 1989
	283	9.3	33	Mitchell and Lerner, 1989
Normal (90–120% of	301	11.0[d]	31	Gormican et al., 1980
standard or BMI	247	12.6	63	Brown et al., 1981
> 19.8–26)	106	10.4	32	Winikoff and Debrovner, 1981
	35	12.6	33	George et al., 1984
	137	10.4	61	Rosso, 1985
	1,535	15.2	31	Abrams and Laros, 1986
	174	13.9	NR	Brown et al., 1986
	868	14.4	39	Muscati et al., 1988
	39	15.8	NR	Haiek and Lederman, 1989
	362	8.4	37	Mitchell and Lerner, 1989
High (120–135% of	901	15.2	35	Abrams and Laros, 1986
standard or BMI				
> 26–29)				
Very high (>135%	224	14.1	55	Abrams and Laros, 1986
of standard or	68	~9.7	NR	Brown et al., 1986
BMI > 29)				

[a] Standards varied among the studies. Weight-for-height tables from Metropolitan Life
Insurance Company (1959) were used most commonly.
[b] BMI = body mass index, metric units.
[c] NR = Not reported.
[d] Weight gain for second and third trimesters only.

and Lerner (1989) found that the gain of women in the low and very
low weight-for-height groups was significantly greater than that of normal-
weight women (9.3 compared with 8.5 kg, or 20.5 versus 19 lb). Brown and
coworkers (1981) did not find any differences in gain between underweight
and normal-weight women. Abrams and Laros (1986) compared the weight
gain of women in low, normal, high, and very high weight-for-height groups.
No statistically significant differences in mean weight gain were found
among women in the four groups, but the total gain of women in the

very overweight group tended to be slightly lower than that of women in the normal and high groups (14.1 compared with 15.2 kg, or 31 versus 33 lb). These investigators noted that the gains of the women in the very overweight category were more variable than those of women in the other groups. Their coefficient of variation for gain was 55% compared with about 31 to 35% in the other three groups. Among the very overweight women in that study, there was a higher percentage of women with low weight gains, which lowered the group average. The very overweight women in this clinic were not told to limit their food intake or to restrict their weight gain.

In these 10 studies, weight gain by women in each of the five groups varied substantially (Table 5-3), and coefficients of variation of gain for women with normal prepregnancy weights ranged from 31 to 63%. This degree of variation in gain after controlling for differences in maternal body size shows that maternal prepregnancy weight-for-height status accounts for only a small part of the variation in weight gain.

An analysis of the 1980 NNS data (Kleinman, 1990, and Table 5-1) showed that as maternal prepregnancy BMI increased from moderate to very high, mean total weight gain fell by about 5 kg (11 lb), and the variation in gain increased. More than 10% of the women in the very overweight group lost weight during gestation, and more than one-third of the women in that group met the criterion for low weight gain, i.e., a gain of less than 6.8 kg (15 lb). The proportion of women with a low total weight gain was about four times greater among women in the very high BMI group than among women in the low and moderate BMI groups. As shown in Figure 5-3, only 25% of those with a low BMI, 20% of those with moderate and high BMIs, and 13% of those with very high BMIs had weight gains close to the gain suggested by Hytten and Leitch (1971), i.e., between 11.8 and 13.6 kg, or 26 and 30 lb. The 1980 NNS study is compatible with the observations of Abrams and Laros (1986) that the gains of very overweight women are lower on average and are more variable than those of other women, but it provided no evidence that underweight women were at an increased risk of low weight gain. This is an interesting finding, and follow-up studies are needed.

There are only a few studies of the effect of prepregnancy body weight on the *pattern* of weight gain. In one recent study, Meserole and coworkers (1984) compared the pattern of gain of underweight, normal, or overweight adolescents (total sample size, 80). The only difference observed was a gain by the normal-weight adolescents in the first trimester in comparison with little or no gain by adolescents in the other two groups, but the methods used to ensure the accuracy of the estimates of prepregnancy weight, and thus of early weight gain, were not described. The rate of gain by the normal-weight adolescents was slightly lower in the second and third trimesters than that of the underweight and overweight adolescents; total weight gains did not differ. There was no further interpretation of these data, and the differences in weight gain pattern were not tested for significance. Results from studies conducted in the 1940s and 1950s of the effect of prepregnancy weight for height on the rate of gain were inconsistent (Robinson et al., 1943; Scott and Benjamin, 1948; Stander and Pastore, 1940; Thomson and Billewicz, 1957).

Maternal Height

In a comprehensive review of the literature, the subcommittee located only one study (Kleinman, 1990) designed to determine whether there is an independent effect of maternal height on total weight gain. In this study, data from the 1980 NNS were analyzed by using multiple linear regression techniques to control for BMI, age and parity, education level, alcohol use, ethnic origin, and cigarette smoking; a significant effect of height on weight gain was observed. Short women (<157 cm, or <62 in.) gained about 1 kg (2 lb) less, on average, than did taller women (>170 cm, or >67 in.), but there was no evidence that short women had an increased risk of low weight gain. An earlier study focused on the relationship between height and the pattern of gain (Thomson and Billewicz, 1957), but no effect was identified. The independent effect of stature on the amount and rate of gain needs further investigation.

Ethnic Origin

Differences in the total amount of weight gained by black and white women during gestation were first reported by Eastman and Jackson (1968) in a study of clinic patients in Baltimore, Maryland, between 1954 and 1961. The total weight gain of the white women averaged 9.9 kg (21.8 lb), whereas that of the black women averaged 9.0 kg (19.8 lb). The statistical significance of this difference was not determined. The reported mean weight gains of the women of both races was the same if the prepregnancy weight was greater than 82 kg (180 lb). In two other large studies of weight gain conducted in the 1950s and 1960s, no difference in weight gain between black and white women was detected (Niswander and Jackson, 1974; Simpson et al., 1975). Both black women and white women in the Collaborative Perinatal Project gained an average of 9.9 kg (21.8 lb) (Niswander and Jackson, 1974). Similar gains were reported for black as well as white wives of military men studied in San Antonio, Texas, between 1946 and 1966 (Simpson et al., 1975). Multivariate analysis was not used in either of these studies to determine whether there was a statistically significant, independent effect of race on gestational weight gain.

More recent studies have focused on the effect of ethnic origin on weight gain in populations including white, black, Southeast Asian, and Hispanic women. In an obstetric clinic for teenagers in San Diego, California, there was no significant difference in the mean weight gain of white, black, and Hispanic mothers (Felice et al., 1986); but Hispanic mothers tended to gain the most weight. In another study, Puerto Rican teenagers in New Jersey gained significantly less than white or black teenagers did (Scholl et al., 1988). In Minnesota, Swenson et al. (1986) studied the weight gains of white, black, Hmong (a Laotian tribe), and other Southeast Asian pregnant adolescents and adults. The total gain of the Hmong and the other Southeast Asian adolescents and adults was about 5 kg (11 lb) less than that of their white and black counterparts. Different attitudes about food practices during pregnancy among Southeast Asian women may contribute to their lower weight gains.

The average weight gain of white women in the 1980 NNS was significantly greater than that of black women (13.2 versus 12.2 kg, or 29.1 versus 26.8 lb) (Taffel, 1986). After controlling for the effects of prepregnancy weight, marital status, education, and age combined with parity, white women still gained about 0.5 kg more than black women did. The gestational period of white women tended to be about 0.5 week longer than that of black women, but this difference only partly explained the higher gains of the white women. The mean weight gain of married Hispanic women and white women did not differ, but the risk of low weight gain was twice as high in Hispanics as it was in whites. Black women also were at a 70% greater risk for low levels of weight gain compared with whites.

In summary, a consistent effect of ethnic origin on gestational weight gain is not apparent in the literature. Black women in the 1980 NNS gained significantly less than white women did. Differences in the gestational period did not account for all this difference. The effect of maternal ethnic origin on the *rate* of weight gain has not been studied.

Age and Parity

There are many reports of weight gain and pregnancy outcome in adolescent women, but most do not control for parity, prepregnancy weight for height, gestational length, ethnic origin, or alcohol and tobacco consumption when evaluating the effect of age on weight gain. The results of nine studies of weight gain among adolescents published since 1970 are summarized in Table 5-4. Adolescent mothers in Lima, Peru, gained from 1 to 7 kg (2 to 15 lb) less than U.S. adolescents on the average (Frisancho et al., 1983), but the study is of value because of the large number of pregnant teenagers of each year of age between 12 and 17. The mean weight gains of the Peruvian teenagers between ages 14 and 17 did not differ. Only 28 girls

TABLE 5-4 Effect of Chronological Maternal Age on Gestational Weight Gain

Reference	Age, yr	Number in Sample	Weight Gain, kg	Coefficient of Variation, %
Ancri et al., 1977	12–17	26	13.4	26
	18–19	22	12.4	31
	20–24	24	11.1	17
	25–32	26	10.7	18
Frisancho et al., 1983	12–13	28	9.0	18
	14	104	9.8	22
	15	296	9.9	26
	16	565	9.7	25
	17	229	10.0	26
	18–25	46	9.7	16
Horon et al., 1983	<16	422	12.5	NR[a]
	20–24	422	12.5	NR
Loris et al., 1985	13–15.9	18	17.2	23
	16–17.9	84	17.1	40
	18–19.9	25	17.3	54
Meserole et al., 1984	13–15	24	14.5	32
	16–17	25	17.9	35
Endres et al., 1985	15–18	46	12.0	NR
	19–30	198	11.0	NR
Muscati et al., 1988	14–17	90	16.5	36
	18–19	135	15.1	36
	20–35	461	13.8	39
Scholl et al., 1988	16.9 ± 1.3 (SD)[b]	696	14.7	39
Haiek and Lederman, 1989	<16	90	14.6	NR
	19–30	90	16.9	NR

[a] NR = Not reported.
[b] SD = Standard deviation.

were between the ages of 12 and 13, but these girls gained about 0.8 kg (1.8 lb) less than the older girls did. This difference was not tested for statistical significance. No consistent relationship between maternal age and weight gain was observed in the six studies of U.S. women. Three groups reported that young mothers gained more weight (Ancri et al., 1977; Endres et al., 1985; Muscati et al., 1988), two reported that young mothers gained less weight (Haiek and Lederman 1989; Meserole et al., 1984), and two found no difference (Horon et al., 1983; Loris et al., 1985). One group reported a relationship between gynecologic age and weight gain; immature girls had lower gains than the more mature girls did (Meserole et al., 1984). This finding, plus the observation that 12- to 13-year-old Peruvian mothers gained less weight (Frisancho et al., 1983), suggests that the weight gains of very young adolescents (<2 years after menarche) may be lower than those of older adolescents. Further research is needed to confirm this conclusion.

Multiple linear regression analysis was used to evaluate the effect of age and parity on weight gain among women who participated in the 1980 NNS (Kleinman, 1990). Primiparous women in all age groups gained about 1 kg (2 lb) more than multiparous women of the same age did, and the risk of low weight gains was about one-third lower among primiparous women. After controlling for parity, differences in weight gain by age were small. Primiparous women of all ages gained more (about 1 kg, or 2 lb) than multiparous women of the same age.

In summary, the limited data suggest that very young mothers have lower gains than other women do. The effect of pregnancy after age 35 or 40 on gestational weight gain has not been studied. Thomson and Billewicz (1957) studied the relationship between maternal age and the pattern of weight gain, and no relationship was found.

Cigarette Smoking

Results of multivariate analysis showed that the mean weight gain of married smokers and nonsmokers in the 1980 NNS were similar, but mothers who smoked cigarettes were 50% likelier to gain less than 6.8 kg (15 lb) than were nonsmoking mothers. Rush (1974) and Davies et al. (1976) reported that female nonsmokers gain less weight than female smokers do, but other investigators have not found this effect (Carruth, 1981; Meyer, 1978; Picone et al., 1982). It appears that smoking has a small effect, if any, on mean gestational weight gain but a larger effect on risk of low weight gain.

Alcohol and Illegal Substances

There are many reports on the effect of maternal alcohol consumption on fetal growth and development, but few on the relationship between alcohol consumption and gestational weight gain. In a study of 204 alcohol abusers and 11,123 alcohol nonabusers (Sokol et al., 1980), no differences were found in maternal prepregnancy weight, height, or gestational weight gain between the two groups. In another study of 270 pregnant women (Tennes and Blackard, 1980), there was no correlation between alcohol use and gestational weight gain. In the 1980 NNS (Kleinman, 1990), alcohol consumption was found to have little effect on mean weight gain. Mean weight gain of moderate users of alcohol (defined as those who drank more than once per month or more than two drinks per drinking occasion) was 0.2 kg (0.4 lb) higher than that of women who consumed no alcohol. The risk of low weight gain was greatest among the nondrinkers.

In a thorough review of the literature, the subcommittee found only one study (Zuckerman et al., 1989) on the relationship between the use of cocaine and marijuana and gestational weight gain. In that study, Zuckerman et al. (1989) compared 202 marijuana users with 895 nonusers and 114 cocaine users with 1,010 nonusers among women attending the prenatal clinic at Boston City Hospital. The mean weight gain of marijuana users was 12.7 kg (28 lb) compared with 14.1 kg (31 lb) for nonusers. The mean gain of cocaine users was 10.5 kg (23 lb) compared with 14.1 kg (31 lb) for nonusers. The use of these substances and other illicit drugs generally is associated with a life-style that is not supportive of good eating and health habits. Therefore, it is not surprising that these women had lower mean weight gains during pregnancy.

Socioeconomic Status

Information about family income was requested on questionnaires that were sent to married mothers in the 1980 NNS (Taffel, 1986). In a bivariate analysis, women from households with incomes above $30,000 per year gained 0.6 kg (1.4 lb) more than did women from households with incomes of less than $9,000 per year. The risk of low weight gain increased nearly twofold as annual household income fell from $30,000 to $9,000. However, these results were not statistically controlled for other variables that could influence weight gain.

Marital status is also linked with socioeconomic status since female-headed households tend to have lower household incomes. On the average, married mothers gained about 1 kg more than unmarried mothers did (Taffel, 1986).

Data on the educational attainment of both married and unmarried mothers were analyzed in the multiple linear regression described by Kleinman (1990). Mean weight gain was similar for women in all educational groups, but compared with mothers with 13 or more years of education, the risk of low weight gain was 50% higher among mothers with <12 years of education and 25% higher among those with 12 years of education.

Work or Physical Activity

Studies on the effect of heavy work or physical activity on weight gain should be interpreted with caution, because high energy expenditure can be offset by increases in energy intake so that energy balance is maintained. Also, it is difficult to determine whether the stress (both physical and psychologic) of work, instead of the increased energy expenditure, may have led to reduced weight gain. Some investigators have reported an elevated risk of preterm delivery among working women (Mamelle and Munoz, 1987; Mamelle et al., 1984), whereas others have failed to identify such a relationship (Berkowitz et al., 1983; Kaminski and Papiernik, 1974;

Zuckerman et al., 1986). If work or physical activity reduced the length of gestation, total weight gain would also be reduced. Measurement of the rate of gain could be used to adjust for differences in the length of gestation.

Although many studies have been conducted on the effects of work on pregnancy (i.e., birth weight, gestational duration, and complications of labor and delivery), those few that provide data on weight gain (Naeye and Peters, 1982; Tafari et al., 1980) provide little useful information about the effect of work on weight gain.

CONCLUSIONS AND RECOMMENDATIONS

Since 1970, most reported average total pregnancy weight gains have ranged between 10 and 15 kg (22 and 33 lb). The mean rate of gain during the last half of gestation ranged from 0.45 to 0.52 kg (~1 lb) per week.

The relatively low energy cost (~4.7 kcal/g) of tissue gain during pregnancy probably reflects the high concentration of water in the lean tissue that is deposited. Hormonal adjustments that induce changes in the efficiency of fuel use for tissue synthesis are possible, but actual measurements of the energy cost for fat or lean tissue synthesis in pregnant women have not been made.

Differences in the physiologic response to pregnancy may account for much of the diversity in gains, but certain maternal factors, e.g., high prepregnancy weight for height, short stature, black or Southeast Asian background, very young age (<2 years after menarche), multiparity, unmarried status, and low income, are important predictors of a risk of low weight gain. Maternal use of alcohol does not appear to affect weight gain significantly. Furthermore, the limited data available do not show that work outside the home or physical activity affects weight gain in U.S. women.

CLINICAL IMPLICATIONS

• Total weight gain during pregnancy varies widely among women with similar ages, weights, heights, ethnic backgrounds, and socioeconomic status. Gestation gains between the 15th and 85th percentiles range from approximately 7 to 18 kg (16 to 40 lb). Therefore, recommended gains should be used only as targets and for identifying individuals who should be evaluated for insufficient or excessive rates of gain.

• The observed rate of gain in the second and third trimesters ranges from 0.3 to 0.7 kg (0.7 to 1.4 lb) per week. The average rate of gain during the second trimester may be slightly higher than that during the third trimester.

- Within a population, the range of gestational weight gains is wider among overweight women than among normal-weight or underweight women.
- Although some investigators have reported different rates of gain among teenagers and members of various minority groups, there is no biologic evidence to justify different recommendations for these women.
- The risk of low weight gain (<6.8 kg, or 15 lb) is higher among unmarried women, black and Hispanic women, cigarette smokers, and women with low levels of education. These women should receive additional nutritional counseling to ensure an adequate weight gain during pregnancy.
- No evidence was found to suggest that work outside the home or regular physical activity increases the risk of low weight gains during pregnancy.

REFERENCES

Abrams, B.F., and R.K. Laros, Jr. 1986. Prepregnancy weight, weight gain, and birth weight. Am. J. Obstet. Gynecol. 154:503-509.

Ancri, G., E.H. Morse, and R.P. Clarke. 1977. Comparison of the nutritional status of pregnant adolescents with adult pregnant women. III. Maternal protein and calorie intake and weight gain in relation to size of infant at birth. Am. J. Clin. Nutr. 30:568-572.

Berkowitz, G.S., J.L. Kelsey, T.R. Holford, and R.L. Berkowitz. 1983. Physical activity and the risk of spontaneous preterm delivery. J. Reprod. Med. 28:581-588.

Brown, J.E., H.N. Jacobson, L.H. Askue, and M.G. Peick. 1981. Influence of pregnancy weight gain on the size of infants born to underweight women. Obstet. Gynecol. 57:13-17.

Brown, J.E., K.W. Berdan, P. Splett, M. Robinson, and L.J. Harris. 1986. Prenatal weight gains related to the birth of healthy-sized infants to low-income women. J. Am. Diet. Assoc. 86:1679-1683.

Carruth, B.R. 1981. Smoking and pregnancy outcome of adolescents. J. Adol. Health Care 2:115-120.

Clapp, J.F., III, B.L. Seaward, R.H. Sleamaker, and J. Hiser. 1988. Maternal physiologic adaptations to early human pregnancy. Am. J. Obstet. Gynecol. 159:1456-1460.

Cummings, H.H. 1934. An interpretation of weight changes during pregnancy. Am. J. Obstet. Gynecol. 27:808-815.

Davies, D.P., O.P. Gray, P.C. Ellwood, and M. Abernethy. 1976. Cigarette smoking in pregnancy: associations with maternal weight gain and fetal growth. Lancet 1:385-387.

Durnin, J.V.G.A. 1987. Energy requirements of pregnancy: an integration of the longitudinal data from the five-country study. Lancet 2:1131-1133.

Eastman, N.J., and E. Jackson. 1968. Weight relationships in pregnancy: I. The bearing of maternal weight gain and pre-pregnancy weight on birth weight in full term pregnancies. Obstet. Gynecol. Surv. 23:1003-1025.

Endres, J.M., K. Poell-Odenwald, M. Sawicki, and P. Welch. 1985. Dietary assessment of pregnant adolescents participating in a supplemental-food program. J. Reprod. Med. 30:10-17.

Felice, M.E., P. Shragg, M. James, and D.R. Hollingsworth. 1986. Clinical observations of Mexican-American, Caucasian, and black pregnant teenagers. J. Adol. Health Care 7:305-310.

Forbes, G.B. 1988. Body composition: influence of nutrition, disease, growth, and aging. Pp. 533-556 in M.E. Shils and V.R. Young, eds. Modern Nutrition in Health and Disease, 7th ed. Lea & Febiger, Philadelphia.

Frisancho, A.R., J. Matos, and P. Flegel. 1983. Maternal nutritional status and adolescent pregnancy outcome. Am. J. Clin. Nutr. 38:739-746.

George, N.N., S.K. Kim, and J.L. Duhring. 1984. Prepregnancy weights and weight gains related to birth weights of infants born to overweight women. J. Am. Diet. Assoc. 84:450-452.

Gormican, A., J. Valentine, and E. Satter. 1980. Relationships of maternal weight gain, prepregnancy weight, and infant birthweight. Interaction of weight factors in pregnancy. J. Am. Diet. Assoc. 77:662-667.

Haiek, L., and S.A. Lederman. 1989. The relationship between maternal weight for height and term birth weight in teens and adult women. J. Adol. Health Care 10:16-22.

Horon, I.L., D.M. Strobino, and H.M. MacDonald. 1983. Birth weights among infants born to adolescent and young adult women. Am. J. Obstet. Gynecol. 146:444-449.

Humphreys, R.C. 1954. An analysis of the maternal and foetal weight factors in normal pregnancy. J. Obstet. Gynaecol. Br. Commonw. 61:764-771.

Husaini, Y.K., M.A. Husaini, Z. Sulaiman, A.B. Jahari, Barizi, S.T. Hudono, and D. Karyadi. 1986. Maternal malnutrition, outcome of pregnancy, and a simple tool to identify women at risk. Food Nutr. Bull. 8:71-76.

Hytten, F.E. 1980a. Nutrition. Pp. 163-192 in F. Hytten and G. Chamberlain, eds. Clinical Physiology in Obstetrics. Blackwell Scientific Publications, Oxford.

Hytten, F.E. 1980b. Weight gain in pregnancy. Pp. 193-233 in F. Hytten and G. Chamberlain, eds. Clinical Physiology in Obstetrics. Blackwell Scientific Publications, Oxford.

Hytten, F.E., and I. Leitch. 1971. The Physiology of Human Pregnancy, 2nd ed. Blackwell Scientific Publications, Oxford. 599 pp.

Kaminski, M., and E. Papiernik. 1974. Multifactorial study of the risk of prematurity at 32 weeks of gestation. II. A comparison between an empirical prediction and a discriminant analysis. J. Perinat. Med. 2:37-44.

Kawakami, S., C. Ishiwata, K. Hayashi, Y. Kawaguchi, N. Kondo, and R. Iizuka. 1977. Alteration of maternal body weight in pregnancy and postpartum. Keio J. Med. 26:53-62.

Kitzmiller, J.L. 1980. The endocrine pancreas and maternal metabolism. Pp. 58-83 in D. Tulchinsky and K.J. Ryan, eds. Maternal-Fetal Endocrinology. W.B. Saunders, Philadelphia.

Kleinman, J.C. 1990. Maternal Weight Gain During Pregnancy: Determinants and Consequences. NCHS Working Paper Series No. 33. National Center for Health Statistics, Public Health Service, U.S. Department of Health and Human Services, Hyattsville, Md. 24 pp.

Kuo, C.C. 1941. Weight gain in normal pregnancy in Chinese patients. Chin. Med. J. 59:278-286.

Loris, P., K.G. Dewey, and K. Poirier-Brode. 1985. Weight gain and dietary intake of pregnant teenagers. J. Am. Diet. Assoc. 85:1296-1305.

Mamelle, N., and F. Munoz. 1987. Occupational working conditions and preterm birth: a reliable scoring system. Am. J. Epidemiol. 126:150-152.

Mamelle, N., B. Laumon, and P. Lazar. 1984. Prematurity and occupational activity during pregnancy. Am. J. Epidemiol. 119:309-322.

Meserole, L.P., B.S. Worthington-Roberts, J.M. Rees, and L.S. Wright. 1984. Prenatal weight gain and postpartum weight loss patterns in adolescents. J. Adol. Health Care 5:21-27.

Metropolitan Life Insurance Company. 1959. New weight standards for men and women. Stat. Bull. Metrop. Life Insur. Co. 40:1-4.

Meyer, M.B. 1978. How does maternal smoking affect birth weight and maternal weight gain? Evidence from the Ontario Perinatal Mortality Study. Am. J. Obstet. Gynecol. 131:888-893.

Mitchell, M.C., and E. Lerner. 1989. Weight gain and pregnancy outcome in underweight and normal weight women. J. Am. Diet. Assoc. 89:634-638.

Muscati, S.K., M.A. Mackey, and B. Newsom. 1988. The influence of smoking and stress on prenatal weight gain and infant birth weight of teenage mothers. J. Nutr. Educ. 20:299-302.

Naeye, R.L., and E.C. Peters. 1982. Working during pregnancy: effects on the fetus. Pediatrics 69:724-727.

Niswander, K., and E.C. Jackson. 1974. Physical characteristics of the gravida and their association with birth weight and perinatal death. Am. J. Obstet. Gynecol. 119:306-313.

NRC (National Research Council). 1970. Maternal Nutrition and the Course of Pregnancy. Report of the Committee on Maternal Nutrition, Food and Nutrition Board. National Academy of Sciences, Washington, D.C. 241 pp.

Picone, T.A., L.H. Allen, M.M. Schramm, and P.N. Olsen. 1982. Pregnancy outcome in North American women. I. Effects of diet, cigarette smoking, and psychological stress on maternal weight gain. Am. J. Clin. Nutr. 36:1205-1213.

Robinson, H.R., A.F. Guttmacher, E.P.H. Harrison, Jr., and J.M. Spence, Jr. 1943. Gain in weight during pregnancy. Child. Dev. 43:131-142.

Rosso, P. 1985. A new chart to monitor weight gain during pregnancy. Am. J. Clin. Nutr. 41:644-652.

Rush, D. 1974. Examination of the relationship between birthweight, cigarette smoking during pregnancy and maternal weight gain. J. Obstet. Gynaecol. Br. Commonw. 81:746-752.

Scholl, T.O., R.W. Salmon, L.K. Miller, P. Vasilenko III, C.H. Furey, and M. Christine. 1988. Weight gain during adolescent pregnancy: associated maternal characteristics and effects on birth weight. J. Adol. Health Care 9:286-290.

Scott, J.A., and B. Benjamin. 1948. Weight changes in pregnancy. Lancet 1:550-551.

Simpson, J.W., R.W. Lawless, and A.C. Mitchell. 1975. Responsibility of the obstetrician to the fetus. II. Influence of prepregnancy weight and pregnancy weight gain on birthweight. Obstet. Gynecol. 45:481-487.

Sokol, R.J., S.I. Miller, and G. Reed. 1980. Alcohol abuse during pregnancy: an epidemiologic study. Alcoholism 4:135-145.

Stander, H.J., and J.B. Pastore. 1940. Weight changes during pregnancy and puerperium. Am. J. Obstet. Gynecol. 39:928-937.

Swenson, I., D. Erickson, E. Ehlinger, S. Swaney, and G. Carlson. 1986. Birth weight, Apgar scores, labor and delivery complications and prenatal characteristics of Southeast Asian adolescents and older mothers. Adolescence 21:711-722.

Tafari, N., R.L. Naeye, and A. Gobezie. 1980. Effects of maternal undernutrition and heavy physical work during pregnancy on birth weight. Br. J. Obstet. Gynaecol. 87:222-226.

Taffel, S.M. 1986. Maternal Weight Gain and the Outcome of Pregnancy: United States, 1980. Vital and Health Statistics, Series 21, No. 44. DHHS Publ. No. (PHS) 86-1922. National Center for Health Statistics, Public Health Service, U.S. Department of Health and Human Services, Hyattsville, Md. 25 pp.

Tennes, K., and C. Blackard. 1980. Maternal alcohol consumption, birth weight, and minor physical anomalies. Am. J. Obstet. Gynecol. 138:774-780.

Thomson, A.M., and W.Z. Billewicz. 1957. Clinical significance of weight trends during pregnancy. Br. Med. J. 1:243-247.

Tompkins, W.T., and D.G. Wiehl. 1951. Nutritional deficiencies as a causal factor in toxemia and premature labor. Am. J. Obstet. Gynecol. 62:898-919.

Venkatachalam, P.S., K. Shankar, and C. Gopalan. 1960. Changes in body-weight and body composition during pregnancy. Indian J. Med. Res. 48:511-517.

Winikoff, B., and C.H. Debrovner. 1981. Anthropometric determinants of birth weight. Obstet. Gynecol. 58:678-684.

Zuckerman, B.S., D.A. Frank, R. Hingson, S. Morelock, and H.L. Kayne. 1986. Impact of maternal work outside the home during pregnancy on neonatal outcome. Pediatrics 77:459-464.

Zuckerman, B., D.A. Frank, R. Hingson, H. Amaro, S.M. Levenson, H. Kayne, S. Parker, R. Vinci, K. Aboagye, L.E. Fried, H. Cabral, R. Timperi, and H. Bauchner. 1989. Effects of maternal marijuana and cocaine use on fetal growth. N. Engl. J. Med. 320:762-768.

6

Body Composition Changes During Pregnancy

In the development of standards for optimum weight gain during pregnancy, or in the use of weight gain to identify suboptimal pregnancies, the variability in the components of weight gain must be recognized. These include the products of conception (fetus, placenta, and amniotic fluid), uterine and breast tissue, extracellular fluid, and maternal fat. These components change over the course of pregnancy and to different extents in different individuals, markedly affecting the interpretation of weight gain.

Although measurement of weight gain can be a clinically useful screening method for identifying some pregnancies that are progressing abnormally, it provides very limited information regarding changes in body composition of an individual pregnant woman, even when weight gain is close to the average for normal pregnancies. Information on body composition would add substantially to understanding of the meaning of a given weight gain. Fetal growth may be influenced more by specific maternal tissue changes, for example, by accretion of lean tissue, fat, or body water, than by total gestational weight gain. Body composition studies in appropriate animals could provide valuable information in this regard. However, even if changes in lean tissue should prove to be more important for fetal outcomes, methods would still be needed to determine accurately the net amount of fat stored during normal pregnancy for estimating energy requirements, since fat is the most calorie-dense substance deposited.

STANDARD METHODS

In the most widely used model for examining body composition, the body is regarded as being composed of only two compartments—fat and lean. In this usage, lean body mass represents a mixture of all the nonfat tissues of the body. Most techniques currently used to estimate body composition are based on measuring the qualities of the lean body tissues. Of the commonly used methods, only density measurements are dependent on both fat and lean tissue, but the fat estimate is still highly influenced by the variability of the lean tissue density. In the two compartment model, the weight of fat is the difference between two large masses—body weight and lean body mass. Therefore, a small relative error in the lean body mass estimation will produce a much larger relative error in calculated body fat.

There are three standard methods for estimating lean body mass: measurement of total body water, determination of total body potassium content, and underwater weighing, which permits estimation of total body density, thereby allowing simultaneous estimation of both fat and lean tissue. Inherent in each of these methods are assumptions relating the actual measurements to specific body compartments. The assumptions are discussed here to assist in later interpretation of the data.

Total Body Water

To calculate lean tissue from total body water, the water content of the lean tissue must be known. Although the *average* percentage of water in lean tissue is known with fair accuracy in adult women, the nonfat tissues added during pregnancy (edema fluid, fetus, amniotic fluid, plasma) contain a high percentage of water. Thus, pregnancy may increase the water content of lean tissue from approximately 72.5% at 10 weeks of gestation to about 75.0% at 40 weeks in women with generalized edema (van Raaij et al., 1988). A difference of this magnitude can cause fat to be underestimated by 50% or more in women gaining 3 to 4 kg of fat.

Since gestational changes in lean tissue *hydration* in individual women have not been measured in body water studies, only approximate corrections are possible. Theoretical corrections for dilution of the lean tissues during pregnancy may improve estimates of body composition changes for a population; lean tissue estimates for an individual (which are important for relating body composition to pregnancy outcome) may still be inexact, although they are useful for identifying markedly aberrant cases. Interpretation of body water changes might be improved with a measure of extracellular water. Variation in extracellular water can be substantial. Hytten (1980) estimated that pregnant women with generalized edema have more than 3 kg (6.6 lb) of additional extracellular fluid compared with that in women with no edema or leg edema only. Extracellular water can be determined either with the use of an extracellular tracer such as bromide or by estimation of intracellular water from measurement of total body potassium and determination of extracellular water by difference from total body water. There have been few studies in which extracellular water has been measured with tracers appropriate for use in pregnant women. Three small studies (Emerson et al., 1975; Forsum et al., 1988; Pipe et al., 1979) combined total body water and total body potassium measurements. These are discussed below.

Underwater Weighing

Underwater weighing is based on the assumption that the weight of fat and lean tissue can be estimated from total body density by using standard values for the average densities of fat and lean tissues. Because of the increased hydration of lean tissue during pregnancy, and especially because added tissue includes little bone, which is dense, the density of the lean body mass is likely to decline during pregnancy. Using theoretical estimates of body composition during pregnancy, Fidanza (1987) estimated that the density of the fat-free body declines from 1.100 kg/m^3 at 10 weeks of gestation to 1.087 at 40 weeks of gestation. If nonpregnancy lean tissue density values are used for pregnant subjects, lean body mass will be underestimated and fat will be overestimated, perhaps by as much as 2.5 kg at term (see van Raaij et al., 1988). In addition, the true mean density of the lean body tissue differs among individuals because of differing proportions of the organs, muscle, and bone comprising the lean body and may also change to varying degrees over the course of pregnancy because of the differential growth of various tissues, especially those with a high water content and no bone.

Total Body Potassium

Measurement of total body potassium can be used to estimate lean body mass if a standard value for the concentration of potassium in the lean tissues is assumed. The vast majority of the body's potassium (approximately 98%) is intracellular; therefore, total body potassium is actually a reflection primarily of the intracellular compartment. Substantial changes in the extracellular compartment can go undetected. For this method to give a good estimate of the weight of total lean tissue, the ratio of intracellular to extracellular tissue must be either close to the norm or assessed independently. This ratio of intra- to extracellular water decreases during pregnancy, resulting in overestimation of fat if not corrected. Independent measures of hydration (total body water, extracellular water) allow correction for individual variation, as has been done in some studies (Forsum et al., 1988; Pipe et al., 1979).

Despite their limitations, total body water, underwater weighing, and total body potassium are the three best methods for studying body composition in pregnant women. However, measurement of total body potassium and underwater weighing require special, large equipment and considerable patient cooperation, and estimation of total body water requires special isotopes that are expensive to use and measure. These considerations have encouraged the use of simpler methods, such as measurement of skinfold thicknesses with calipers.

SKINFOLD THICKNESS MEASUREMENT

Changes in skinfold thickness have been widely used to estimate changes in the fat content of pregnant women. Skinfold thickness measurements suggest that more maternal fat is accumulated centrally than peripherally (Taggart et al., 1967). Skinfold thickness can be measured quickly with relatively inexpensive equipment. As one early researcher cautioned, however, ". . . skinfold measurements are relatively inaccurate and . . . a high degree of standardization is required to obtain reliable comparisons, even with one observer" (Taggart et al., 1967, p. 441). Proper use requires extensive training and monitoring to consistently achieve reproducible measurements.

To convert skinfold thickness measurements to estimates of body fat, standard regression equations are used. Generally, these are based on studies correlating skinfold thickness to body fat measured by total body water, body density, or total body potassium. Of special importance is the fact that the most widely used regression equations for interpreting skinfold thicknesses in pregnant women (Durnin and Womersley, 1974) have been developed in studies of nonpregnant subjects. Longitudinal studies of skinfold thickness in pregnant women (Taggart et al., 1967) suggest that skinfold thickness in late pregnancy may be increased by water retention. Therefore, an observed increase in skinfold thickness may not indicate an increase in body fat. The magnitude of this hydration effect may also vary from one measurement site to another, as indicated by a decrease in some skinfold thicknesses between the final weeks of pregnancy and the first month post partum. This has been studied by Adair et al. (1984) in Taiwan, by Taggart et al. (1967) in Scotland, and by Forsum et al. (1989) in Sweden. Thus, especially during late pregnancy, skinfold thickness measurements may be less indicative of body fat content. Because skinfold measurements are used (despite their limitations) in many clinical settings, it would be of great value to develop calibration equations derived from pregnant women whose body fat was estimated with the best methods and models available. The applicability of the equations may also be affected by differences in age, ethnic background, and exercise patterns of the reference and study populations. The usefulness of a regression equation depends in part on the comparability of the measurement techniques used in the population under study and in the reference population from which the equation was derived. Different or less experienced workers in the same research group may obtain different values or measurement variabilities (Taggart et al., 1967). Therefore, even very exact regression equations obtained by one group of investigators may give less accurate estimates of body fat when applied in a new study.

DIRECT COMPARISONS OF SKINFOLD THICKNESS MEASUREMENTS

In several studies, skinfold thickness values themselves have been used without calculating body fat content. In this approach, investigators used either individual skinfold thicknesses (Frisancho et al., 1977; Maso et al., 1988; Viegas et al., 1987) or a sum of several different skinfold thicknesses (Arroyo et al., 1978; Lawrence et al., 1984; Prentice et al., 1981; Taggart et al., 1967), but they did not assume that all the measured change reflects changes in body fat. This approach may be conceptually more justifiable than relating skinfold thicknesses to body fat. Furthermore, by combining skinfold thickness measurements with arm circumference measurements, it is possible to estimate arm muscle area, which reflects the amount of lean tissue. This could be of value, since it is not known whether maternal fat or lean tissue increments are more important for fetal growth. Frisancho et al. (1977) observed that maternal arm fat in Peruvian women was related to infant fatness but not birth weight, whereas arm muscle area was related to infant length. In contrast, Maso et al. (1988) observed that arm fat area and arm circumference changes between weeks 22 and 32 of gestation were correlated with birth weight in a U.S. black population, but arm muscle area was not.

Changes in total body water and plasma volume also reflect components of the lean tissue. Both these measurements have been related to birth weight (Duffus et al., 1971). Thus, although fat changes may contribute most to gestational calorie needs, lean tissue may influence important aspects of fetal growth. Clearly, better understanding of the importance of lean tissue changes during pregnancy is needed. Development of this understanding will require further study of total body water, total body potassium, extracellular water, and plasma volume and their relationship to pregnancy outcome.

NUTRITIONAL STATUS AND WEIGHT GAIN

TABLE 6-1   Changes in Total Body Water from Studies Covering
Different Periods of Gestation

Country and Reference	Number of Subjects	Change in Total Body Water, liters	Period of Gestation, wk	Comments on Study Subjects
Scotland	82–91	$7.74 \pm 2.63 \ (SD)^a$	10 to 38	Mixed parities
Hytten et al.,	84	1.88	10 to 20	
1966	82	2.80	20 to 30	
	91	3.03	30 to 38	
Scotland	48	7.3	10 to 38	Estimated from their
Taggart et				reported dry
al., 1967[b]				weight
Scotland	35	3.2	30–32 to 36–39	Primiparous, under
Duffus et al.,				age 30
1971				
United States	5	4.4	20 to 40	Four subjects
(Boston)				restricted their
Emerson				food intake; one
et al., 1975				was obese
England	27	7.2	10–14 to 36–38	Normal
Pipe et al.,		3.3	10–14 to 24–28	prepregnancy
1979		3.9	24–28 to 36–38	weight for height
Scotland	81	3.8	30 to 38	Obese women
Campbell,				
1983				
Sweden	22	5.7^c	Prepregnancy	Twenty-one
Forsum			to 36 weeks	multiparous
et al., 1988		4.2	16–18 to 30	
		2.0	30 to 36	

[a] SD = Standard deviation.

[b] It is not clear whether the patients in the study by Taggart et al. (1967) are a subset of those in the study by Hytten et al. (1966). Hytten's group had 39 primiparas and 54 multiparas and Taggart's group had 23 and 25, respectively, drawn from the same research site, at about the same time, with the same coauthors.

[c] All other studies used deuterium oxide dilution to determine total body water. This study used water labeled with [18]oxygen.

Several newer methods (e.g., total body electrical conductivity, bioimpedance analysis, and computerized axial tomography) for measuring fat or lean tissue may produce accurate results quickly and relatively easily. Some have gained acceptance by being validated against more familiar methods. However, there are no formal reports of their application to pregnant women for consideration by this subcommittee.

TABLE 6-2 Estimated Total Maternal Weight Gain, Corrected to 40 Weeks of Gestation,[a] from Six Studies

Reference	Reported Mean Weight Gain, kg ± SD	Period of Gestation, wk	Total Weight Gain, kg (corrected to 40 weeks of gestation)
Hytten et al., 1966	11.15 ± 3.34	10–38	13.0
Taggart et al., 1967[b]	11.0[c]	10–38	12.8
Emerson et al., 1975	9.2[c]	NR[d]	9.2[e]
Pipe et al., 1979	10.4[c]	10–14 to 36–38	12.0
Campbell, 1983	9.2[c]	20–38	13.8
Forsum et al., 1988	13.6 ± 3.0	Prepregnancy to delivery	13.6

[a] See text for method used to correct to 40 weeks of gestation.
[b] See footnote b in Table 6-1.
[c] Standard deviations (SD) were not reported.
[d] NR = Not reported.
[e] Not adjusted. Mean of "maximum gain" as reported by the authors, based on reported prepregnancy weights. Some of the five subjects were limiting their food intake.

RESULTS OF STUDIES

Total Body Water

Table 6-1 presents data from studies of total body water during pregnancy. The tabulated results illustrate the interpretive problems: wide variations in weight gains among studies (see Table 6-2), different periods used to compute the gestational increment in body water, and small sample sizes.

A better comparison of the tabulated studies, which cover different gestational periods, can be made by normalizing all the weight gain figures to 40 weeks of gestation (Table 6-2). A graph of maternal weight gain (Hytten and Leitch, 1971) was used to estimate the weight that would have been gained before and after the measurement periods listed in Table 6-2. On the basis of this standard, expected additional weight gains are 0.5 kg (1.1 lb) before 5 weeks, 1 kg (2.2 lb) before 10 weeks, 4 kg (8.8 lb) before 20 weeks, 1.3 kg (2.9 lb) after 37 weeks, and 0.8 kg (1.8 lb) after 38 weeks of gestation. Table 6-2 shows the estimated total weight gains for six studies. These numbers suggest a consistency in average weight gain among the studies, whereas the values given for the various periods actually measured did not.

The data provided by Pipe et al. (1979) and Hytten et al. (1966), which include measurements at three and four gestational periods, respectively,

TABLE 6-3   Estimations of Fat Gain from Body Water Studies

Study	Number of Subjects	Change in Body Water, kg ± SD[a,b]	Equivalent in Lean Mass,[c] kg	Change in Body Weight, kg	Fat Gain Estimate, kg
Hytten et al., 1966	75	7.74 ± 2.63	8.5	11.15[a]	2.65
Taggart et al., 1967	48	7.3[d]	8.0	11.0[a]	3.0
Emerson et al., 1975	5	6.3[d] (2.0 kg added for 10–20 wk)	6.9	8.2[e]	1.3
Pipe et al., 1979	27	7.2[d] (10–12 to 36–38 wk)	7.9	10.4	2.5
Campbell, 1983	81	8.5[d] (4.7 kg added for 10–30 wk)	9.3	12.8[e]	3.5
Forsum et al., 1988	22	5.7[d,f]	6.3	11.7	5.4

NOTE: All data are normalized to a period ranging from 10 to 38 weeks or more of gestation and are corrected for the extra hydration of pregnancy.
[a] From 10 to 38 weeks of gestation.
[b] SD = Standard deviation.
[c] Assuming 91.1% water in added lean tissues at term; see van Raaij et al. (1988). This corrects for the added hydration of pregnancy, which would otherwise result in an underestimation of fat.
[d] Standard deviation not reported or not applicable.
[e] One kilogram was subtracted from the estimate of weight gain for the entire pregnancy to eliminate gains before 10 weeks of gestation.
[f] The values for body water and pregnancy weight gain are the reported values from prepregnancy to 36 weeks of gestation.

provide a means of evaluating the body water values obtained in the other studies. Both data sets show a larger increment of body water later in pregnancy than early in pregnancy. In general, other studies that provide fewer longitudinal data are in agreement (Campbell, 1983; Duffus et al., 1971). The early increments obtained by Pipe et al. (1979) or Hytten et al. (1966) can be used in combination with data from studies that only provide measurements for the last half of gestation to estimate total increases in body water and body fat. Table 6-3 presents the results of six studies, along with estimations where needed.

The highest estimate for fat gain was obtained by Forsum et al. (1988). Their result was influenced by the value they found for body water increments, which was much lower than those reported by Hytten et al. (1966) and Campbell (1983). Of these three studies, only the one reported by Forsum and colleagues involved the use of water labeled with the isotope [18]oxygen, rather than deuterium, and saliva, rather than blood, to monitor dilution of the isotopically labeled water. Unless a correction is made, the use of deuterium oxide will lead to a higher estimate of body water compared with that from the use of ^{18}oxygen water (which is considered the more accurate method), because deuterium exchanges with nonaqueous hydrogen to a small extent. These methodologic differences may contribute to the lower body water values obtained by Forsum and colleagues. However, since deuterium oxide values are corrected for hydrogen exchange, it is unlikely that this factor completely explains the reported differences.

Nevertheless, the study by Forsum and colleagues is provocative, because it is the first longitudinal body water study that includes actual prepregnancy measurements. In addition, both the body water and total body potassium values they obtained suggest a loss of lean tissue in early pregnancy, as discussed below. Other considerations suggest that caution be exercised in accepting the data of Forsum and colleagues. For example, Clapp et al. (1988) showed an increase of both fat and lean tissue during the first 7 weeks of gestation and from weeks 7 to 15 of gestation (based on skinfold thicknesses). Taggart et al. (1967), however, reported no increase in skinfold thicknesses in a group of women followed from before conception through early pregnancy. The finding by Forsum et al. (1988) that total body water at 6 months post partum is lower than the prepregnancy value, while body fat is 3.2 kg (7 lb) above prepregnancy levels, is surprising. It is difficult to accept the fact that women were retaining so much fat while they lost enough weight to place them *below* their prepregnancy weight. van Raaij et al. (1988) found that a 1.7-kg (3.7 lb) increase in weight from the prepregnancy to the postpartum period was associated with a 1.5-kg (3.3 lb) increase in fat, as determined by densitometry. Further studies will be needed to provide certainty about the changes that occur during early pregnancy.

Body Density (by Underwater Weighing)

Body density has been measured in two studies of pregnant women. In the most recent study (van Raaij et al., 1988), a new approach was used to interpret the measurements, correcting for changing density as pregnancy advances. This approach can also be applied to the earlier study by Seitchik et al. (1963), who reported individual values.

When consistent methods of calculation are used, the two studies on body density are in excellent agreement (Table 6-4). All the differences in fat gain could be due to the differences in weight gains and gestation periods studied. These two studies give corrected fat estimates that are within the range of values obtained from total body water measurements.

Total Body Potassium

Results from studies of total body potassium in adult pregnant women are shown in Figure 6-1. Comparison of the three data sets reveals large differences in the absolute values obtained for total body potassium, espe-

TABLE 6-4 Estimated Change in Total Body Fat During Pregnancy

Number of Subjects	Period of Gestation, wk	Body Weight, kg	Body Density, ($\times 10^3$ kg/m^3)	Total Body Fat,[a] kg	Change in Weight, kg	Change in Fat, kg	Reference
42	11	61.70	1.0342	17.51			van Raaij et al., 1988
	23	66.10	1.0295	19.70	9.1 (11–35 wk)	2.3 (11–35 wk)	
	35	70.85	1.0298	19.80[b]			
	9 wk postpartum	63.3	1.0308	19.12			
21	7–15	58.8	1.026	18.94			Seitchik et al., 1963
	16–23	61.4	1.022	20.50			
	24–31	64.6	1.020	21.50			
	37–40	68.4	1.020	21.72	9.6 (11–38 wk)	2.8 (11–38 wk)	
	6 wk postpartum	59.7	1.020	21.07			

NOTE: Total body fat change was calculated from body density measurements and body weight and corrected for the change in lean tissue density during pregnancy.

[a] Fat values were calculated from the equations of van Raaij et al. (1988), which adjust for changing density of lean tissue during pregnancy. The equations were for weeks 10, 20, 30, and 40.

[b] For the 35-week data, the calculation was done with the equations for weeks 30 and 40 and by averaging the results obtained.

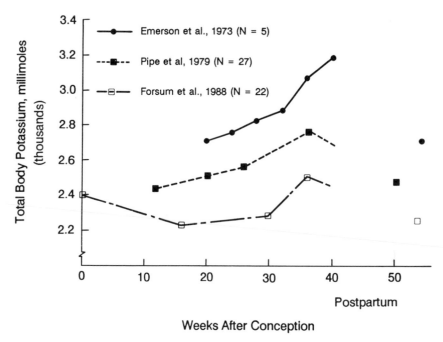

FIGURE 6-1 Changes in total body potassium during pregnancy based on data from three studies.

cially in late pregnancy—differences that do not correspond to the reported differences in body weight. For example, weight gain was lowest in the report of Emerson et al. (1975), but total body potassium changes were the highest.

Comparison of the incremental gestational changes in total body potassium also reveals substantial differences among the studies. The incremental value of Forsum and colleagues (1988) from early to late pregnancy is approximately one-third that of the other two studies. The total body potassium data provided by Forsum's group, if correct, also suggest the loss of lean tissue during early pregnancy. In fact, the reported increment from prepregnancy to term is so low that it is insufficient to account for the amount of potassium others have estimated to be required for the contribution of the conceptus alone. However, all three studies show postpartum figures that are very close to their early pregnancy figures. If one ignores the prepregnancy figures of Forsum and colleagues, the pattern of the data is more consistent with those from the other studies.

The total body potassium value and an estimate of the conceptus contribution to it (i.e., 169 mmol of potassium at 36 to 38 weeks of gestation; Pipe et al., 1979) can be used to calculate the amount of potassium gained by the mother herself. In turn, this value can be used to estimate the change in maternal lean tissue in the three studies, assuming that the incremental lean tissue has 92 mmol of potassium per kilogram (Pipe et al., 1979). The results indicate a maternal gain of 1.2 to 2.1 kg (2.6 to 4.6 lb) of lean tissue between early and late pregnancy, excluding the conceptus. This would include blood, mammary gland, and uterine increments. Subtracting this estimate of the mother's lean tissue gain and an estimate of the weight of the conceptus from the weight gained during the corresponding period provides an estimate of the increment in maternal stores, largely fat, gained by the mother. This method of estimation indicated a loss of 1.6 kg (3.5 lb) of fat (weeks 20 to 40 of gestation) in the study of five women who were restricting food intake (Emerson et al., 1975); these women may have gained weight earlier. When data from the other two studies and total body potassium changes are used, the estimated maternal stores are 3.6 kg (7.9 lb) (Forsum et al., 1988) or 4.6 kg (10.1 lb) (Pipe et al., 1979). Both groups of workers have combined their data on total body water and their data on total body potassium to calculate a corrected value for total body fat. In this approach, changes in hydration are taken into consideration in computing lean tissue from the total body potassium. Their corrected fat estimates were 1.6 kg (3.5 lb) (Forsum et al., 1988) and 1.87 kg (4.1 lb) (Pipe et al., 1979) from early to late pregnancy, which are quite different from the uncorrected values calculated from the total body potassium value only. The values for fat increments in women on unrestricted diets estimated from the three standard methods suggest very different calorie requirements for fat storage—i.e., nearly a 30,000-kcal difference between the low and high values. This represents a substantial portion of the estimated energy requirement for pregnancy and indicates the need for a better definition of the changes that occur in calorie requirements and energy partitioning in successful pregnancies.

Skinfold Thicknesses

Skinfold thicknesses have been used to describe normal body fat changes throughout gestation, to determine whether skinfold thickness is associated with fetal outcome or with supplementation in undernourished women, to identify women with unusually small or large changes in body fat during pregnancy, and to estimate the initial body fat content. Measured mean triceps values range from a low of approximately 10 mm (at term in Taiwanese women; Adair et al., 1984) to a high of 18.9 mm (at 22 weeks of gestation, in black teenagers having appropriate-for-gestational-age newborns; Maso et al., 1988). Mean values for the sum of triceps, biceps, subscapular, and suprailiac skinfold thicknesses ranged from a low of 31.3 mm (4 to 6 weeks post partum; Gambian data reported by Durnin,

TABLE 6-5   Estimations of Total Body Fat and Increase in Fat During Gestation Based on Skinfold Thickness Measurements and the Equation of Durnin and Womersley (1974)

Study and Country	Estimated Total Body Fat in First Trimester, kg ± SD[a]	Fat Increment, kg
Pipe et al., 1979 England	15.4 ± 2.9	2.8[b]
Dibblee and Graham, 1983 England	14.1 ± 3.9	4.4[b]
Langhoff-Roos et al., 1987 Sweden	Not available	4.0[c]
Durnin, 1987		
Scotland	15.1 ± 4.6	2.3[d]
The Netherlands	17.7 ± 4.9	2.0[d]
The Gambia	10.3 ± 2.5	0.6[d]
Thailand	11.3 ± 2.8	1.4[d]
Philippines	11.2 ± 3.4	1.3[d]

[a] SD = Standard deviation.
[b] Fat gain from first to last trimester.
[c] Fat gain from weeks 17 to 37 of gestation.
[d] Fat gain from week 10 of gestation to 4 to 6 weeks postpartum.

1987) to a high of 64.8 mm (at 17 weeks of gestation in Swedish women; Langhoff-Roos et al., 1987). Differences of this magnitude may partly reflect methodologic differences.

Table 6-5 shows the values obtained for body fat in the four studies in which the regression equation of Durnin and Womersley (1974) was used to compute body fat changes from skinfold thickness measurements. In light of the fact that the equation was derived from data on nonpregnant women, the general consistency of these findings with those from more complex methods is reassuring. The values for women from industrialized countries are in the same range as those found by the methods discussed previously, but there is nearly a twofold difference between the highest and lowest estimates of body fat content changes. The range is even wider if the values for women from developing countries are included. The data presented by Durnin (1987) are based on skinfold thicknesses measured 4 to 6 weeks post partum. This may partly explain why they are lower than the values from the other studies. For example, Dibblee and Graham (1983) estimated a 4.4 kg (9.7 lb) fat increment between the first and third trimesters, based on skinfold thickness changes. Yet, only 1.3 kg (2.9 lb) of that estimated fat gain was retained at 4 weeks post partum. Although some fat may be lost post partum, it is likely that the increase in body water contributes to the increase in skinfold thickness during pregnancy;

the water loss post partum may contribute to the decrease in the skinfold thickness.

A study by Clapp et al. (1988) has provided some information on changes in skinfold thickness that occur very early in pregnancy. Six skinfold thicknesses were measured serially in 20 women, starting before pregnancy. The data indicate that body weight increased by 2 kg (4.4 lb) and body fat increased by 1.54 kg (3.4 lb) between the prepregnancy measurement and the seventh week of pregnancy. Thus, this study supports the possibility that maternal fat may already be increased above prepregnancy levels by the time most studies of body composition during pregnancy are begun. If so, then when measurements begin after the first trimester, increments in total body fat may be underestimated. Alternatively, these findings may indicate that the relationship between skinfold thickness and total body fat is altered very early in pregnancy. This possibility cannot be evaluated until more studies using serial measurements of total body water, total body density, or total body potassium are done during the periconceptional period.

SUMMARY

Issues to consider when examining results of pregnancy body composition studies include the following:

• Each body composition method is based on underlying assumptions, and correction factors are needed to adjust for changes in the lean body during pregnancy. Without these corrections, total body water tends to underestimate total body fat and both underwater weighing and total body potassium tend to overestimate it.

• In the future, multicompartment models of body composition need to be used in studies of larger numbers of pregnant women. Attention must also be given to differences in the gestational period studied, weight gain, initial weight, maternal age, ethnic background, and parity.

• Skinfold thickness may be useful for research purposes, but the currently used reference equations may not permit calculation of actual total body fat changes. Because of its potential for clinical as well as research use, measurement of skinfold thickness needs to be standardized against reference methods in a large number of pregnant women.

• For the development of dietary and weight gain recommendations, more information is needed on the relationship of weight gain to body fat gain in individual women. Studies of the effects of composition changes on other outcomes are also needed.

REFERENCES

Adair, L.S., E. Pollitt, and W.H. Mueller. 1984. The Bacon Chow study: effect of nutritional supplementation on maternal weight and skinfold thicknesses during pregnancy and lactation. Br. J. Nutr. 51:357-369.

Arroyo, P., D. García, C. Llerena, and S.E. Quiroz. 1978. Subcutaneous fat accumulation during pregnancy in a malnourished population. Br. J. Nutr. 40:485-489.

Campbell, D.M. 1983. Dietary restriction in obesity and its effect on neonatal outcome. Pp. 243-250 in D.M. Campbell and M.D.G. Gillmer, eds. Nutrition in Pregnancy: Proceedings of the Tenth Study Group in the Royal College of Obstetricians and Gynaecologists, September, 1982. The Royal College of Obstetricians and Gynaecologists, London.

Clapp, J.F., III, B.L. Seaward, R.H. Sleamaker, and J. Hiser. 1988. Maternal physiologic adaptations to early human pregnancy. Am. J. Obstet. Gynecol. 159:1456-1460.

Dibblee, L., and T.E. Graham. 1983. A longitudinal study of changes in aerobic fitness, body composition, and energy intake in primigravid patients. Am. J. Obstet. Gynecol. 147:908-914.

Duffus, G.M., I. MacGillivray, and K.J. Dennis. 1971. The relationship between baby weight and changes in maternal weight, total body water, plasma volume, electrolytes and proteins, and urinary oestriol excretion. J. Obstet. Gynaecol. Br. Commonw. 78:97-104.

Durnin, J.V.G.A. 1987. Energy requirements of pregnancy: an integration of the longitudinal data from the five-country study. Lancet 2:1131-1133.

Durnin, J.V.G.A., and J. Womersley. 1974. Body fat assessed from total body density and its estimation from skinfold thickness: measurements on 481 men and women aged from 16 to 72 years. Br. J. Nutr. 32:77-97.

Emerson, K., Jr., E.L. Poindexter, and M. Kothari. 1975. Changes in total body composition during normal and diabetic pregnancy. Obstet. Gynecol. 45:505-511.

Fidanza, F. 1987. The density of fat-free body mass during pregnancy. Int. J. Vitam. Nutr. Res. 57:104.

Forsum, E., A. Sadurskis, and J. Wager. 1988. Resting metabolic rate and body composition of healthy Swedish women during pregnancy. Am. J. Clin. Nutr. 47:942-947.

Forsum, E., A. Sadurskis, and J. Wager. 1989. Estimation of body fat in healthy Swedish women during pregnancy and lactation. Am. J. Clin. Nutr. 50:465-473.

Frisancho, A.R., J.E. Klayman, and J. Matos. 1977. Influence of maternal nutritional status on prenatal growth in a Peruvian urban population. Am. J. Phys. Anthropol. 46:265-274.

Hytten, F.E. 1980. Weight gain in pregnancy. Pp. 193-233 in F. Hytten and G. Chamberlain, eds. Clinical Physiology in Obstetrics. Blackwell Scientific Publications, Oxford.

Hytten, F.E., and I. Leitch. 1971. The Physiology of Human Pregnancy, 2nd ed. Blackwell Scientific Publications, Oxford. 599 pp.

Hytten, F.E., A.M. Thomson, and N. Taggart. 1966. Total body water in normal pregnancy. J. Obstet. Gynaecol. Br. Commonw. 73:553-561.

Langhoff-Roos, J., G. Lindmark, and M. Gebre-Medhin. 1987. Maternal fat stores and fat accretion during pregnancy in relation to infant birthweight. Br. J. Obstet. Gynaecol. 94:1170-1177.

Lawrence, M., F. Lawrence, W.H. Lamb, and R.G. Whitehead. 1984. Maintenance energy cost of pregnancy in rural Gambian women and influence of dietary status. Lancet 2:363-365.

Maso, M.J., E.J. Gong, M.S. Jacobson, D.S. Bross, and F.P. Heald. 1988. Anthropometric predictors of low birth weight outcome in teenage pregnancy. J. Adol. Health Care 9:188-193.

Pipe, N.G.J., T. Smith, D. Halliday, C.J. Edmonds, C. Williams, and T.M. Coltart. 1979. Changes in fat, fat-free mass and body water in human normal pregnancy. Br. J. Obstet. Gynaecol. 86:929-940.

Prentice, A.M., R.G. Whitehead, S.B. Roberts, and A.A. Paul. 1981. Long-term energy balance in child-bearing Gambian women. Am. J. Clin. Nutr. 34:2790-2799.

Seitchik, J., C. Alper, and A. Szutka. 1963. Changes in body composition during pregnancy. Ann. N.Y. Acad. Sci. 110:821-829.

Taggart, N.R., R.M. Holliday, W.Z. Billewicz, F.E. Hytten, and A.M. Thomson. 1967. Changes in skinfolds during pregnancy. Br. J. Nutr. 21:439-451.

van Raaij, J.M.A., M.E.M. Peek, S.H. Vermaat-Miedema, C.M. Schonk, and J.G.A.J. Hautvast. 1988. New equations for estimating body fat mass in pregnancy from body density or total body water. Am. J. Clin. Nutr. 48:24-29.

Viegas, O.A.C., T.J. Cole, and B.A. Wharton. 1987. Impaired fat deposition in pregnancy: an indicator for nutritional intervention. Am. J. Clin. Nutr. 45:23-28.

7

Energy Requirements, Energy Intake, and Associated Weight Gain During Pregnancy

Optimal maternal and fetal outcomes of pregnancy are contingent upon nutrient intakes sufficient to meet maternal and fetal requirements. Energy is the major nutrient determinant of gestational weight gain, although specific nutrient deficiencies may restrict that gain. Clinical and public health interventions designed to improve gestational weight gain may be directed at energy intake or expenditure (see Figures 2-2 and 2-3 in Chapter 2). Effective dietary intervention, however, requires an understanding of the energy requirements of pregnancy and the relationship between energy intake and gestational weight gain. The subcommittee reviewed energy intakes in the context of gestational weight gain, the effectiveness of energy supplementation on weight gain, and net energy balance during pregnancy.

Extra energy is required during pregnancy for the growth and maintenance of the fetus, placenta, and maternal tissues. Basal metabolism increases because of the increased mass of metabolically active tissues; maternal cardiovascular, renal, and respiratory work; and tissue synthesis. Energy requirements are greatest between 10 and 30 weeks of gestation, when relatively large quantities of maternal fat normally are deposited. Substantial fetal demands (56 kcal/kg per day) are offset in the last quarter of pregnancy by the near cessation of maternal fat storage (Sparks et al., 1980). Hytten (1980) estimated the energy cost of pregnancy to be 85,000 kcal, or 300 kcal/day, based on theoretical calculations that assumed a 3.4-kg infant, deposition of 0.9 kg (2.0 lb) of protein and 3.8 kg (8.4 lb) of fat, and an increase in basal metabolism (Table 7-1). No allowance was made for the increased energy cost of moving a heavier maternal body

TABLE 7-1   Theoretical Cumulative Energy Cost of Pregnancy and Its Components[a]

| Component | Energy Cost, kcal/day (Mean Daily Increments of Protein and Fat, g/day) by Period of Gestation, wk | | | | Cumulative Total, kcal (g) |
	0–10	10–20	20–30	30–40	
Protein deposition	3.6 (0.64)[b]	10.3 (1.84)	26.7 (4.76)	34.2 (6.1)	5,186 (925)
Fat deposition	55.6 (5.85)	235.6 (24.80)	207.6 (21.85)	31.3 (3.3)	36,329 (3,825)
Increase in basal metabolism	44.8	99.0	148.2	227.2	35,717
Total net energy	104.0	344.9	382.5	292.7	77,234
Additional energy required from food (total net energy + 10%)	114.0	379.0	421.0	322.0	84,957

[a] From Hytten (1980), with permission from Blackwell Scientific Publications, Inc.
[b] Heat of combustion defined as 5.6 kcal/g for protein and 9.5 kcal/g for fat.

mass; it was assumed that this expenditure was compensated by a reduction in physical activity. The validity of these estimates has been challenged, as described later in this chapter.

On the basis of theoretical calculations, recommended allowances for energy intake during pregnancy have been set at 200 to 300 kcal/day (FAO/WHO/UNU, 1985; NRC, 1989) above nonpregnant levels; however, few dietary studies of pregnant women corroborate increments of this magnitude. Hytten (1980) suggested that the increased needs of pregnancy could be met by reductions in physical activity.

RELATIONSHIP BETWEEN ENERGY INTAKE AND GESTATIONAL WEIGHT GAIN

Tables 7-2A and 7-2B list studies in which the relationship between energy intake and gestational weight gain was described. Longitudinal studies of well-nourished pregnant women indicated a slight, although not always statistically significant and not universal, increase in energy intake during pregnancy. One study showed that the energy consumption of Scottish women increased gradually through the second and third trimesters to the extent that energy consumption at parturition was approximately 150 kcal/day higher than intake before pregnancy (Durnin, 1987; Durnin et al., 1986). In a study of well-nourished Dutch women, energy intake was unchanged throughout the first two trimesters and increased in the third trimester by approximately 47 kcal/day (van Raaij et al., 1986, 1987). In an

139

TABLE 7-2A Studies Relating Energy Intake and Weight Gain During Pregnancy in Industrialized Countries

Country and Reference	Population	Mean Energy Intake, kcal/day ± SD, Gestation Period (GP), and Number of Subjects	Mean Weight Gain, kg ± SD, by Gestation Period	Mean Birth Weight, g ± SD, by Gender	Reported Correlations or Significance Level for Total Study Population
Scotland Thomson, 1959	Normal and abnormal pregnancies including preeclamptic toxemia and hypertension	<1,800[a] GP = 2nd & 3rd trimesters N = 38	0.35/wk[a] GP = 20 to 36 wk	3,090,[a] both sexes	Energy intake with weight gain, R = .30 Energy intake with birth weight, R = .05
		1,800–2,200[a] GP = 2nd & 3rd trimesters N = 94	0.43/wk[a] GP = 20 to 36 wk	3,190,[a] both sexes	
		2,200–2,600[a] GP = 2nd & 3rd trimesters N = 131	0.45/wk[a] GP = 20 to 36 wk	3,210,[a] both sexes	
		2,600–3,000[a] GP = 2nd & 3rd trimesters N = 93	0.49/wk[a] GP = 20 to 36 wk	3,210,[a] both sexes	
		>3,000[a] GP = 2nd & 3rd trimesters N = 56	0.56/wk[a] GP = 20 to 36 wk	3,330,[a] both sexes	
United States Beal, 1971	Private patients, mean weight and height of 54 kg and 164.5 cm, respectively	1,887[a] GP = entire N = 95	10.7[a] GP = entire	3,260,[a] males 3,230,[a] females	Energy intake with weight gain: R = .29, p < .01 (second trimester); R = .20, NS[b] (entire pregnancy) Energy intake with birth weight, NS

Table 7-2A continues

TABLE 7-2A—Continued

Country and Reference	Population	Mean Energy Intake, kcal/day ± SD, Gestation Period (GP), and Number of Subjects	Mean Weight Gain, kg ± SD, by Gestation Period	Mean Birth Weight, g ± SD, by Gender	Reported Correlations or Significance Level for Total Study Population
United States King et al., 1972	Teenagers, 14–18 years old	1,871 ± 474 GP = 3rd trimester N = 18	12.3 ± 4.1 GP = entire	3,030 ± 534, both sexes	Weight gain with birth weight: R = .20, males, NS; R = .37, females, p < 0.05
		1,682 ± 373 GP = 3rd trimester N = 34	13.6 ± 4.1 GP = entire	3,318 ± 559, both sexes	Energy intake with weight gain, NS Energy intake with birth weight, NS Weight gain with birth weight, p < .01
United States Ancri et al., 1977	12–17 years old	2,189 ± 615 GP = 3rd trimester N = 26	13.4 ± 3.4 GP = entire	3,281 ± 272, both sexes	Energy intake with weight gain, NS Energy intake with birth weight, NS
	18–19 years old	2,254 ± 637 GP = 3rd trimester N = 22	12.4 ± 3.8 GP = entire	2,986 ± 602, both sexes	Weight gain with birth weight, NS
	20–24 years old	1,922 ± 380 GP = 3rd trimester N = 24	11.2 ± 1.8 GP = entire	3,381 ± 525, both sexes	
	25–32 years old	2,007 ± 552 GP = 3rd trimester N = ?6	10.7 ± 2.0 GP = entire	3,473 ± 477, both sexes	

					Correlations
Canada Haworth et al., 1980	Private patients, nonsmokers	2,421 ± 701 GP = 3rd trimester N = 175	Measured, not reported	NR	Energy intake with weight gain, R = .16, p < .01 Weight gain with birth weight, R = .19, p < .001
	Private patients, smokers	2,587 ± 736 GP = 3rd trimester N = 208			
United States Picone et al., 1982a,b	Low weight gain nonsmokers	1,617 ± 459 GP = 2nd & 3rd trimesters N = 10	2.4 ± 3.2 GP = entire	3,060 ± 512 mean for both sexes, both groups	Energy intake with weight gain, R = .44, p < .02 Weight gain with birth weight, R = .57, p < .001
	Average weight gain nonsmokers	1,905 ± 322 GP = 2nd & 3rd trimesters N = 18	14.9 ± 3.2 GP = entire		Energy intake with birth weight, R = .34, p < .05
France Papoz et al., 1982	Never smoked	2,151[a] GP = 1st trimester N = 334	11.4 ± 3.6 GP = entire	3,260 ± 457, both sexes	Energy intake with weight gain, NS Weight gain with birth weight, R = .25, p < .001
	Exsmokers	2,189[a] GP = 1st trimester N = 97	12.4 ± 3.9 GP = entire	3,270 ± 404, both sexes	
	Persistent smokers	2,242[a] GP = 1st trimester N = 103	12.7 ± 4.0 GP = entire	3,190 ± 355, both sexes	
England Abraham et al., 1985	Harrow Asians	2,010 ± 532 GP = 2nd trimester N = 813	0.462/wk[a] GP = entire	NR	NR
	Europeans	2,013 ± 636 GP = 2nd trimester N = 54	0.458/wk[a] GP = entire	NR	

Table 7-2A continues

TABLE 7-2A—Continued

Country and Reference	Population	Mean Energy Intake, kcal/day ± SD, Gestation Period (GP), and Number of Subjects	Mean Weight Gain, kg ± SD, by Gestation Period	Mean Birth Weight, g ± SD, by Gender	Reported Correlations or Significance Level for Total Study Population
United States Endres et al., 1985	Adolescent WIC[d] participants	1,908 ± 749 GP = 2nd trimester N = 46	12.0[a] GP = entire	NR	NR
	Adolescents requesting WIC certification	1,927 ± 895 GP = 2nd trimester N = 19	10.2[a] GP = entire	NR	
	Adult WIC participants	1,904 ± 806 GP = 2nd trimester N = 204	11.0[a] GP = entire	NR	
United States Loris et al., 1985	Adolescents 13–20 years old	2,822 ± 1,035 GP = 2nd & 3rd trimesters N = 132	17.2 ± 7.1 GP = entire	3,425 ± 437, both sexes	Weight gain with birth weight, $R = .26$, $p < .001$
England Anderson and Lean, 1986	Healthy women	2,065 ± 441 GP = 3rd trimester N = 49	11.2[a] GP = entire	NR	Weight gain ≤ 8 kg; mean energy intake of 1,770 ± 452 kcal (SD) Weight gain > 8 kg; mean energy intake of 2,115 ± 425 kcal (SD)
Scotland Durnin, 1987; Durnin et al., 1986	Healthy women, mean weight and height, 57 ± 8 kg and 162 ± 6 cm, respectively	2,250[a] GP = 3rd trimester 2,120 ± 334 GP = 1st trimester N = 88	11.7 ± 3.2 GP = entire	3,370 ± 404, both sexes	NR

Reference	Subjects				
United States Endres et al., 1987	Adolescents, 15–18 years old	1,876[d] GP = 2nd trimester N = 526	9.5[a] GP = 32 wk	NR	NR
	Older women, >35 years old	1,512[a] GP = 2nd trimester N = 63	7.6[a] GP = 34 wk	NR	
Sweden Langhoff-Roos et al., 1987	Healthy women	2,201 ± 399 GP = 2nd trimester 2,266 ± 406 GP = 3rd trimester N = 56	Measured, not reported	NR	Energy intake with weight gain, NS Energy intake with birth weight, NS
The Netherlands van Raaij et al., 1986, 1987	Healthy women, mean weight and height, 62 ± 8 kg and 169 ± 7 cm, respectively	2,140 ± 461 GP = 1st trimester 2,119 ± 392 GP = 2nd trimester 2,187 ± 426 GP = 3rd trimester 2,140 ± 461 GP = entire N = 57	11.6[a] GP = entire	3,458 ± 527, both sexes	NR
Australia Truswell et al., 1988	Healthy women, mean weight and height, 57 ± 7 kg and 164 ± 6.4 cm, respectively	2,113 ± 483 GP = 1st trimester 2,127 ± 434 GP = 2nd trimester 2,127 ± 532 GP = 3rd trimester N = 49	12.4 ± 3.7 GP = entire	3,540 ± 473, both sexes	NR

[a] Standard deviation (SD) not applicable or not reported.
[b] NS = Not significant.
[c] NR = Not reported.
[d] WIC = Supplemental Food Program for Women, Infants, and Children.

TABLE 7-2B Studies Relating Energy Intake and Weight Gain During Pregnancy in Developing Countries

Country and Reference	Population	Mean Energy Intake, kcal/day ± SD, Gestation Period (GP), and Number of Subjects	Mean Weight Gain, kg ± SD, by, Gestation Period	Mean Birth Weight, g ± SD, by Gender	Reported Correlations or Significance Level for Total Study Population
The Gambia Paul et al., 1979	Keneba women in dry season	1,524[a] GP = 3rd trimester N = 19	2.95 ± 1.57 GP = 3rd trimester	3,000 ± 441, both sexes	Energy intake with birth weight: $R = .50$, $p < .05$ Maternal energy balance affected weight gain
	Keneba women in wet season	1,435[a] GP = 3rd trimester N = 6	0.37 ± 0.86 GP = 3rd trimester	2,920 ± 449, both sexes	
Ethiopia Tafari et al., 1980	Women engaged in hard work	1,540 ± 488 GP = 2nd & 3rd trimesters N = 64			NR[b]
	Early pregnancy weight <49 kg		6.9[a] GP = entire	3,096 ± 313, both sexes	
	Early pregnancy weight 49–58 kg		6.5[a] GP = entire	3,034 ± 342, both sexes	
	Early pregnancy weight >58 kg		4.7[a] GP = entire	3,129 ± 534, both sexes	

				NR
Women engaged in light work	1,641 ± 367 GP = 2nd & 3rd trimesters N = 66			
Early pregnancy weight <49 kg		10.1[a] GP = entire	3,300 ± 386, both sexes	
Early pregnancy weight 49–58 kg		9.2[a] GP = entire	3,198 ± 361, both sexes	
Early pregnancy weight >58 kg		8.5[a] GP = entire	3,345 ± 419, both sexes	
Jamaica de Benoist et al., 1985	Healthy, middle-income, primaparous women	1,864 ± 294 GP = 1st trimester N = 6	10.0 ± 2.2 GP = entire	3,200 ± 490, both sexes
		2,271 ± 527 GP = 2nd trimester N = 6	11.2 ± 2.9 GP = entire	3,200 ± 245, both sexes
		2,366 ± 235 GP = 3rd trimester N = 6	13.7 ± 2.9 GP = entire	3,500 ± 490, both sexes

Table 7-2B continues

TABLE 7-2B—Continued

Country and Reference	Population	Mean Energy Intake, kcal/day ± SD, Gestation Period (GP), and Number of Subjects	Mean Weight Gain, kg ± SD, by Gestation Period	Mean Birth Weight, g ± SD, by Gender	Reported Correlations or Significance Level for Total Study Population
Thailand Thongprasert and Valaysevi, 1986; Thongprasert et al., 1987	Healthy women from 12 rural villages	1,932 ± 358 GP = 1st trimester 2,279 ± 380 GP = 2nd trimester 2,201 ± 350 GP = 3rd trimester N = 44	8.9 ± 2.9 GP = entire	2,980 ± 358, both sexes	NR
	Women engaged in light work	1,641 ± 367 GP = 2nd & 3rd trimesters N = 66			

	Early pregnancy weight <49 kg		10.1[a] GP = entire	3,300 ± 386, both sexes	
	Early pregnancy weight 49–58 kg		9.2[a] GP = entire	3,198 ± 361, both sexes	
	Early pregnancy weight >58 kg		8.5[a] GP = entire	3,345 ± 419, both sexes	
					NR
Philippines Tuazon et al., 1986, 1987	Rural women, mean weight and height, 44 ± 6 kg and 151 ± 5 cm, respectively	1,760 ± 347 GP = 1st trimester 1,773 ± 412 GP = 2nd trimester 1,680 ± 382 GP = 3rd trimester 1,750 ± 352 GP = total N = 51	8.4 ± 2.4 GP = entire	2,885 ± 395, both sexes	
Mexico Hunt et al., 1987	Women attending one of two clinics, mean weight and height, 56 ± 10 kg and 155 ± 5 cm, respectively	1,831 ± 623 GP = 2nd trimester 1,750 ± 481 GP = 3rd trimester N = 44	0.4 ± 0.2 kg/wk GP = 19 to 35 wk	3,381 ± 456, both sexes	NR

[a] Standard deviation (SD) not applicable or not reported.
[b] NR = Not reported.

Australian study, energy intake did not increase during pregnancy (Truswell et al., 1988). Minor, but not consistent, changes in energy intake have been reported in other studies of well-nourished pregnant women (King et al., 1987). Failure to detect significant trends in energy intake may be due to the substantial variability in food intake, the cross-sectional design of many studies, and measurement sensitivity and error.

Results of energy intake studies in pregnant women subsisting on low energy intakes in developing countries are inconsistent. In one study from Thailand, energy intake progressively increased during pregnancy (Thongprasert et al., 1987). In studies conducted in the Philippines and Mexico, a slight, but insignificant, *decline* in energy intake was observed in the third trimester (Hunt et al., 1987; Tuazon et al., 1986, 1987). If energy intake does not increase in chronically undernourished women during pregnancy, fetal and maternal tissue accretion may be restricted to that which can be achieved by adjustments in nutrient utilization.

Statistically significant correlations between energy intake and gestational weight gain have been reported by some investigators (Beal, 1971; Haworth et al., 1980; Picone et al., 1982a,b; Thomson, 1959) but not by others (Ancri et al., 1977; King et al., 1972; Langhoff-Roos et al., 1987; Papoz et al., 1982). Thomson (1959) cited a correlation coefficient (R) of .30 between these two variables. Beal (1971) noted a significant negative correlation between preconceptional energy intake and weight gain, but positive relationships throughout pregnancy $(R = .05$ to $.29)$; statistical significance was demonstrated in the second trimester only. In a large sample, Haworth et al. (1980) detected a significant relationship between energy intake and weight gain $(R = .16)$. Picone et al. (1982a) reported a relatively high correlation for nonsmokers only $(R = .44)$, possibly the result of clustering of subjects at the extremes of the range of weight gains. During the first trimester, a positive correlation was observed between the increase in food intake and weight gain $(R = .17)$ (Papoz et al., 1982). Associations between energy intake and weight gain were evident in other studies, but no correlation analyses were reported (Anderson and Lean, 1986; de Benoist et al., 1985; Endres et al., 1987; Paul et al., 1979).

The relatively weak correlation may accurately reflect or may underestimate the actual relationship between energy intake and gestational weight gain. Assessment of the relationship between these two variables is problematic (Kramer, 1987). Precise and accurate measurement of energy intake is difficult, particularly over the 9-month gestational period. High variability in food intake by pregnant women, as is found in general in the United States, was reported in all studies.

The relationship between energy intake and weight gain is confounded by intervening variables such as physical activity and body size. Because weight gain or loss is determined by net energy balance, an evaluation of the impact of energy intake on weight gain requires information about or control of energy expenditure. An accurate measurement of energy expenditure by indirect calorimetry throughout pregnancy is technically difficult. Application of the doubly labeled water method to pregnant women should refine estimates of the energy available for weight gain. The energy cost of weight gain may be overestimated by excessive extracellular fluid expansion, which occurs at negligible energy cost to the pregnant woman. Toward the end of pregnancy, the rate of weight gain often decreases; thus, differences in the length of gestation between individuals may be confounding. Imprecise quantification of energy intake, gestational weight gain, and modifiers such as physical activity would decrease the probability of detecting a statistically significant relationship, even if one exists.

Alternatively, the actual association between energy intake and gestational weight gain may be weak. Variation in energy intake among pregnant women is determined largely by body size and the level of physical activity— not by gestational weight gain. The failure to achieve statistical significance in the majority of studies reviewed in Tables 7-2A and 7-2B may have been due to insufficient statistical power. The sample size required to detect a significant correlation of .1, .3, or .5 would be 784, 195, or 86, respectively, at a significance level of .05 and a power of .8.

Gestational weight gain is unquestionably a function of energy intake, although the strength of the relationship is confounded by intervening factors. Maternal weight gain, skinfold thickness, and birth weight have been reduced by iatrogenic dietary restriction during pregnancy (Campbell and MacGillivray, 1975). Acute maternal deprivation during the Dutch famine of 1944-1945 in the western part of The Netherlands provided a dramatic demonstration of the impact of energy intake on the course and outcome of pregnancy (Stein and Susser, 1975a,b). Pregnant women were subjected to 6 months of gradually increasing deprivation ($\sim$670 to 1,414 kcal/day), followed by rapid rehabilitation ($\sim$3,200 kcal/day). Birth weights were reduced substantially (-300 g) at the height of the famine and rebounded ($+400$ g above the famine nadir) after the famine. Detrimental effects on birth weight were confined to women who consumed fewer than 1,500 kcal/day during the third trimester. The limited data indicate that postpartum maternal weight declined 4.3% during the famine and rose 10.5% above famine levels during rehabilitation.

Some studies, particularly those conducted in nutritionally vulnerable populations, have shown that energy supplementation results in increased gestational weight gain and birth weight (Bhatnagar et al., 1983; Herrera et al., 1980; Iyenger, 1967; Kardjati et al., 1988; Tontisirin et al., 1986). The compilation of studies in Tables 7-2A and 7-2B indicates that energy intakes by adult pregnant women living in industrialized countries are generally greater than 1,900 kcal/day, and their gestational weight gain exceeds 10 kg (22 lb). The energy intakes by women in developing countries are generally less than 1,900 kcal/day, and associated weight gains are less than 10 kg.

STUDIES OF ENERGY SUPPLEMENTATION DURING PREGNANCY

Energy intake is one determinant of pregnancy outcome amenable to experimental intervention; studies that evaluated the effectiveness of energy supplementation on weight gain during pregnancy and on birth weight are summarized in Tables 7-3A and 7-3B. The subcommittee reviewed the findings and limitations of intervention studies conducted in both developing (Table 7-3A) and industrialized countries (Table 7-3B). The likelihood of demonstrating the effectiveness of energy supplementation during pregnancy is enhanced in nutritionally vulnerable populations. This explains the focus on developing countries in this review. Although not without exception, the studies in developing countries represented more poorly nourished women than did studies conducted in industrialized countries.

The subcommittee focused on the impact of energy supplementation on gestational weight gain and fetal growth. Information regarding other fetal or maternal outcomes was not consistently provided in reports of the supplementation studies.

Supplementation Studies of Pregnant Women in Developing Countries

In the following discussion, women are described as chronically undernourished, malnourished, or marginally nourished. Different investigators used different criteria to categorize the women based on customary dietary intake or anthropometric measurements.

Guatemala

Chronically undernourished women from four Guatemalan villages were offered either a protein-energy supplement (Atole) or a low-energy supplement (Fresco) (Delgado et al., 1982a,b; Lechtig et al., 1975a,b, 1978). Initially, the study was designed to test the effect of protein supplementation, but the investigators discarded the initial design on the premise that the effects of energy supplementation might be masked, because no advantage of the Atole over the Fresco supplement was evident. Therefore, post hoc analyses were performed in which women were categorized according to self-selected levels of energy intake (Table 7-3A). The mean monthly rate of gestational weight gain was 1.2 kg (2.6 lb); the adjusted correlation between supplemented calories and monthly weight gain was .213 ($N=$ 137) (Lechtig et al., 1978). The greater the level of energy supplementation, the lower the proportion of mothers with low gestational weight gains, defined as less than 0.5 kg (1.1 lb) per month. Birth weight was significantly related to energy intake over the course of gestation (29-g increment in birth weight per 10,000 kcal from the supplement). Comparison of the high energy intake group (>20,000 kcal) and the low energy intake group (<20,000 kcal) indicated that a net increment of 149 kcal/day was associated with an 111-g increase in birth weight and reductions in the incidence of low-birth-weight (LBW) infants and preterm births. The major limitations of this study included subject self-selection and exclusion of 38% of the sample because of missing birth weights.

Colombia

Poor women at risk of undernutrition were randomly assigned to supplementation or control groups for the third trimester of pregnancy (Mora et al., 1979). Energy supplementation (net increment of 155 kcal/day) had a significant effect ($p < .05$) on the birth weight of male infants only (+95 g). Weight gain of the women who were supplemented for 13 weeks or more and had male children was also higher (+140 g/week) than that of controls, suggesting that improved maternal nutrition influenced birth weight. The gender-specific effect of supplementation may have been due to the achievement of the greater fetal growth potential in males. Post hoc stratification of the sample by maternal weight-for-height ratio at 6 months of gestation revealed that supplementation had a significant impact on the birth weights of infants of both sexes (+181 g) among women with lower weight-for-height ratios (Herrera et al., 1980).

Taiwan

A group of rural Taiwanese women was given a protein-energy supplement (800 kcal/day) or a low-energy supplement (80 kcal/day) from 3 weeks after the birth of their first (male) child until the end of the lactation period for the second child of either sex (Adair and Pollitt, 1983; Adair et al., 1983, 1984; McDonald et al., 1981). Supplementation prior to and during the second pregnancy had no effect on anthropometric measurements (gestational weight gain, body weight, or skinfold thickness) of these women whose usual diet was only marginally adequate. Maternal weight gain averaged 7.6 kg (16.7 lb). Comparisons of outcomes of the second pregnancies (birth weight, incidence of LBW infants, and fetal deaths) revealed no statistical differences between the two groups. Within the supplemented group, however, male infants born after a nutrient-supplemented pregnancy had significantly higher birth weights than those of first-born males (+162 g).

These findings suggest that some infants benefited from maternal supplementation, even though maternal anthropometric measurements did

TABLE 7-3A Supplementation Studies During Pregnancy: Relationships Between Energy Intake, Maternal Weight Gain, and Pregnancy Outcomes—Studies of Pregnant Women from Developing Countries

Location and Reference	Population and Customary Daily Intake	Study Design and Intervention	Mean Energy Intake ± SD,[a] kcal/day	Mean Weight Gain ± SD	Mean Birth Weight ± SD, g	Associations Between Variables
Hyderabad, India Iyenger, 1967	Women of low socioeconomic status engaged in manual labor during pregnancy; 1,400 kcal, 40 g of protein	Unsupplemental matched controls, N = 26		0.35 ± 0.17 kg/mo	2,707 ± 122	NR[b]
		Supplement: 2,450 kcal + 95 or 60 g of protein given during hospitalization in the third trimester, N = 25	2,450[c]	1.25 ± 0.13 kg/mo	3,028 ± 415	NR
Guatemala Delgado et al., 1982a,b; Lechtig et al., 1975a,b	Rural women in four villages; 1,450 kcal, 40 g of protein	Nonrandom, supplemented over entire pregnancy				Energy intake with maternal weight: $R = .213$, $p < .05$
		Fresco: 59 kcal/180 ml ad libitum, N = 389	1,492[c]	NR	3,077 ± 334	Energy intake with birth weight: $R = .135$, $p < .01$
		Atole: 163 kcal ± 11 g of protein/180 ml ad libitum, N = 441	1,580[c]	NR	3,027 ± 461	
		Post hoc analysis:				
		Low supplementation (<20,000 kcal total) N = 235	1,458 ± 444	NR	2,994[c]	Increase (+29 g) in birth weight per 10,000 supplemental kcal
		High supplementation (>20,000 kcal total) N = 170	1,607 ± 380	NR	3,105[c]	

153

Location/Reference	Population	Design/Supplementation	Intake	Weight gain	Birth weight	Results
Bogata, Colombia Herrera et al., 1980; Mora et al., 1979	Poor urban women with malnourished preschool children; 1,600 kcal, 35 g of protein	Random assignment, unblinded. Unsupplemented. Net take home supplement: 155 kcal + 20 g of protein/day during third trimester	1,556 ± 641 1,766 ± 570	NR NR	2,953 ± 311 3,003 ± 355	Increase (+95 g) in birth weight of males
Taiwan Adair et al., 1983, 1984; McDonald et al., 1981	Married women with one prior male child living in 14 rural villages; 1,200 kcal, < 40 g of protein	Unsupplemented: 80 kcal. Supplemented: 800 kcal + 40 g of protein	Trimester:[c] 1, 1,217 2, 1,235 3, 1,167 Trimester:[c] 1, 1,606 2, 1,666 3, 1,678	7.75 ± 2.51 kg total 7.52 ± 2.77 kg total	M[d]: 3,160[c] F[e]: 2,981[c] M: 3,216[c] F: 3,012[c]	Increase (+162 g) from first to second pregnancy in birth weight of male infants born to supplemented mothers: $p < .05$. Weight gain with birth weight: $R = .38$
New Delhi, India Bhatnagar et al., 1983	Women from urban slum area; 1,200 kcal, 40 g of protein	Unsupplemented matched controls, N = 170. Supplement: 300 kcal + 16 g of protein from week 24 of gestation, N = 140	1,166 ± 142 1,500[c]	3.57 ± 0.85 kg total; M only 4.28 ± 0.95 kg total; M only	2,580 ± 330 2,750 ± 300	Significant effect of supplementation on weight gain ($p < .001$) and on birth weight ($p < .001$). Weight gain with birth weight: $R = .92$ to $.95$
Rajchaburi, Bangkok Tontisirin et al., 1986	Rural women; 1,437 kcal, 52 g of protein	Unsupplemented randomized controls, N = 15	NR	0.28 ± 0.01 kg/wk	2,853 ± 248	

Table 7-3A continues

TABLE 7-3A—Continued

Location and Reference	Population and Customary Daily Intake	Study Design and Intervention	Mean Energy Intake ± SD,[a] kcal/day	Mean Weight Gain ± SD	Mean Birth Weight ± SD, g	Associations Between Variables
		Supplement A: 350 kcal + 13 g of protein, N = 14	NR	0.45 ± 0.03 kg/wk	3,089 ± 308	Significant effect of supplementation on weight gain (p < .005) and on birth weight (p < .02)
		Supplement B: 350 kcal + 13 g of protein, N = 14	NR	0.46 ± 0.04 kg/wk	3,104 ± 259	
Keneba, The Gambia Prentice et al., 1987	Rural women engaged in seasonal subsistence farming; 1,467 kcal	Unsupplemented retrospective controls, N = 182	1,467[c]	NR	W[f]: 2,808 ± 400 D[g]: 2,944 ± 401	Significant effect of maternal weight, height, and third-trimester weight gain on birth weight
		Supplement: 673 kcal (1980–1982), 616 kcal (1982–1984) (net supplement of 400 kcal), N = 197	1,898[c]	6.8 kg[c] total	W: 3,033 ± 398 D: 2,946 ± 405	Supplementation had no effect on weight gain during wet or dry seasons Supplementation increased birth weight in wet but not in dry season; overall effect = +124 g, p < .005

155

				Subgroup by degree of compliance			
East Java, Indonesia Kardjati et al., 1988	Nutritionally vulnerable housewives and productive laborers; 1,500 kcal, 41 g of protein	Randomized	Supplement A: 52 kcal + 6.2 g of protein, N = 265	1: 1,616 ± 515 2: 1,645 ± 447 3: 1,543 ± 388	6.4 kg[c] total for all three subgroups	2,948 ± 392	Energy supplementation did not affect birth weight
			Supplement B: 465 kcal + 7.1 g of protein, N = 272	1: 1,717 ± 516 2: 1,590 ± 457 3: 1,582 ± 440	7.1 kg[c] total for all three subgroups	2,908 ± 397	
Santiago, Chile Mardones-Santander et al., 1988	Low-income urban women; 2,115 kcal, 41 g of protein	Randomized	Supplement A: 498 kcal + 27.9 g of protein	2,301[c]	11.5 ± 5.6 kg total	3,220 ± 363	Fortified supplement associated with higher weight gain ($p < .05$) and birth weight ($p < .05$)
			Supplement B: 470 kcal + 14.5 g of protein, fortified with vitamins and minerals	2,292[c]	12.4 ± 4.7 kg total	3,283 ± 360	

[a] SD = Standard deviation.
[b] NR = Not reported.
[c] Standard deviation not reported.
[d] M = Male.
[e] F = Female.
[f] W = Wet season.
[g] D = Dry season.

TABLE 7-3B Supplementation Studies During Pregnancy: Relationships Between Energy Intake, Maternal Weight Gain, and Pregnancy Outcomes—Studies of Pregnant Women from Industrialized Countries

Location and Reference	Population and Customary Daily Intake	Study Design and Intervention	Mean Energy Intake ± SD,[a] kcal/day	Mean Weight Gain ± SD	Mean Birth Weight ± SD, g	Associations Between Variables
San Francisco, USA Adams et al., 1978	Women enrolled in prepaid medical plan deemed at risk for delivering a low-birth-weight infant; 1,995 kcal, 80 g of protein	Randomized Unsupplemented controls, N = 43	1,844 ± 484	NR[b]	3,272 ± 500	No association between energy intake, weight gain, or prepregnancy weight and birth weight
		Supplement A: 470 kcal + 40 g of protein, N = 23	2,194 ± 594	NR	3,227 ± 500	
		Supplement B: 320 kcal + 6 g of protein, N = 36 (supplemented from 21 to 27 wk onward)	1,859 ± 462	NR	3,364 ± 545	
National WIC[c] Evaluation, USA Edozien et al., 1979	WIC participants from 14 states; 1,729 kcal, 66 g of protein	No controls Vouchers to buy food providing 900 to 1,000 kcal + 40 to 50 g of protein, N = 4,125	NR	11.1 kg[d]	3,225 ± 605	Compared with initial values, WIC supplementation did not result in different energy intakes or weight gain, but did increase birth weight ($p < .02$)

Study	Population	Treatment	Birth weight	Weight gain		Comments
New York City, USA Rush et al., 1980	Urban poor black women at risk for delivery of a low-birth-weight infant; 2,065 kcal, 79 g of protein	Randomized Unsupplemented controls, $N = 264$	2,065[d]	9.8[d]	2,970 ± 535	Weight gain with energy intake: $R = .10$, $p < .01$
		Supplement A: 470 kcal + 40 g of protein, $N = 248$	2,326[d]	10.6 kg[d]	2,938 ± 611	Supplement A: increased prematurity, neonatal deaths, and growth retardation up to wk 39
		Supplement B: 322 kcal + 6 g of protein, $N = 256$	2,272[d]	10.6 kg[d]	3,011 ± 508	Supplement B: increased gestational duration, decreased low birth weight, nonsignificant 41-g increase in birth weight

Table 7-3B continues

TABLE 7-3B—Continued

Location and Reference	Population and Customary Daily Intake	Study Design and Intervention	Mean Energy Intake ± SD,[a] kcal/day	Mean Weight Gain ± SD	Mean Birth Weight ± SD, g	Associations Between Variables
Montreal, Canada Rush, 1981	Public patients in prenatal supplementation program; usual intake not reported	Unsupplemented (retrospective matched controls), N = 1,212	NR	11.4 kg[d]	3,251[d]	Birth weight greater by 40 g in supplemented group (p < .05)
		Supplement: milk, eggs, and oranges, N = 1,213	NR	11.5 kg[d]	3,291[d]	
Birmingham, England Viegas et al., 1982	Asian mothers identified as nutritionally adequate (A) or at risk (B); usual intake not reported	Unsupplemented, A: N = 85	NR	506 g/wk[d]	3,077[d]	Supplemental energy + protein + vitamins associated with higher birth weight (p < .05)
		Supplemented, B: vitamins, N = 14	NR	312 g/wk[d]	3,020 ± 260	
		Supplemented, B: 425 kcal + vitamins, N = 17	NR	304 g/wk[d]	2,900 ± 660	
		Supplemented, B: 425 kcal + 40 g of protein + vitamins, N = 14	NR	480 g/wk[d]	3,350 ± 470	
Aberdeen, Scotland Campbell-Brown, 1983	Primigravid women at risk for delivering a low-birth-weight infant; 2,062 kcal, 70 g of protein	Unsupplemented, matched controls, N = 90	2,043 ± 393	0.35 ± 0.12 kg/wk	2,995 ± 395	As total amount of supplement supplied increased, the difference in birth weight between matched pairs increased (p < .03)
		Supplement: 300 kcal + 15 to 20 g of protein during the third trimester, N = 90	2,217 ± 463	0.36 ± 0.11 kg/wk	3,032 ± 372	

Study	Diet	Groups				Effect of WIC participation on birth weight
Massachusetts, USA Kennedy and Kotelchuck, 1984	Non-WIC and WIC participants; usual intake not reported	Nonparticipants, N = 418 Participants, N = 418	NR NR	NR NR	3,148[d] 3,255[d]	Effect of WIC participation on birth weight (p = .01), gestational duration (p = .001), and incidence of low birth weight (p = .059)
Oklahoma, USA Metcoff et al., 1985	Non-WIC and WIC participants; 2,000 28 kcal/kg, 1.1 g of protein/kg	Nonparticipants, N = 172 Participants, N = 238	NR NR	14.7 kg[d] 16.1 kg[d]	NR NR	Supplementation effect on adjusted birth weight (+168 g) found in heavy smokers only (p < .017)
Second National WIC Evaluation, USA Rush et al., 1988	Non-WIC and WIC participants; 2,000 kcal, 80 g of protein	Nonparticipants, N = 497 Participants, N = 2,708	1,905[d] 2,016[d]	NR NR	3,285[d] 3,292[b]	WIC associated with improvement of weight gain in early pregnancy, but with lower late-pregnancy skinfold thickness; no effect on birth weight

[a] SD = Standard deviation.
[b] NR = Not reported.
[c] WIC = Supplemental Food Program for Women, Infants, and Children.
[d] Standard deviation not reported.

not differ between the supplemented and unsupplemented women. The weight gain of approximately one-third of all these women during lactation suggested, however, that their usual energy intake was adequate. Weight gain during pregnancy and maternal weight for height may have been almost optimal for these women. The potential to increase birth weights in this population was limited, because pregnancy outcomes were already favorable: the mean birth weight was >3 kg and the proportion of LBW infants was <6%. A positive energy balance was maintained throughout gestation and lactation in this group of women who reported low usual energy intakes (1,200 kcal). Estimates of energy intake were seriously flawed, however. No information was collected on between-meal food consumption or preintervention dietary intake. Thus, it was impossible to determine the extent to which the feeding program supplemented home diets. The original design to study supplementation of marginally nourished women was not achieved for two reasons: indiscriminate subject selection and failure to quantify the intervention variable.

The Gambia

Rural Gambian women received an energy-dense dietary supplement (net increment of ~400 kcal/day) throughout pregnancy (Prentice et al., 1987). Since all pregnant women in the community were included in the experimental group, it was necessary to use retrospective controls. Supplementation had no impact on weight gain or fat changes (as measured by triceps skinfold thickness) in either the wet season, when food shortages and agricultural work caused negative energy balances, or the dry season. Stratification of the mothers by height, weight, or weight for height did not indicate an advantage of supplementation for the more undernourished women. Supplementation was highly effective in augmenting birth weight (+225 g) in the wet season, but was ineffective in the dry season. The proportion of LBW infants decreased significantly from 23.7 to 7.5% in the wet season. There appeared to be a threshold above which birth weight was protected from the acute effects of malnutrition; birth weight was compromised when the women were in negative energy balance. The mechanism by which birth weight increased during the wet season but maternal weight gain did not change is unclear; the authors suggest that the supplement shortened the otherwise long overnight period when women took no food and thereby increased glucose availability to the fetus.

Theories of adaptation have evolved to explain how these active pregnant women existed on energy intakes that barely exceeded estimated basal requirements. Subsequent studies on the energy expenditure of pregnant Gambian women, however, have cast doubt on the energy intake records of the earlier investigations (Lawrence et al., 1986). In the later studies, mean daily energy expenditures during pregnancy exceeded previous estimates of energy intake by approximately 950 kcal. It is believed that this large discrepancy between energy intake and expenditure resulted from an underestimation of energy intake. Although understanding of the energy balance of these Gambian women is incomplete, the major impact of supplementation on birth weight and the incidence of LBW infants during the wet season was undeniable.

Chile

The effects of supplemental powdered milk (498 kcal/day) on maternal nutritional status and birth weight were compared with those of a milk-based product fortified with minerals and vitamins (470 kcal/day) in a group of underweight pregnant women (Mardones-Santander et al., 1988). The supplements were distributed from approximately 14 weeks of gestation onward. For full-term births without complications, the fortified product was associated with statistically higher maternal weight gain (+0.9 kg, or 2.0 lb) and birth weight (+63 g). The relatively high increment in birth weight relative to maternal weight gain (74-g birth weight per kilogram of maternal weight gain) may have resulted from the increased supply of micronutrients. Greater rates of weight gain in those with similar energy intakes may have been caused by greater maternal fluid retention and plasma expansion. The lack of randomly assigned unsupplemented controls precluded evaluation of the overall effect of supplementation on weight gain and birth weight. Supplements were distributed monthly; sharing of part of the supplement with other family members was acknowledged, but the amount was not quantitated.

Supplementation Studies of Pregnant Women in Industrialized Countries

Canada

A retrospective matched-pair analysis was performed on pregnant women who had received nutritional counseling and, if it was deemed necessary, dietary supplementation at the Montreal Diet Dispensary (Rush, 1981). A small and nonsignificant increase in weight gain (+0.3 kg, or 0.7 lb) was observed. A significant increase in birth weight (53 g more than that of controls) was limited to infants born to women who weighed less than 63 kg (139 lb) at the time of conception. The proportion of LBW infants was not statistically different.

Scotland

A group of primagravid women ($N = 90$) was selected for energy supplementation on the basis of poor nutritional status associated with a high risk of delivering an LBW infant (Campbell-Brown, 1983). At 20 weeks of gestation, women classified into the lowest quartile for weight, height, or rate of weight gain qualified for supplementation (300 kcal/day during the third trimester). Maternal weight gain and birth weight were greater in the supplemented group than in the matched control group, but the differences were not statistically significant.

United States

Reports of intervention trials and evaluations of the Special Supplemental Food Program for Women, Infants, and Children (WIC) often omit consideration of program effects on gestational weight gain; evaluation of the program effects on birth weight are conflicting. A fundamental problem germane to these studies is the selection of unsupplemented controls. The use of women enrolled in WIC postnatally as control subjects tends to lead to overestimates of the impact of food supplementation, since one criterion for postnatal WIC enrollment is delivery of an LBW infant. Alternatively, control subjects recruited from the community tend to be at lower risk of an adverse perinatal outcome compared with WIC recipients.

In a nationwide evaluation of WIC, food supplementation for longer than 3 months was associated with an increase in weight gain and in mean birth weight (+68 g for 3 to 6 months and +136 g for more than 6 months of program participation) (Edozien et al., 1979). The duration of gestation was 5 to 6 days longer for women who were enrolled for more than 6 months. A major limitation of this evaluation was the small number (41) of non-WIC participants used as controls.

In a prospective, randomized, controlled evaluation of WIC conducted in Oklahoma (Metcoff et al., 1985), women eligible for WIC were randomly assigned to WIC or to an unsupplemented control group. The WIC group had neither greater mean weight gains nor infants with higher birth weights compared with controls. Food supplementation was reported to be beneficial among smokers (+168 g increase in infant birth weight) but not among nonsmokers.

A longitudinal study was designed to overcome some limitations of previous investigations of the effectiveness of WIC supplementation (Rush et al., 1988). In this study, WIC participation was associated with increased energy intake, normalization of weight gain that had been low in early pregnancy, and decreased triceps skinfold thickness late in pregnancy. There was no apparent relationship between WIC supplementation and birth weight. The failure to demonstrate any positive effects of WIC supplementation on birth weight may have resulted from the small size of the control sample or from insufficient adjustment for differences in social factors between WIC participants and controls. Lower frequencies of early delivery (<33 weeks of gestation) and of preterm delivery (<37 weeks) among the WIC participants did not reach statistical significance. In a New York City trial, women at risk of preterm delivery were given one of three specially formulated supplements: high protein-energy, balanced protein-energy, or vitamin-minerals (Rush et al., 1980). Weight gain in this study was significantly related to energy and protein intakes. The balanced protein-energy supplement was associated with increases in the duration of gestation and higher mean birth weights (+41 g), although the differences were not statistically significant. The proportion of LBW infants was decreased in this group. The high-protein supplement was associated with significantly depressed birth weights among preterm infants; associations with an increased number of early preterm deliveries and neonatal deaths were both of borderline statistical significance. Women who entered the treatment group early and had a history of previous LBW deliveries were especially adversely affected by the high-protein supplement. Total weight gain and the average rate of weight gain (unadjusted) tended to be markedly depressed among the women who delivered preterm infants.

Interpretive Summary

Despite their dissimilar experimental designs, important inferences can be drawn from published supplementation trials. The basic premise of prenatal energy supplementation programs is that birth weight can be increased by greater energy intake and that this effect is associated with increased maternal weight gain. Few experimental designs discerned the specific, independent effect of supplementation, since most supplements used in the experiments provided not only energy but essential nutrients as well. Also, the relationship between energy intake and gestational weight gain is confounded by several other intervening factors, such as physical activity and body size. Few supplementation trials confirmed the direct link between energy intake, weight gain, and birth weight. It remains unclear whether the effects of energy intake on birth weight are a result of changes in gestational weight gain. Energy supplementation studies of undernourished women demonstrating a statistically significant impact on birth weight showed that gestational weight gain was increased, except in Gambian and Taiwanese women. In these studies, birth weight was increased with no apparent change in maternal weight gain. In the energy supplementation trials of more adequately nourished women, only minor changes in weight gain were observed. Gestational weight gain before intervention was substantially higher in women in developed countries (~12 kg) compared with that in women in developing countries (~7 kg).

The impact of energy supplementation on birth weight appeared to be influenced by the nutritional vulnerability of the pregnant women and the extent to which the supplement diminished the deficit between usual energy intakes and requirements. In the series of reports of undernourished women in developing countries, customary intakes averaged approximately 1,500 kcal/day, net supplementation in field trials ranged from 118 to 511 kcal/day, and mean increments in birth weight in the supplemented groups ranged between 50 and 321 g (−40 g in one trial). In the reports of more adequately nourished women in developed countries, usual intakes were approximately 2,000 kcal/day; supplements added between 15 and 261 kcal/day and differences in birth weights in the supplemented groups ranged between −177 and +273 g. The potential for improvement in birth weight was greater in the undernourished populations, in which birth weight before intervention averaged approximately 2,900 g, in comparison with approximately 3,100 g in better-nourished populations, and the incremental increase in energy intake was higher.

The proportion of LBW infants was effectively reduced by prenatal energy supplementation, especially in chronically malnourished populations (Table 7-3A). Modest reductions were demonstrated in better-nourished populations. Except for the studies of Delgado et al. (1982a) and Kennedy and Kotelchuck (1984), energy supplementation was shown to have no effect on the duration of gestation. The supplementation of more adequately nourished women at risk of delivering LBW infants produced meager or even negative results if high-protein supplements were used. The lower the nutritional status of the pregnant women, the greater the probability of detecting a statistically significant effect of energy supplementation.

In several studies, stratification of the study sample by maternal or environmental factors revealed that energy supplementation had significant effects on weight gain and birth weight. Discriminating factors included weight-for-height ratio in Bogota, Colombia (Herrera et al., 1980), socioeconomic status and height in Guatemala (Lechtig et al., 1975a,b), triceps skinfold thickness in Birmingham, United Kingdom (Viegas et al., 1982), season in The Gambia (Prentice et al., 1987), and prepregnancy weight in New York City and Montreal (Rush, 1981; Rush et al., 1980).

Fundamental problems with research design may have prevented the detection of significant effects of energy supplementation in some studies. Effectiveness of supplementation may have been underestimated by imperfect matching of control subjects or inadequate sample size. Randomization to include control groups was sometimes ruled out for ethical reasons related to the population's nutritional need. The amount of supplement consumed may have been insufficient, because it was shared with other family members, because of noncompliance, or because subjects replaced their customary diet with the supplement. Subjects may not have been undernourished, and intrauterine growth retardation in the population may have resulted from factors other than undernutrition.

FACTORS INFLUENCING ENERGY BALANCE DURING PREGNANCY

Weight gain during pregnancy is a direct consequence of energy balance, that is, the difference between energy intake and energy expenditure. The basic components of energy expenditure—basal metabolism, thermogenesis, and physical activity—are discussed below in relation to pregnancy.

Basal Metabolism

Longitudinal measurements of basal metabolic rate (BMR) or resting metabolic rate (RMR) have been made to ascertain the degree to which metabolism is increased during pregnancy (Table 7-4). Basal metabolism is measured in the morning after awakening, whereas resting metabolism may be measured at any time during the day after resting for at least 30 minutes. Resting metabolism tends to be about 10% higher than basal metabolism. Both are related to the amount of lean body mass. Since lean and fat tissues are increased in obese women, their basal requirements are higher than those of women of normal weight.

Although all reports indicate a net increase in basal or resting metabolism, the magnitude of change differed considerably between populations (Banerjee et al., 1971; Blackburn and Calloway, 1976a; Durnin et al., 1986; Forsum et al., 1985; Illingworth et al., 1987; Lawrence et al., 1986; Nagy and King, 1983; Thongprasert and Valyasevi, 1986; Tuazon et al., 1986; van Raaij et al., 1986). The reported increase in RMR by the third trimester ranged from 5% in unsupplemented Gambian women to 39% in well-nourished women in the United States. The increase was generally greater in pregnant women from developed countries (27%) than it was in those from developing countries (15%). Compared with the nonpregnant state, the total increment in resting metabolism for the entire pregnancy ranged from a reduction of 10,700 kcal in unsupplemented Gambian women to an increase of 46,500 kcal in well-nourished Swedish women. The increase in total resting metabolism in women from developing countries was lower than the theoretical value (36,000 kcal), in part as a consequence of their smaller size, but possibly also the result of metabolic adaptations.

Thermogenesis

The thermic effect of feeding refers to the increase in energy expenditure above basal metabolism following the ingestion of food. It is due mainly to the energy costs of digestion, absorption, transport, and storage and averages approximately 10% of the energy intake. A reduction in the thermic effect of feeding during pregnancy could minimally conserve energy.

TABLE 7-4 Resting Metabolic Rate (RMR) of Pregnant Women[a]

Country or Area (No. of Subjects)	Nonpregnancy RMR, kcal/min	Pregnancy RMR, by Trimester, kcal/min			Total Increment in Resting Metabolism, kcal	Reference
		1st (10-20 wk)	2nd (20-30 wk)	3rd (30-40 wk)		
Theoretical[b]	1.07	1.14	1.17	1.23	36,000	Hytten, 1980
Industrialized countries						
United States (6-16)	0.79	NR[c]	0.96	1.10	NR	Blackburn and Calloway, 1976a[d]
United States (5)	0.86	NR	1.01	1.15	NR	Nagy and King, 1983
Scotland (88)	0.93	0.94	1.03	1.21	30,100	Durnin et al., 1986[e]
Sweden (19)	0.93	0.97	1.13	1.22	46,500	Forsum et al., 1985
The Netherlands (55)	1.00	1.07	1.07	1.19	34,700	van Raaij et al., 1986[e]
United Kingdom (7)	1.00	1.01	1.04	1.08	NR	Illingworth et al., 1987
Developing countries						
Asia (42)	0.84	NR	NR	1.07	NR	Banerjee et al., 1971
The Gambia						
Unsupplemented (21)	0.98	0.90	0.92	1.03	-10,700	Lawrence et al., 1986[e]
Supplemented (29)	0.95	0.92	0.94	1.02	+ 1,000	Lawrence et al., 1986[e]
Thailand (44)	0.89	0.90	1.01	1.09	24,034	Thongprasert and Valyasevi, 1986[d]
Philippines (40)	0.86	0.83	0.89	0.98	21,200	Tuazon et al., 1986[d]

[a] Based on King et al. (1987), with permission from S. Karger AG.
[b] NA = Not applicable.
[c] NR = Not reported.
[d] Values represent BMR (basal metabolic rate) data, not RMR data. Prepregnancy data are postpartum measurements of lactating and nonlactating women.
[e] Values represent BMR data, not RMR data.

The thermic effect of feeding was measured in seven primigravid women at 12 to 15, 25 to 28, and 34 to 36 weeks of gestation and after the cessation of lactation (Illingworth et al., 1987). The metabolic response to a 533 ± 41-kcal (standard deviation) liquid test meal was significantly reduced by 28% (5 kcal) in the second trimester compared with postpartum values. The response was reduced by 15% in the third trimester, but the reduction failed to reach statistical significance.

In a contrasting report, the thermic response to a 750-kcal meal was not different among six women in early pregnancy (10 to 20 weeks of gestation), four women in late pregnancy (30 to 40 weeks of gestation), and six nonpregnant subjects studied cross-sectionally (Nagy and King, 1984).

Physical Activity

Assuming that increased energy costs of pregnancy were compensated by a reduction in physical activity, Hytten (1980), in his theoretical estimates of energy requirements, did not include an allowance for the energy cost associated with movement of a heavier body mass. Studies of activity patterns of North American pregnant women do not indicate reduced activity (Blackburn and Calloway, 1974, 1976b). Women from industrialized societies tend to have sedentary life-styles but they do not become even less active during pregnancy; reductions in recreational activities during pregnancy are slight. Subtle changes in physical activity, i.e., less walking and more sitting, by pregnant Scottish and Dutch women were noted in two reports (Durnin et al., 1986; van Raaij et al., 1986).

Women in developing countries are generally more active and may have more latitude in adjusting their level of physical activity during pregnancy. For example, pregnant women in The Gambia conserved energy by reducing the amount of heavy farm work and housework they performed (Roberts et al., 1982). In New Guinea, they decreased the intensity and duration of arduous tasks (Durnin, 1980). Thai and Philippine women increased their sitting time and decreased the heavy agricultural and household tasks they performed during gestation (Thongprasert and Valyasevi, 1986; Tuazon et al., 1986). Despite these adjustments, food scarcity combined with hard work during the rainy season in The Gambia was detrimental to fetal growth (Prentice et al., 1987). The rates of weight gain in Ethiopian pregnant women who engaged in hard work were lower, and the birth weights of their children were compromised, compared with women with lighter work demands (Tafari et al., 1980). Lower energy intake and lower weights during early pregnancy in the Ethiopian women may have been contributory factors.

The energy cost of physical activities has been measured at progressive stages of pregnancy (Durnin et al., 1986; Emerson et al., 1972; King et al.,

1987; Seitchik, 1967; Torún et al., 1982). The energy cost of non-weight-bearing activities, such as cycling, was not increased during pregnancy. In absolute terms, the energy expended in sedentary activities such as sitting and standing was 15 to 30% higher in pregnant women, but was not different if standardized by body weight. The energy expenditure of weight-bearing activities such as walking was increased in proportion to gestational weight gain; however, the energy expenditure of treadmill walking expressed per unit of body mass did not differ between pregnant and nonpregnant women. Because of their higher weight for height, obese women expend more energy during physical activity than do lighter women.

In contrast to these findings, results of the Dutch, Thai, and Gambian studies suggested greater energy efficiency for weight-bearing activities during pregnancy. When expressed per kilogram of body weight, the energy cost of walking on a treadmill at a fixed speed was reduced by approximately 5% in late pregnancy compared with prepregnancy or early pregnancy values (Thongprasert and Valyasevi, 1986; van Raaij et al., 1986). No increase in the energy cost of 40 activities was found in pregnant Gambian women, despite substantial weight gain (Lawrence et al., 1985, 1986). Rates of energy expenditure, normalized by body weight, were reported to be less than those of nonpregnant Gambian women, suggesting higher levels of work efficiency. However, walking (nonstandardized and at a set pace on a treadmill) displayed the expected increase in energy expenditure in Gambian women. Various investigators have reported that pregnant women reduce the pace and intensity of certain activities (Banerjee et al., 1971; Blackburn and Calloway, 1974; van Raaij et al., 1986). Pregnant women may expend less energy per unit of time performing a task, but they take longer to complete the task.

Although activity patterns and work intensity can be adjusted to conserve energy in pregnant woman, the energy expenditure of weight-bearing activities increases in most populations in proportion to weight gain. The impact of physical activity on the energy requirements of pregnancy depends on the proportion of time spent in such activities.

Total Daily Energy Expenditure

The total energy requirements of pregnancy have been estimated to be 2,115, 2,275, and 2,356 kcal/day for the three successive trimesters. The mean ratio of total expenditure to basal energy expenditure was 1.5 (Blackburn and Calloway, 1976b). The doubly labeled water technique has been applied to three pregnant women in Britain to estimate their total daily energy expenditures (Prentice et al., 1985). Total energy expenditures of 1,912, 2,490, and 3,009 kcal/day were equivalent to 1.40, 1.39, and 1.77

times the basal expenditure, respectively, emphasizing the considerable individual variation in physical activity. The total energy expenditure of rural Gambian women has been estimated from time-motion studies (Lawrence and Whitehead, 1988). Total daily energy expenditure declined from 2,400 kcal/day in early pregnancy to 2,200 kcal/day at term. When adjusted for stage of pregnancy or lactation, total daily energy expenditure averaged 2,300 kcal/day, or 1.68 times the basal expenditure in the dry season, and 2,700 kcal/day, or 1.97 times the basal expenditure in the wet season.

Energy Balance During Pregnancy

The mean total energy cost of pregnancy computed from data derived from five diverse populations (Table 7-5) was approximately 55,000 kcal for all groups except the Gambian women (Durnin, 1987). Small differences between the Scottish, Dutch, Thai, and Philippine women may be due primarily to variable amounts of fat deposition, which ranged between 1.3 and 2.3 kg (2.9 to 5.1 lb). Although the ranges of weight gains (8.5 to 11.7 kg, or 18.7 to 25.7 lb) and fat gains (1.3 to 2.3 kg) were wide, variability diminished when these rates of fat gain were expressed as a percentage of initial weight (2.9 to 4.0% of initial weight). Total weight gain was from 17 to 20% of initial weight. The Gambian women had exceptionally low weight gain (7.3 kg, or 16 lb), fat storage (0.6 kg, or 1.3 lb), and cumulative increase in basal energy expenditure (1,900 kcal). Chronically undernourished Gambian women apparently adapted to their pregnancy by decreased basal metabolism and activity and mobilization of adipose tissue; energy supplementation partially reversed these changes by increasing the BMR and fat deposition. In all countries, the estimation of the energy cost of pregnancy was subject to error, specifically in the estimation of maternal body fat and nonpregnant baseline values of BMR, but their estimates were all substantially lower than the theoretical estimates of Hytten (1980).

Increases in energy intake recorded for these populations did not approach the estimated energy costs of pregnancy, except for the Thai women. Apparent energy deficits may be explained by an underestimation of energy intake or by undetected compensatory reductions in physical activity. With the exception of the Gambian study, the investigators were confident of their food intake records. There was some question in the Thai study as to whether the energy intakes recorded at 10 weeks of gestation underestimated prepregnancy intakes and resulted in inflated estimates of increased intake during pregnancy. Underreporting of food intake in the Gambian study was strongly suspected. The investigators fully recognized the limitations of the techniques used to derive energy balance values. The methods used to measure energy intake and energy expenditure during pregnancy were not sufficiently accurate to discriminate to levels of 150

TABLE 7-5   Energy Requirements of Pregnancy as Estimated by the
Five-Country Study[a]

Factor	Energy Cost and Additional Intake During Pregnancy, kcal, by Country				
	Scotland	Holland	The Gambia	Thailand	Philippines
Energy cost					
Fetus	8,110	8,230	7,140	7,140	6,900
Placenta	730	740	560	600	600
Maternal tissues	2,890	2,950	2,480	2,480	2,410
Maternal fat	25,230	14,300	6,600	15,400	14,300
Basal metabolism	30,100	34,500	1,900	24,000	19,000
Total energy cost	67,060	60,720	18,680	49,620	43,210
Additional energy intake	21,000	5,200	NR[b]	56,900	0
Discrepancy in energy balance	−46,060	−55,520	NR	− 7,280	−43,210

[a] Adapted from Durnin (1986).
[b] NR = Not reported.

to 200 kcal/day—the expected net increment. Although the absolute cost of pregnancy is uncertain for such diverse populations, strong scientific evidence suggests that the energy cost of pregnancy is less than previous theoretical estimations.

SUMMARY

Effective public health intervention aimed at improving gestational weight gain, and thus birth weight, requires an understanding of energy requirements during pregnancy. The total energy cost of pregnancy is now believed to be approximately 55,000 kcal.

Prenatal energy supplementation may increase birth weight through greater rates of gestational weight gain. The impact of energy supplementation appears to be influenced by the nutritional vulnerability of pregnant women and the extent to which the supplement diminishes the deficit between usual energy intakes and requirements.

Gestational weight gain is a function of energy intake, although this relationship can be modified by the extent to which basal metabolism changes, by increased work efficiency, by compensatory reductions in physical activity, and by the composition of accumulated maternal and fetal tissue. Within the limitations of these physiologic and metabolic adaptations, gestational weight gain may be affected by changes in energy intake.

CLINICAL APPLICATIONS

• Extra dietary energy is ordinarily required to meet the increased growth needs during pregnancy.

• Women who remain physically active at weight-bearing activities during pregnancy are likely to have energy requirements higher than those of sedentary women.

• Because of their larger body mass, obese women require energy intakes higher than those of normal-weight women.

• Gestational weight gain is a function of energy intake, although the strength of the relationship is confounded by intervening factors.

• Prenatal energy supplementation may increase birth weight through greater rates of gestational weight gain; however, the effectiveness is conditional upon the nutritional vulnerability of the pregnant woman. Energy supplementation is most likely to improve the gestational weight gain of women whose usual diet is low in calories (e.g., below about 1,900 kcal/day).

REFERENCES

Abraham, R., M. Campbell-Brown, A.P. Haines, W.R.S. North, V. Hainsworth, and I.R. McFadyen. 1985. Diet during pregnancy in an Asian community in Britain—energy, protein, zinc, copper, fibre and calcium. Hum. Nutr.: Appl. Nutr. 39A:23-35.

Adair, L.S., and E. Pollitt. 1983. Seasonal variation in pre- and postpartum maternal body measurements and infant birth weights. Am. J. Phys. Anthropol. 62:325-331.

Adair, L.S., E. Pollitt, and W.H. Mueller. 1983. Maternal anthropometric changes during pregnancy and lactation in a rural Taiwanese population. Hum. Biol. 55:771-787.

Adair, L.S., E. Pollitt, and W.H. Mueller. 1984. The Bacon Chow study: effect of nutritional supplementation on maternal weight and skinfold thicknesses during pregnancy and lactation. Br. J. Nutr. 51:357-369.

Adams, S.O., G.D. Barr, and R.L. Huenemann. 1978. Effect of nutritional supplementation in pregnancy. I. Outcome of pregnancy. J. Am. Diet. Assoc. 72:144-147.

Ancri, G., E.H. Morse, and R.P. Clarke. 1977. Comparison of the nutritional status of pregnant adolescents with adult pregnant women. III. Maternal protein and calorie intake and weight gain in relation to size of infant at birth. Am. J. Clin. Nutr. 30:568-572.

Anderson, A.S., and M.E.J. Lean. 1986. Dietary intake in pregnancy. A comparison between 49 Cambridgeshire women and current recommended intake. Hum. Nutr.: Appl. Nutr. 40A:40-48.

Banerjee, B., K.S. Khew, and N. Saha. 1971. A comparative study of energy expenditure in some common daily activities of non-pregnant Chinese, Malay and Indian women. J. Obstet. Gynaecol. Br. Commonw. 78:113-116.

Beal, V.A. 1971. Nutritional studies during pregnancy. II. Dietary intake, maternal weight gain, and infant size. J. Am. Diet. Assoc. 58:321-326.

Bhatnagar, S., N.S. Dharamshaktu, K.R. Sundaram, and V. Seth. 1983. Effect of food supplementation in the last trimester of pregnancy and early post-natal period on maternal weight and infant growth. Indian J. Med. Res. 77:366-372.

Blackburn, M.W., and D.H. Calloway. 1974. Energy expenditure of pregnant adolescents. J. Am. Diet. Assoc. 65:24-30.

Blackburn, M.W., and D.H. Calloway. 1976a. Basal metabolic rate and work energy expenditure of mature, pregnant women. J. Am. Diet. Assoc. 69:24-28.

Blackburn, M.W., and D.H. Calloway. 1976b. Energy expenditure and consumption of mature, pregnant and lactating women. J. Am. Diet. Assoc. 69:29-37.

Campbell, D.M., and I. MacGillivray. 1975. The effect of a low calorie diet or a thiazide diuretic on the incidence of pre-eclampsia and on birth-weight. Br. J. Obstet. Gynaecol. 82:572-577.

Campbell-Brown, D.M. 1983. Protein energy supplements in primigravid women at risk of low birthweight. Pp. 85-100 in D.M. Campbell and M.D.G. Gillmer, eds. Nutrition in Pregnancy: Proceedings of the Tenth Study Group in the Royal College of Obstetricians and Gynaecologists, September, 1982. The Royal College of Obstetricians and Gynaecologists, London.

de Benoist, B., A.A. Jackson, J. St E. Hall, and C. Persaud. 1985. Whole-body protein turnover in Jamaican women during normal pregnancy. Hum. Nutr.: Clin. Nutr. 39C:167-179.

Delgado, H., R. Martorell, E. Brineman, and R.E. Klein. 1982a. Nutrition and length of gestation. Nutr. Res. 2:117-126.

Delgado, H.L., V.E. Valverde, R. Martorell, and R.E. Klein. 1982b. Relationship of maternal and infant nutrition to infant growth. Early Hum. Dev. 6:273-286.

Durnin, J.V.G.A. 1980. Food consumption and energy balance during pregnancy and lactation in New Guinea. Pp. 86-95 in H. Aebi and R. Whitehead, eds. Maternal Nutrition during Pregnancy and Lactation. Hans Huber, Bern.

Durnin, J.V.G.A. 1986. Energy requirements of pregnancy. An integrated study in 5 countries: background and methodology. Pp. 33-38 in Nestlé Foundation Annual Report 1986. Nestlé Foundation, Lausanne, Switzerland.

Durnin, J.V.G.A. 1987. Energy requirements of pregnancy: an integration of the longitudinal data from the five-country study. Lancet 2:1131-1133.

Durnin, J.V.G.A., F.M. McKillop, S. Grant, and G. Fitzgerald. 1986. Energy requirements of pregnancy. A study on 88 Glasgow women. Pp. 39-52 in Nestlé Foundation Annual Report 1986. Nestlé Foundation, Lausanne, Switzerland.

Edozien, J.C., B.R. Switzer, and R.B. Bryan. 1979. Medical evaluation of the Special Supplemental Food Program for Women, Infants, and Children. Am. J. Clin. Nutr. 32:677-692.

Emerson, K., Jr., B.N. Saxena, and E.L. Poindexter. 1972. Caloric cost of normal pregnancy. Obstet. Gynecol. 40:786-794.

Endres, J.M., K. Poell-Odenwald, M. Sawicki, and P. Welch. 1985. Dietary assessment of pregnant adolescents participating in a supplemental-food program. J. Reprod. Med. 30:10-17.

Endres, J., S. Dunning, S. Poon, P. Welch, and H. Duncan. 1987. Older pregnant women and adolescents: nutrition data after enrollment in WIC. J. Am. Diet. Assoc. 87:1011-1019.

FAO/WHO/UNU (Food and Agriculture Organization/World Health Organization/United Nations University). 1985. Energy and Protein Requirements. Report of a Joint FAO/WHO/UNU Expert Consultation. Technical Report Series No. 724. World Health Organization, Geneva. 206 pp.

Forsum, E., A. Sadurskis, and J. Wager. 1985. Energy maintenance cost during pregnancy in healthy Swedish women. Lancet 1:107-108.

Haworth, J.C., J.J. Ellestad-Sayed, J. King, and L.A. Dilling. 1980. Fetal growth retardation in cigarette-smoking mothers is not due to decreased maternal food intake. Am. J. Obstet. Gynecol. 137:719-723.

Herrera, M.G., J.O. Mora, B. de Paredes, and M. Wagner. 1980. Maternal weight/height and the effect of food supplementation during pregnancy and lactation. Pp. 252-263 in H. Aebi and R. Whitehead, eds. Maternal Nutrition during Pregnancy and Lactation. Hans Huber, Bern.

Hunt, I.F., N.J. Murphy, P.M. Martner-Hewes, B. Faraji, M.E. Swendseid, R.D. Reynolds, A. Sanchez, and A. Mejia. 1987. Zinc, vitamin B_6, and other nutrients in pregnant women attending prenatal clinics in Mexico. Am. J. Clin. Nutr. 46:563-569.

Hytten, F.E. 1980. Nutrition. Pp. 163-192 in F. Hytten and G. Chamberlain, eds. Clinical Physiology in Obstetrics. Blackwell Scientific Publications, Oxford.

Illingworth, P.J., R.T. Jung, P.W. Howie, and T.E. Isles. 1987. Reduction in postprandial energy expenditure during pregnancy. Br. Med. J. 294:1573-1576.

Iyengar, L. 1967. Effects of dietary supplements late in pregnancy on the expectant mother and her newborn. Indian J. Med. Res. 55:85-89.

Kardjati, S., J.A. Kusin, and C. de With. 1988. Energy supplementation in the last trimester of pregnancy in East Java: I. Effect on birthweight. Br. J. Obstet. Gynaecol. 95:783-794.

Kennedy, E.T., and M. Kotelchuck. 1984. The effect of WIC supplemental feeding on birth weight: a case-control analysis. Am. J. Clin. Nutr. 40:579-585.

King, J.C., S.H. Cohenour, D.H. Calloway, and H.N. Jacobson. 1972. Assessment of nutritional status of teenage pregnant girls. I. Nutrient intake and pregnancy. Am. J. Clin. Nutr. 25:916-925.

King, J.C., M.N. Bronstein, W.L. Fitch, and J. Weininger. 1987. Nutrient utilization during pregnancy. World Rev. Nutr. Diet. 52:71-142.

Kramer, M.S. 1987. Determinants of low birth weight: methodological assessment and meta-analysis. Bull. W.H.O. 65:663-737.

Langhoff-Roos, J., G. Lindmark, E. Kylberg, and M. Gebre-Medhin. 1987. Energy intake and physical activity during pregnancy in relation to maternal fat accretion and infant birthweight. Br. J. Obstet. Gynaecol. 94:1178-1185.

Lawrence, M., and R.G. Whitehead. 1988. Physical activity and total energy expenditure of child-bearing Gambian village women. Eur. J. Clin. Nutr. 42:145-160.

Lawrence, M., J. Singh, F. Lawrence, and R.G. Whitehead. 1985. The energy cost of common daily activities in African women: increased expenditure in pregnancy? Am. J. Clin. Nutr. 42:753-763.

Lawrence, M., F. Lawrence, W.A. Coward, T.J. Cole, and R.G. Whitehead. 1986. Energy expenditure and energy balance during pregnancy and lactation in The Gambia. Pp. 77-103 in Nestlé Foundation Annual Report 1986. Nestlé Foundation, Lausanne, Switzerland.

Lechtig, A., J.P. Habicht, H. Delgado, R.E. Klein, C. Yarbrough, and R. Martorell. 1975a. Effect of food supplementation during pregnancy on birthweight. Pediatrics 56:508-520.

Lechtig A., C. Yarbrough, H. Delgado, J.P. Habicht, R. Martorell, and R.E. Klein. 1975b. Influence of maternal nutrition on birth weight. Am. J. Clin. Nutr. 28:1223-1233.

Lechtig, A., R. Martorell, H. Delgado, C. Yarbrough, and R.E. Klein. 1978. Food supplementation during pregnancy, maternal anthropometry and birth weight in a Guatemalan rural population. J. Trop. Pediatrics. 24:217-222.

Loris, P., K.G. Dewey, and K. Poirier-Brode. 1985. Weight gain and dietary intake of pregnant teenagers. J. Am. Diet. Assoc. 85:1296-1305.

Mardones-Santander, F., P. Rosso, A. Stekel, E. Ahumada, S. Llaguno, F. Pizarro, J. Salinas, I. Vial, and T. Walter. 1988. Effect of a milk-based food supplement on maternal nutritional status and fetal growth in underweight Chilean women. Am. J. Clin. Nutr. 47:413-419.

McDonald, E.C., E. Pollitt, W. Mueller, A.M. Hsueh, and R. Sherwin. 1981. The Bacon Chow study: maternal nutritional supplementation and birth weight of offspring. Am. J. Clin. Nutr. 34:2133-2144.

Metcoff, J., P. Costiloe, W.M. Crosby, S. Dutta, H.H. Sandstead, D. Milne, C.E. Bodwell, and S.H. Majors. 1985. Effect of food supplementation (WIC) during pregnancy on birth weight. Am. J. Clin. Nutr. 41:933-947.

Mora, J.O., B. de Paredes, M. Wagner, L. de Navarro, J. Suescum, N. Christiansen, and M.G. Herrera. 1979. Nutritional supplementation and the outcome of pregnancy. I. Birth weight. Am. J. Clin. Nutr. 32:455-462.

Nagy, L.E., and J.C. King. 1983. Energy expenditure of pregnant women at rest or walking self-paced. Am. J. Clin. Nutr. 38:369-376.

Nagy, L.E., and J.C. King. 1984. Postprandial energy expenditure and respiratory quotient during early and late pregnancy. Am. J. Clin. Nutr. 40:1258-1263.

NRC (National Research Council). 1989. Recommended Dietary Allowances, 10th ed. Report of the Subcommittee on the Tenth Edition of the RDAs, Food and Nutrition Board, Commission on Life Sciences. National Academy Press, Washington, D.C. 284 pp.

Papoz, L., E. Eschwege, G. Pequignot, J. Barrat, and D. Schwartz. 1982. Maternal smoking and birth weight in relation to dietary habits. Am. J. Obstet. Gynecol. 142:870-876.

Paul, A.A., E.M. Muller, and R.G. Whitehead. 1979. The quantitative effects of maternal dietary energy intake on pregnancy and lactation in rural Gambian women. Trans. R. Soc. Trop. Med. Hyg. 73:686-692.

Picone, T.A., L.H. Allen, M.M. Schramm, and P.N. Olsen. 1982a. Pregnancy outcome in North American women. I. Effects of diet, cigarette smoking, and psychological stress on maternal weight gain. Am. J. Clin. Nutr. 36:1205-1213.

Picone, T.A., L.H. Allen, P.N. Olsen, and M.E. Ferris. 1982b. Pregnancy outcome in North American women. II. Effects of diet, cigarette smoking, stress, and weight gain on placentas, and on neonatal physical and behavioral characteristics. Am. J. Clin. Nutr. 36:1214-1224.

Prentice, A.M., W.A. Coward, H.L. Davies, P.R. Murgatroyd, A.E. Black, G.R. Goldberg, J. Ashford, M. Sawyer, and R.G. Whitehead. 1985. Unexpectedly low levels of energy expenditure in healthy women. Lancet 1:1419-1422.

Prentice, A.M., T.J. Cole, F.A. Foord, W.H. Lamb, and R.G. Whitehead. 1987. Increased birthweight after prenatal dietary supplementation of rural African women. Am. J. Clin. Nutr. 46:912-925.

Roberts, S.B., A.A. Paul, T.J. Cole, and R.G. Whitehead. 1982. Seasonal changes in activity, birth weight and lactational performance in rural Gambian women. Trans. R. Soc. Trop. Med. Hyg. 76:668-678.

Rush, D. 1981. Nutritional services during pregnancy and birthweight: a retrospective matched pair analysis. Can. Med. Assoc. J. 125:567-576.

Rush, D., Z. Stein, and M. Susser. 1980. A randomized controlled trial of prenatal nutritional supplementation in New York City. Pediatrics 65:683-697.

Rush, D., N.L. Sloan, J. Leighton, J.M. Alvir, D.G. Horvitz, W.B. Seaver, G.C. Garbowski, S.S. Johnson, R.A. Kulka, M. Holt, J.W. Devore, J.T. Lynch, M.B. Woodside, and D.S. Shanklin. 1988. The National WIC Evaluation: evaluation of the Special Supplemental Food Program for Women, Infants, and Children. V. Longitudinal study of pregnant women. Am. J. Clin. Nutr. 48:439-483.

Seitchik, J. 1967. Body composition and energy expenditure during rest and work in pregnancy. Am. J. Obstet. Gynecol. 97:701-713.

Sparks, J.W., J.R. Girard, and F.C. Battaglia. 1980. An estimate of the caloric requirements of the human fetus. Biol. Neonate 38:113-119.

Stein, Z., and M. Susser. 1975a. The Dutch famine, 1944-1945, and the reproductive process. I. Effects on six indices at birth. Pediatr. Res. 9:70-76.

Stein, Z., and M. Susser. 1975b. The Dutch famine, 1944-1945, and the reproductive process. II. Interrelations of caloric rations and six indices at birth. Pediatr. Res. 9:76-83.

Tafari, N., R.L. Naeye, and A. Gobezie. 1980. Effects of maternal undernutrition and heavy physical work during pregnancy on birth weight. Br. J. Obstet. Gynaecol. 87:222-226.

Thomson, A.M. 1959. Diet in pregnancy. 3. Diet in relation to the course and outcome of pregnancy. Br. J. Nutr. 13:509-525.

Thongprasert, K., and A. Valyasevi. 1986. The energy requirements of pregnant rural Thai women. Pp. 105-112 in Nestlé Foundation Annual Report 1986. Nestlé Foundation, Lausanne, Switzerland.

Thongprasert, K., V. Tanphaichitre, A. Valyasevi, J. Kittigool, and J.V.G.A. Durnin. 1987. Energy requirements of pregnancy in rural Thailand. Lancet 2:1010-1012.

Tontisirin, K., U. Booranasubkajorn, A. Hongsumarn, and D. Thewtong. 1986. Formulation and evaluation of supplementary foods for Thai pregnant women. Am. J. Clin. Nutr. 43:931-939.

Torún, B., J. McGuire, and R.D. Mendoza. 1982. Energy cost of activities and tasks of women from a rural region of Guatemala. Nutr. Res. 2:127-136.

Truswell, A.S., S. Ash, and J.R. Allen. 1988. Energy intake during pregnancy. Lancet 1:49.

Tuazon, P.A.G., C.V.C. Barba, J.M.A. van Raaij, M.E.M. Peek, and J.G.A.J. Hautvast. 1986. Maternal energy requirements during pregnancy of rural Philippine women. Pp. 113-146 in Nestlé Foundation Annual Report 1986. Nestlé Foundation, Lausanne, Switzerland.

Tuazon, M.A.G., J.M.A. van Raaij, J.G.A.J. Hautvast, and C.V.C. Barba. 1987. Energy requirements of pregnancy in the Philippines. Lancet 2:1129-1131.

van Raaij, J.M.A., M.E.M. Peek, and J.G.A.J. Hautvast. 1986. Maternal energy requirements in pregnancy in Dutch women. Pp. 53-75 in Nestlé Foundation Annual Report 1986. Nestlé Foundation, Lausanne, Switzerland.

van Raaij, J.M.A., S.H. Vermaat-Miedema, C.M. Schonk, M.E.M. Peek, and J.G.A.J. Hautvast. 1987. Energy requirements of pregnancy in The Netherlands. Lancet 2:953-955.

Viegas, O.A.C., P.H. Scott, T.J. Cole, P. Eaton, P.G. Needham, and B.A. Wharton. 1982. Dietary protein energy supplementation of pregnant Asian mothers at Sorrento, Birmingham. II. Selective during third trimester only. Br. Med. J. 285:592-595.

8

Effects of Gestational Weight Gain on Outcome in Singleton Pregnancies

The subcommittee reviewed the evidence concerning the effects of gestational weight gain on short-term fetal, infant, and maternal health outcomes, as well as maternal factors that could modify those effects. The following outcomes were considered: fetal and neonatal mortality, fetal growth, gestational duration, spontaneous abortion (miscarriage), congenital anomalies, maternal mortality, complications of pregnancy, lactation performance, and postpartum obesity. The concepts and terms illustrated in Figure 2-1 were used to analyze and review published studies of human populations bearing on these potential consequences of maternal weight gain. Particular attention was given to controlling for other maternal factors that could confound the relationship between weight gain and pregnancy outcome. Animal studies were considered only when the clinical and epidemiologic literature was too sparse or contradictory to permit reasonable inferences (e.g., for lactation performance). The discussion here is restricted to singleton pregnancies; twin pregnancies are considered in Chapter 9.

The subcommittee focused on the links between gestational weight gain and short-term pregnancy outcomes because data relating weight gain to long-term outcomes are relatively scanty, and there is no strong evidence indicating that weight gain affects long-term outcomes directly, i.e., without first affecting shorter-term outcomes. For example, several reports (Naeye and Chez, 1981; Singer et al., 1968; Tavris and Read, 1982) have linked maternal weight gain to subsequent cognitive development in the offspring, but none has shown that such effects occur independently of the effects on

176

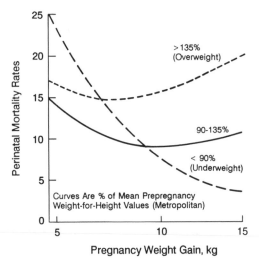

FIGURE 8-1 Perinatal mortality as a function of maternal weight gain. From Naeye (1979) with permission.

fetal (including brain) growth. The long-term child health consequences of preterm birth and intrauterine growth retardation (IUGR) are reviewed briefly later in this chapter. Links between other short-term and longer-term outcomes for both mothers and children (see Figure 2-3) are discussed in Chapter 10, along with other general issues regarding the entire causal pathway.

FETAL AND INFANT OUTCOMES

Mortality

Fetal and infant mortality rates have been used extensively to track progress in improving infant health and, indeed, to reflect the overall health status of the nation. Because these rates are quite low (approximately 1%), however, very large numbers of births are required to study the relationship between weight gain and fetal and infant deaths. Thus, few such studies have been conducted. Two exceptions are the Collaborative Perinatal Project (Naeye, 1979) and a National Center for Health Statistics (NCHS) study linking data from the 1980 National Fetal Mortality Survey and the 1980 National Natality Survey (Taffel, 1986).

Data from the Collaborative Perinatal Project (Figure 8-1) indicate that the relationship between gestational weight gain and perinatal mortality is strongly influenced by maternal prepregnancy nutritional status; i.e., there is evidence for important *effect modification* (see Chapter 2). For women who were underweight prior to pregnancy, the greater the gestational weight gain, the lower the perinatal mortality. However, for women with desirable prepregnancy weight for height (based on the 1959 Metropolitan Life Insurance Company's tables), perinatal mortality began to rise with gestational weight gains in excess of 11.4 kg (25 lb), which might be partially explained by a rise in the rate of high birth weight and a corresponding increased risk for shoulder dystocia and other complications of labor and delivery (see below). For weight gains above 6.8 to 7.3 kg, (15 to 16 lb) the highest perinatal mortality rates occurred among overweight women (i.e., those with prepregnancy weights greater than 135% of standard weight for height). Data shown in Figure 8-1 may be biased (because women who deliver preterm infants will have had less time to gain weight, and preterm infants are at increased risk for perinatal death). Nevertheless, other data in the same report indicate similar trends even when gestational weight gain was considered as a percentage of a gestational age-adjusted "optimum" gain. According to Naeye, the effects shown were not confounded by maternal age, parity, race, family income, number of prenatal care visits, cigarette smoking, or prior pregnancy history.

The NCHS study (Taffel, 1986) focused on late fetal deaths ($\geq$ 28 weeks of gestational age). The results, stratified by gestational age (Figure 8-2), are consistent with those from the Collaborative Perinatal Project. The trend toward higher fetal deaths per 1,000 live births for women with lower weight gains (below 11.8 kg, or 26 lb) was most marked among women with low prepregnancy weights and persisted after stratification (one variable at a time) for maternal age, education, and cigarette smoking.

Beyond this direct evidence, there is a fairly strong link between fetal growth and mortality (see discussion below). Because of this strong relationship, it is also reasonable to assume, even in the absence of abundant direct evidence, that any effects of gestational weight gain on intrauterine growth will be reflected by corresponding, albeit smaller, effects on mortality.

Fetal Growth

Importance of Birth Weight as a Pregnancy Outcome

Infant size at birth is a key determinant of child health, especially in early infancy, but even beyond (see the review by McCormick, 1985). As shown in Figure 8-3A, for example, neonatal mortality decreases sharply with increasing birth weight up to 2,700 or 2,800 g, declines more slowly up to 3,500 g, is relatively flat from 3,500 to 4,250 g, and then begins to rise slightly (Hogue et al., 1987). A similar but less pronounced trend is seen for postneonatal mortality (Figure 8-3B).

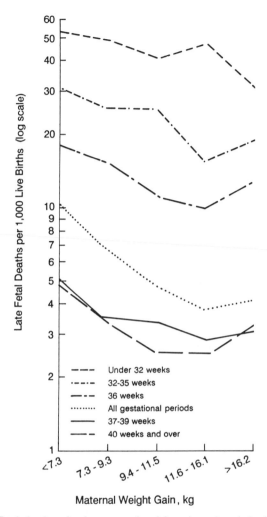

FIGURE 8-2 Fetal death ratios by maternal weight gain and period of gestation in the United States, based on data from the 1980 National Natality and National Fetal Mortality Surveys. From Taffel (1986).

In an attempt to identify those infants at highest risk, many researchers and policymakers have compared infants with low birth weights (LBWs), i.e., <2,500 g, with infants who weigh more. This dichotomy is crude but provides striking contrasts in outcomes: compared with infants who weigh ≥2,500 g, LBW babies are nearly 40 times as likely to die during the neonatal period, and those that survive are five times as likely to die during the postneonatal period. Of those who survive infancy, LBW babies are

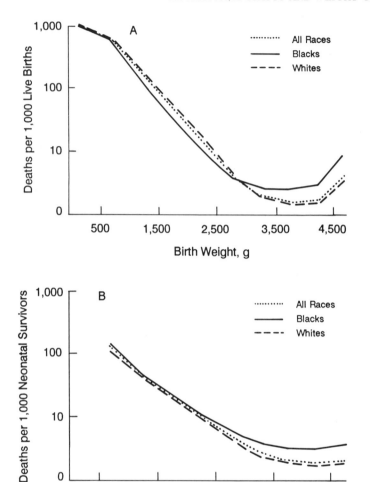

FIGURE 8-3 (A) Neonatal mortality risks by race and birth weight, United States, 1980 live birth cohort. (B) Postneonatal mortality risks by race and birth weight, United States, neonatal survivors of 1980 live-birth cohorts. From Hogue et al. (1987).

about 50% more likely to have serious developmental problems or other illnesses (Shapiro et al., 1980).

Further subdivisions based on birth weight have been used to refine risk categories. For example, the LBW group is often subdivided into very low birth weight (VLBW), i.e., <1,500 g, and moderately LBW, i.e., 1,500 to 2,499 g. The VLBW infants are at much greater risk of death and disability than are infants in the moderately LBW group (Kleinman and Kessel, 1987). At the other end of the scale, high-birth-weight (>4,000 g) infants, especially those weighing >4,500 g, are also at higher risk than normal-weight infants (2,500 to 4,000 g) for adverse outcomes, including mortality (but less so than for the moderately LBW group; see Figure 8-3A), meconium aspiration, clavicular fracture, brachial plexus injury, and birth asphyxia (Boyd et al., 1983; Koff and Potter, 1939; Modanlou et al., 1980).

Birth weight is a composite of two outcomes: the rate of fetal growth and gestational duration. Thus, the use of birth weight often hides more than it reveals. For example, survival among VLBW infants with the same birth weights is considerably higher among those who are small for gestational age (SGA) than it is among those who have a lower gestational age but are larger for their age (Arnold et al., 1988).

A combined classification based on both birth weight and gestational age provides a more discriminating basis for etiologic and prognostic distinctions. It is possible to distinguish those LBW infants who are small because they are born preterm (gestational age <37 weeks) from those with IUGR (also referred to as SGA), which is usually defined as a birth weight below the 10th percentile for gestational age. This definition obviously depends on the choice of reference population.

Birth weight and gestational age have independent effects on fetal and neonatal mortality (Erhardt et al., 1964; Hoffman et al., 1977; Koops et al., 1982; Lubchenco et al., 1972; Yerushalmy et al., 1965). Both IUGR and, to a greater extent, preterm infants have an increased risk of developing cerebral palsy (Ellenberg and Nelson, 1979). Preterm infants (especially those born extremely early) have a far greater risk of developing respiratory distress syndrome, apnea, intracranial hemorrhage, sepsis, retrolental fibroplasia, and other conditions related to physiologic immaturity.

IUGR infants appear to have increased risks of hypoglycemia, hypocalcemia, polycythemia, and birth asphyxia (Arora et al., 1987; Kramer et al., 1989; Ounsted et al., 1988; Usher, 1970). The extent to which these neonatal complications are responsible for the increased risk of mortality or later neurocognitive deficits (see below) is not clear. Some degree of deficit in both stature and head circumference may persist (Babson, 1970; Babson and Phillips, 1973; Fancourt et al., 1976; Fitzhardinge and Inwood, 1989; Fitzhardinge and Steven, 1972; Hill et al., 1984; Low et al., 1982; Neligan et al., 1976; Ounsted and Taylor, 1971; Villar et al., 1984; Walther, 1988; Walther and Ramaekers, 1982; Westwood et al., 1983). Long-term deficits in neurocognitive performance have been observed in IUGR infants (Fitzhardinge and Steven, 1972; Neligan et al., 1976; Ounsted et al., 1984; Rubin et al., 1973; Westwood et al., 1983; Ylitalo et al., 1988). However, since asphyxia is a frequent concomitant of growth retardation and studies have not been limited to nonasphyxiated infants (Westwood et al., 1983), the magnitude of neurocognitive deficits due to growth retardation may be somewhat less than is generally reported.

Heterogeneity of IUGR

Several methodologic issues should be kept in mind before considering the relationship between gestational weight gain and fetal growth. Problems include measurement of gestational age, as discussed in Chapter 4, and the definition of retarded fetal growth (IUGR). Growth-retarded infants represent a highly heterogeneous group in terms of etiology, severity, and body proportionality. A number of chromosomal and other congenital anomalies associated with growth retardation may lead to prognoses much worse than those for infants without those anomalies. Major congenital anomalies affect only a small percentage of IUGR infants but account for a disproportionate number of deaths. For example, Ounsted et al. (1981) reported that 6.9% of the IUGR infants in their study had such anomalies but represented 62% of the total deaths.

It would be quite surprising if two full-term infants, one weighing 2,000 g and the other weighing 2,800 g, had the same prognosis for subsequent morbidity and mortality. Yet, follow-up studies have not subdivided their IUGR cohorts by severity of growth retardation. Thus, little is known about the magnitude of such prognostic distinctions.

In recent studies, IUGR infants have been subdivided according to their body proportions, especially as defined by Rohrer's ponderal index (birth weight divided by the length cubed). Those with low ponderal indices are said to be *disproportional* (also referred to as *asymmetric* or *wasted*). Several investigators have reported higher neonatal mortality rates among disproportional IUGR infants (Guaschino et al., 1986; Haas et al., 1987; Hoffman and Bakketeig, 1984), but better early catch-up growth and better prognoses for long-term growth and development than for those among proportional IUGR infants (Fancourt et al., 1976; Harvey et al., 1982; Hill et al., 1984; Villar et al., 1984). Unfortunately, most studies in this area have not controlled for the severity of IUGR, with which disproportionality appears to be associated (Kramer et al., 1989), nor have they ensured accurate measurements of gestational age or controlled for confounding by short maternal stature or the postnatal nutritional and other environmental influences listed in Figure 2-2.

Other Methodologic Caveats

Interpretation of the literature relating gestational weight gain to fetal growth requires adequate consideration of several other factors: problems in measurement of length of gestation and gestational weight gain (Chapter

4), differences in components of the gain (Chapter 6), and maternal factors that might either confound or modify the relationship (Chapter 5).

The subcommittee emphasizes that use of total weight gain leads to overstatements of the association between gestational weight gain and fetal growth. That is, if the baby's weight is not subtracted from the mother's weight gain, the association is biased by a part-whole correlation problem (i.e., y is being correlated with $x + y$). Net gain avoids this problem by subtracting the baby's weight.

Overstatements of the association of gestational weight gain and fetal growth are also expected unless birth weight is adjusted for gestational age, either by dividing net weight gain by the number of weeks of gestation or by using analytic methods to adjust for the expected gain at each week of gestation. The most appropriate measure of weight gain would be based on serial measurements of weight gain (i.e., the *pattern* of weight gain) during the course of normal pregnancies.

Effects on Birth Weight (for Gestational Age)

Despite the methodologic caveats discussed in the preceding section, the published data concerning the effect of gestational weight gain on fetal growth are quite convincing. Methodologically acceptable studies have been virtually unanimous in reporting a positive relationship of gestational weight gain with gestational age-adjusted birth weight and with the risk for IUGR. Based on a meta-analysis (Kramer, 1987) of 61 English- and French-language studies published between 1970 and 1984, the average magnitude of the effect on mean birth weight in women with adequate prepregnancy weight for height is approximately 20 g/kg of total weight gain. The relative risk for IUGR in women with low (<7 kg, or 15 lb) total gestational weight gain is approximately 2.0. Given the prevalence of low weight gain, the etiologic fraction (population attributable risk) in women with average prepregnancy weight for height in developed countries is approximately 14%. In other words, low weight gain can account for about one in seven cases of IUGR. All these quantitative estimates are likely to be inflated, because they are based on total weight gain and thus reflect some degree of part-whole correlation. The effect on mean birth weight, for example, appears to be reduced by about one-third (from 20 to 13 g/kg) when based on net gain rather than total gain (Kramer et al., 1989).

Investigators who have examined the effect of a given gestational weight gain in women with different prepregnancy weight-for-height status have been virtually unanimous in concluding that the two factors strongly interact (i.e., that prepregnancy weight for height is an *effect modifier*) (see Chapter 2). Miller and Merritt (1979), for example, showed a clear trend for increasing rates of IUGR with decreasing prepregnant weight

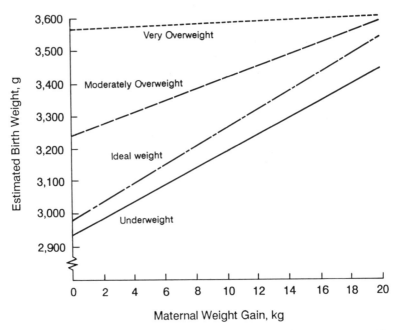

FIGURE 8-4 Birth weight as a function of maternal weight and prepregnancy weight for height. Adapted from Abrams and Laros (1986) with permission.

for height among women with low gestational weight gain. Similar results were reported in several studies investigating mean birth weight (Abrams and Laros, 1986; Frentzen et al., 1988; Mitchell and Lerner, 1989; Naeye, 1981b,d; Seidman et al., 1989; Winikoff and Debrovner, 1981). Illustrative data from Abrams and Laros (1986), as adapted by B. Abrams (University of California at Berkeley, personal communication, 1989), are shown in Figure 8-4. Thus, underweight women appear to derive a greater benefit from a given gestational weight gain than do those with adequate or excessive weights.

Nonetheless, prepregnancy weight for height is itself a determinant of fetal growth above and beyond the effect of gestational weight gain (Kramer, 1987). Women who are thinner before pregnancy tend to have smaller babies than do heavier women with the same weight gain. Thus, desirable weight gains in thin women are higher than those in normal-weight women, despite the effect modification, and desirable weight gains for overweight and obese women are lower.

The effect of gestational weight gain on fetal growth is weak, or perhaps even absent, in obese women (>35% of standard prepregnancy weight for height) (Abrams and Laros, 1986; Brown et al., 1986; Frentzen et al., 1988; Harrison et al., 1980; Luke et al., 1981; Mitchell and Lerner, 1987; Naeye, 1981b; Rosso, 1985; Winikoff and Debrovner, 1981). Nonetheless, obese women clearly have infants that are larger than those of nonobese women for the same weight gain (Kramer, 1987). It seems prudent to recommend that obese women gain a minimum equivalent to the weight of the products of conception (6.8 kg, or 15 lb), although lower weight gains in such women are often compatible with optimal birth weights. The subcommittee has not identified an upper limit for this group.

The evidence for other effect modifiers is not nearly as strong as that for prepregnancy weight for height. Recent data indicate that the relationship of gestational weight gain to fetal growth is similar in adolescents and older women after controlling for prepregnancy weight for height and other potentially confounding differences (Scholl et al., 1988), although one recent Israeli study reported a substantially (but nonsignificantly) reduced relationship in women under age 20 (Seidman et al., 1989). These data are concordant with the results of several earlier studies indicating no significant differences in fetal growth in adolescents (even those within 1 or 2 years of menarche), once differences in gestational weight gain, prepregnancy weight, and other confounders have been controlled (Duenhoelter et al., 1975; Horon et al., 1983; Scholl et al., 1984), thus undermining the notion of a competition between the adolescent's own requirements for growth and those of the fetus.

Research findings have not been unanimous on this point, however, especially for younger adolescents (≤16 years). In an analysis of young, black adolescent mothers in the Collaborative Perinatal Project, Naeye (1981d) found significantly lower mean birth weights among infants born at 38 to 44 weeks of gestation to nonsmokers who were not obese prior to pregnancy. This was particularly true in those aged 10 to 14, in whom deficits averaged approximately 150 to 200 g. However, potential differences in alcohol or drug use were not controlled. In a study of poor, young, urban Peruvian mothers, Frisancho et al. (1985) reported a birth weight deficit of approximately 200 g in young adolescents (<15 years) compared with that in older women (17 to 25 years), even after controlling for gestational weight gain. But these results were not controlled for potentially confounding differences in parity or socioeconomic status. A recent study from New York City (Haiek and Lederman, 1989) showed large (200 to 400 g) deficits in birth weight among full-term infants born to young adolescents (≤15 years) compared with those born to 19- to 30-year-old women, even after stratification by weight for height at full-term, unless the adolescents had achieved 140% of their standard (nonpregnant) weight for height.

Potentially confounding differences in cigarette, alcohol, and drug use were not controlled.

Even those studies showing reduced fetal growth in young adolescents do not necessarily demonstrate a true effect modification of weight gain by age. Even if the infants of young teenage mothers have lower birth weights for gestational age after controlling for gestational weight gain (and a variety of potential confounders), this may not indicate a smaller effect of a given weight gain on fetal growth. The lower birth weights might reflect true biologic differences in potential for fetal growth (perhaps related to the young adolescents' own nutritional requirements for growth (Scholl et al., 1989) or to other, unknown mechanisms) in fetal growth or unmeasured or inadequately controlled confounding factors. Of the three studies cited above (Frisancho et al., 1985; Haiek and Lederman, 1989; Naeye, 1981d), only Frisancho et al. present data that directly bear on effect modification. Although the regression coefficients (adjusted slopes) for gestational weight gain in that study decrease with lower maternal age (13 to 15 years), the absolute magnitude of the slopes for 16 year olds (44.4-g birth weight per kilogram of total gestational weight gain) and 17 to 25 year olds (52.2 g/kg) is far higher than the usual effect size of approximately 20 g/kg cited above and, therefore, is difficult to accept at face value, even considering the poor, potentially undernourished population under study. These extremely large effect sizes strongly suggest the existence of residual confounding by socioeconomic or other differences. But lower birth weights seen in infants of young adolescents compared with those seen in infants of older women with the same weight gain, even in the absence of effect modification, argue for promotion of weight gains toward the upper end of the range recommended for older women with a similar weight for height.

The subcommittee was able to locate only a single study (Seidman et al., 1989) bearing on possible effect modification by older age (i.e., >35 years). That study reported a slightly but significantly *increased* effect of gestational weight gain in Israeli women over age 30 as compared with those between the ages of 20 and 30, after controlling for prepregnancy weight for height and other potential confounding variables. (The reported effect was 16.6- compared with 14.0-g birth weight per kilogram of gestational weight gain, respectively.) In addition, since weight does increase with age, older women might be protected to some degree against the adverse effects of low weight gains.

Few data are available concerning differences in the effect of weight gain on fetal growth among women of different racial or ethnic backgrounds. Analysis of the 1980 National Natality Survey (Taffel, 1986), however, indicates similar effects of gestational weight gain on mean birth weight among white as well as black women. But as with the case of young teenagers, black infants tend to be smaller than white infants for the same weight gain of the mother (Kramer, 1987; Taffel, 1986). Black women should therefore strive for weight gains toward the upper end of the ranges recommended for white women with similar prepregnancy weights for height.

The evidence also indicates that women with large gestational weight gains are at increased risk for high-birth-weight infants (Ounsted and Scott, 1981; Scholl et al., 1988; Udall et al., 1978), which can secondarily lead to dysfunctional labor, midforceps delivery, cesarean delivery, shoulder dystocia, meconium aspiration, clavicular fracture, brachial plexus injury, and asphyxia (Acker et al., 1985; Boyd et al., 1983; Koff and Potter, 1939; Modanlou et al., 1980; Sandmire and O'Halloin, 1988).

Most studies cited previously are based on nonrepresentative samples. Thus, their results are of uncertain generalizability. Moreover, few have based their measurements of gestational weight gain on net gain or rate of net gain, so that many of the reported effect sizes may be inflated.

A recent analysis of the 1980 National Natality Survey offers an important advance regarding both of these methodologic issues (Kleinman, 1990). This survey, described in Chapter 5, oversampled LBW infants and included both a physician's and a mother's questionnaire (Taffel and Keppel, 1986). The analysis focused on the risk for full-term LBW (<2,500 g and $\geq$37 weeks of gestational age) among married, white, non-Hispanic women who responded to the mother's questionnaire. (The term LBW is a reasonable proxy for one class of IUGR, since infants born at full-term who weigh <2,500 g are clearly growth-retarded. Infants weighing $\geq$2,500 g at birth who also fall below the 10th percentile are not included by this definition, however.) The analysis uses multiple logistic regression techniques to control for the following potentially confounding maternal variables: age (<20, 20 to 29, and $\geq$30 years), total birth order (1 versus $\geq$2), the interaction of age with birth order, high birth order ($\geq$3 if age <20, $\geq$4 if age $\geq$20), education (<12, 12, and $\geq$13 years), height (<160, 160 to 168, and >168 cm, or <63, 63 to 66, $\geq$67 inches), cigarette smoking (yes or no), and alcohol consumption (none, light—two drinks or less once a month or less, moderate—more than once a month or more than 2 drinks when they drink). Maternal weight for height was measured by using the body mass index (BMI; i.e., weight in kilograms divided by height in meters squared) in three groups: low (BMI <19.8), moderate (BMI 19.8 to 26.0), and high (BMI >26.0). The cutoff at 19.8 corresponds to the lowest quartile of BMI among the survey subjects, whereas the cutoff at 26.0 closely approximates 120% of the 1959 Metropolitan Life Insurance Company's standards for women with a medium frame (Metropolitan Life Insurance Company, 1959). Because most other studies of weight gain have found

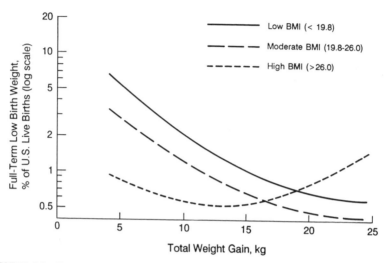

FIGURE 8-5   Full-term low birth weight of live-born singleton infants by total maternal weight gain and prepregnancy BMI of white, non-Hispanic married mothers in the United States in 1980. From Kleinman (1990).

different effects, depending upon the mother's prepregnancy weight (see above), the effects of all weight gain measures were assessed separately for each BMI group.

Three measures of maternal weight gain were used: total gain, net gain, and the rate of net gain. The effect of weight gain on LBW was assumed to have a quadratic rather than a linear form. That is, weight gain and its square were entered in the logistic regression models.

Figures 8-5 to 8-7 show the percentage of full-term LBW infants (on a logarithmic scale) as a function of each weight gain measure, with separate curves for each of the three prepregnancy BMI strata. In each figure, the effect of gestational weight gain is largest (i.e., the slope is steepest) in the low BMI group and least in the high BMI group. For all three groups, however, the effect is greatly attenuated in moving from total weight gain to net weight gain to net weight gain per week.

Table 8-1 compares the full-term LBW odds ratios for women with low weight gain by prepregnancy BMI according to each weight gain measure (e.g., total and net weight gain). The cutoff for low weight gain was the 25th percentile for each measure among all women. The effects were similar among women with low and moderate prepregnancy BMIs; those with total weight gains of ≤10 kg (22 lb) were three to four times as likely to have a full-term LBW baby as those with a gain of >10 kg. However, if either the net weight gain or the net weight gain per week measure is used instead (adjusting the cutoff for low weight gain), the relative odds are reduced to

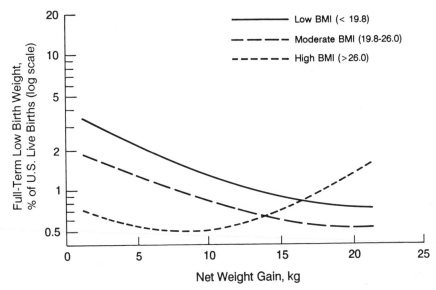

FIGURE 8-6 Full-term low birth weight of live-born singleton infants by net weight gain and prepregnancy BMI of white, non-Hispanic married mothers in the United States in 1980. From Kleinman (1990).

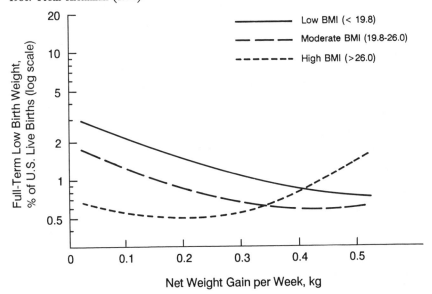

FIGURE 8-7 Full-term low birth weight of live-born singleton infants by net weight gain per week and prepregnancy BMI of white, non-Hispanic married mothers in the United States in 1980. From Kleinman (1990).

TABLE 8-1   Full-Term Low-Birth-Weight Odds Ratios for Low Maternal Weight Gain,[a] by Prepregnancy Body Mass Index (BMI)[b,c]

Weight Gain Measure	Odds Ratios (95% Confidence Intervals), by Prepregnancy BMI		
	Low (<19.8)	Moderate	High (>26.0)
Total weight gain, ≤10 vs >10 kg (≤22 vs >22 lb)	2.4 (1.5, 4.0)	3.1 (2.2, 4.5)	1.3 (0.6, 2.8)
Net weight gain, ≤6.8 vs >6.8 kg (≤15 vs >15 lb)	1.4 (0.8, 2.4)	2.0 (1.4, 2.9)	1.0 (0.4, 2.3)
Net weight gain per week ≤0.17 vs >0.17 kg/wk (≤0.375 vs >0.375 lb/wk)	1.4 (0.8, 2.3)	1.7 (1.1, 2.5)	0.9 (0.4, 2.1)

[a] Odds of full-term low birth weight (<2,500 g and ≥37 weeks of gestation) for mothers with low weight gain (below 25th percentile) compared to other mothers. Based on live births in single deliveries to white non-Hispanic married mothers. Adjusted for maternal age, parity, height, cigarette smoking, and education.

[b] BMI expressed in metric units.

[c] From Kleinman (1990).

1.5 or 2 (i.e., an estimated increased risk of 50 to 100%). Regardless of which measure of weight gain is used, the association is weakest (relative odds near 1.0) and becomes nonsignificant (i.e., the 95% confidence interval around the odds ratio includes 1.0) among women with high prepregnancy BMIs. In fact, among those with the highest prepregnancy BMIs, there is an increased risk of a full-term LBW infant among those who gain more than 15.0 kg (35 lb) total (Figure 8-5), 11.4 kg (25 lb) net (Figure 8-6), or 0.27 net kg (0.6 net lb) per week (Figure 8-7).

Finally, the survey data also permit an analysis of weight gains associated with optimal fetal growth, defined here as a birth weight of 3,000 to 4,000 g and a gestational age of 39 to 41 weeks. The range for optimal fetal growth is based on a balance between lower infant mortality and higher birth weight at full-term and high rates of meconium aspiration, birth trauma, and asphyxia for infants with weights above 4,000 g. In this analysis, a fourth very high BMI (>29) group, which approximates 135% of the 1959 Metropolitan Life Insurance Company standards for women of medium frame, has been split off from the high (BMI >26 to 29) group. As shown in Figure 8-8, the distribution of total weight gains among women giving birth to optimally-grown infants is extremely wide for all four BMI groups. In the middle 70% (i.e., those between the 15th and 85th percentiles), mothers with low or moderate prepregnancy BMIs had total gains of between 7.3 and 18.2 kg (16 and 40 lb). For mothers in the high and very high BMI groups, the corresponding ranges were somewhat wider:

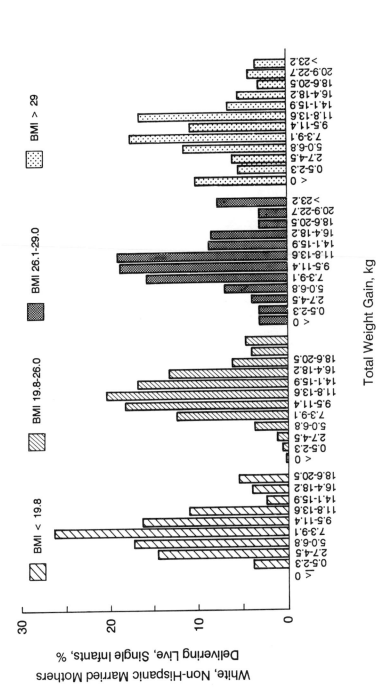

FIGURE 8-8 Distribution of maternal weight gain among white, non-Hispanic married mothers delivering live infants weighing between 3,000 and 4,000 g at 39 to 41 weeks of gestation in the United States in 1980. From Kleinman (1990).

5.0 to 18.2 kg (11 to 40 lb) and 0.5 to 15.9 kg (1 to 35 lb), respectively. Mean ± standard deviation gains in the low and moderate BMI groups were about 13.6 ± 5 kg (30 ± 11 lb). For the high-BMI group, the mean was somewhat lower (12.3 kg, or 27 lb), but the standard deviation was considerably higher (6.8 kg, or 15 lb). Very high BMI mothers had an even lower mean (9.5 kg, or 21 lb) and higher standard deviation (8.2 kg, or 18 lb).

Effect of Weight Gain Pattern

Few investigators have examined the relationship between the pattern of weight gain and fetal growth. Because comparatively little weight is gained in the first trimester, one would expect second- and third-trimester weight gains to have the largest impact on fetal growth. This theoretical argument is supported by the results of the Dutch famine study (Stein et al., 1975) and those of supplementation trials, in which caloric supplements were usually begun in the second or third trimester (Lechtig et al., 1975; Mora et al., 1979; Prentice et al., 1983; Viegas et al., 1982).

Several investigations of weight gain patterns are consistent with this evidence. For example, Thomson and Billewicz (1957) reported that low weight gains during weeks 20 to 30 or weeks 30 to 36 of gestation were associated with an increased risk of LBW. Picone et al. (1982) found that birth weight was significantly correlated with weight gain during the second and third trimesters, but not the first. Hediger et al. (1989) reported that adolescents with low weight gains either before or after 24 weeks of gestation were at increased risk of delivering an IUGR infant. In a recent case-control study (Lawton et al., 1988), women giving birth to IUGR infants were found to have only half the average weight gain between 28 and 32 weeks of gestation as that of women giving birth to non-IUGR infants (other specific gestational periods were not examined).

The first trimester of weight gain may also be important, however. Tompkins and colleagues (Tompkins and Wiehl, 1951; Tompkins et al., 1955) found elevated rates of LBW associated with low first- or second-trimester weight gains, even after stratification by prepregnancy weight. In France, Lazar (1981) reported that correlations between maternal weight gain and sex- and gestational age-adjusted birth weights were low and did not increase with advancing length of gestation. In fact, the ultimate average difference in gestational weight gain of approximately 2 kg (4.4 lb) between mothers giving birth to IUGR and large-for-gestational-age infants appeared to be established by midgestation. Finally, a recent study (Gross et al., 1989) of pregnancy outcome in women with hyperemesis gravidarum (generally associated with improved outcomes) reported impaired fetal growth in those who lost more than 3.6 kg (8 lb) of their prepregnant weight. (Most of this loss presumably occurred during the first trimester, although details of the timing were not provided.) Given the small amount of new maternal tissue (lean or fat) that accumulates during the first trimester, any relationship between early weight gain and fetal growth may reflect expansion of plasma volume or even noncausal mechanisms.

Effect of Weight Gain Composition

The importance of the composition of tissues gained is far from clear. Studies in Peru (Frisancho et al., 1977) and Sweden (Langhoff-Roos et al., 1987) suggest that increases in lean body mass may be more important than fat accretion for intrauterine growth. Similarly, data collected by Pipe et al. (1979) at 10 to 14 weeks of gestation and later analyzed by Campbell-Brown and McFadyen (1985) showed correlation coefficients (R) between birth weight and maternal fat-free mass, height, weight, and skinfold thickness of .44, .24, .22, and .07, respectively. In Senegal, Briend (1985) found a *negative* correlation between maternal triceps skinfold thickness at full-term and birth weight in full-term infants after controlling for maternal weight (also at full-term), parity, and sex of the infant. Although Briend interpreted these data to indicate that maternal energy reserves do not limit fetal growth, they are equally compatible with the inference that mobilization of fat stores in late pregnancy results in improved fetal growth.

Data from two recent studies suggest that an increase in maternal fat stores (as approximated by skinfold thicknesses) may enhance fetal growth. Viegas et al. (1987) found that infants born to mothers with a ≤ 0.02-mm weekly increase in triceps skinfold thickness between 18 and 28 weeks of gestation not only had a lower mean birth weight but also a smaller head circumference and mid-upper arm circumference. Similarly, Maso et al. (1988) reported anthropometric changes between 22 and 32 weeks of gestation in 100 black teenage mothers. The 10 women who gave birth to LBW infants (8 of the 10 were preterm) had significantly smaller increases in their mid-upper arm circumferences, and actual decreases in their triceps skinfold thicknesses. However, the results are difficult to interpret because of the small number of LBW infants and the failure to control for other potentially confounding differences between the two groups.

Differences in gestational weight gain may also reflect changes in nonnutritional body components, especially those due to body water content and plasma volume. Several studies indicate that changes in body water may affect intrauterine growth independently of the nutritional aspects of maternal weight gain (Campbell and MacGillivray, 1975; Duffus et al., 1971). It has long been recognized that edema alone (i.e., not accompanied by proteinuria or hypertension) is associated with improved fetal growth (Billewicz and Thomson, 1970; Naeye, 1981a,c; Thomson et al., 1967).

The beneficial effect is seen even in women with dependent (leg) edema only, despite the absence of any increase in total body water (Hytten and Thomson, 1976).

Effects on Birth Length and Head Circumference

The term *fetal growth* should be interpreted as indicating more than merely birth weight or birth weight for gestational age. In particular, other dimensions of fetal growth, especially body length and head circumference, have often been used as indices of pregnancy outcome. Although few data directly link gestational weight gain to infant length, head circumference, or body proportionality, IUGR infants tend to be shorter and have smaller heads than those of infants with a normal weight for gestational age (Kramer et al., 1989). There does appear to be some degree of head and length sparing, however, such that the relative shapes of infants change with successive degrees of growth retardation. The well-controlled observational study by Miller and Merritt (1979) of women in the Kansas City area showed that rates of short-for-date infants and, to a far lesser extent, infants with small head circumferences both increased with low gestational weight gain. This trend was especially marked in women with low prepregnancy weights for height.

Studies of nutritional deprivation and energy supplementation support these overall findings. For example, the Dutch famine study (Stein et al., 1975) demonstrated a significant reduction of 1.3 cm in length and 1.0 cm in head circumference among infants born to women exposed to famine conditions in the third trimester. Conversely, a supplementation trial of poorly nourished women in Colombia (Herrera et al., 1980) suggested positive effects of supplementation on birth length and head circumference. Larger head circumferences were also reported among infants born to supplemented women in The Gambia (Prentice et al., 1983); no data on birth length were provided in that study.

Gestational Duration

Compared with the extensive amount of literature on fetal growth, there are relatively few published reports on the relationship between maternal weight gain and gestational duration. Papiernik and Kaminski (1974) found a significantly increased risk of subsequent preterm birth to mothers with either low (<5 kg, or 11 lb) or high (>9 kg, or 20 lb) weight gains up to 32 weeks of gestation; however, these results were based on bivariate (i.e., potentially confounded) associations. A companion report (Kaminski and Papiernik, 1974) showed that low weight gain by 32 weeks of gestation significantly discriminated between subsequent low (<2,500 g)-

and normal ($\geq$2,500 g)-birth-weight infants, but a specific relationship with preterm birth (as opposed to IUGR) was not examined. Miller and Merritt (1979) reported a higher rate of preterm birth among 108 white women who gained less than 227 g/week during the last two trimesters, but no such effect was seen among the 70 black women with low weight gains.

Berkowitz (1981) reported a fourfold increased risk of preterm delivery in women with inadequate weight gains compared with that in women with adequate gains. No details were provided, however, on the criteria used for assessing adequacy other than a general statement that the assessment was based on "a schedule . . . which adjusted for pregnancy duration," p. 87. Hingson et al. (1982) found a significant positive partial correlation (i.e., simultaneously adjusted for multiple potential confounding variables) between total weight gain and mean gestational age, but this result was based on total gain, rather than rate of gain, and may therefore reflect a reverse causal influence of gestational duration on total weight gain. Mitchell and Lerner (1989) found an increased risk of preterm delivery in women with both normal and subnormal prepregnancy relative weights and total weight gains of <9 kg (20 lb). Here, too, the increase in total weight gain does not permit firm inferences to be made about causal direction.

Picone et al. (1982) compared women with predicted low ($\leq$6.8 kg, or 15 lb) and adequate (>6.8 kg) total weight gains. They based their predictions on weight gains of <3.6 kg, or $\geq$3.6 kg (<8 or $\geq$8 lb) at 20 weeks of gestation. There was no difference in mean gestational age between the two groups when based on the mother's last menstrual period (LMP), but there was a slightly shorter (38.5 compared with 39.2 weeks of gestation; p <.01) gestational age when based on neonatal (Dubowitz) examination. These results are even more difficult to interpret in light of the fact that the investigators reclassified two of the women whose total weight gains did not agree with their predictions at 20 weeks of gestation.

van den Berg and Oechsli (1984) reported a highly significant increased risk of preterm birth (based on LMP) in women with weight gains averaging <0.23 kg/week (<0.5 lb/week) after 20 weeks of gestation in the large Child Health and Development Studies conducted in the San Francisco Bay area. These results are closely paralleled by those in a recent study by Abrams et al. (1989), who observed an increased risk of preterm delivery in women with a low (<0.27 kg/week, or 0.6 lb/week) rate of weight gain (a 60% increase in risk over women gaining 0.27 to 0.52 kg/week, or 0.6 to ~1 lb/week). The magnitude of elevated risk reported by Abrams and colleagues was not materially altered when the analysis was restricted to preterm births of infants whose gestational ages had been confirmed by ultrasound examination before 28 weeks of gestation. Two other reports of a recent study among adolescents (Hediger et al., 1989; Scholl et al., 1989) also indicated an association between low rate of weight gain during gestation and preterm delivery. The magnitude of the increased risk varied from 50 to 75%, depending on whether the gestational age was based on the LMP or an "obstetric" (undefined) estimate. The risk appeared to be even higher if the low gain occurred both before and after 24 weeks of gestation.

Data from the 1980 National Natality Survey (Kleinman, 1990) were also reviewed by the subcommittee. Preterm LBW (<2,500 g at <37 weeks of gestation) was examined as a function of maternal weight gain. Stratification of prepregnancy BMI and the three different weight gain measures used were the same as those in the analysis for full-term LBW infants. As shown in Figures 8-9 to 8-11, women in the lowest BMI group generally had the highest rates of preterm LBW infants. The apparent effect of weight gain in women in all three BMI groups diminished markedly, however, in moving from total weight gain to net weight gain to net weight gain per week. In fact, Figure 8-11 indicates little or no effect of net weight gain per week, except perhaps for a slight reduction in LBW with higher gains in the low BMI group. That the results differ so markedly according to which weight gain measure is used strongly suggests that the apparent effect of total (or even net) gain is due to reverse causality; i.e., women who deliver their infants preterm will have had less time to gain weight.

Table 8-2 shows the preterm LBW odds ratios for women with low

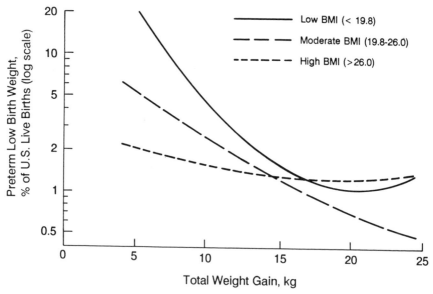

FIGURE 8-9 Preterm low birth weight of live-born singleton infants by total maternal weight gain and prepregnancy BMI of white, non-Hispanic married mothers in the United States in 1980. From Kleinman (1990).

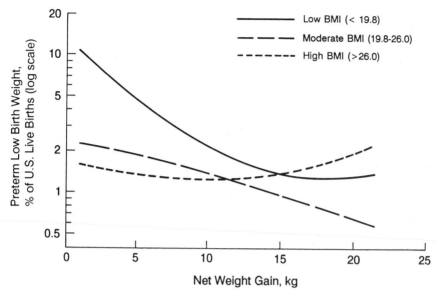

FIGURE 8-10 Preterm low birth weight of live-born singleton infants by net maternal weight gain and prepregnancy BMI of white, non-Hispanic married mothers in the United States in 1980. From Kleinman (1990).

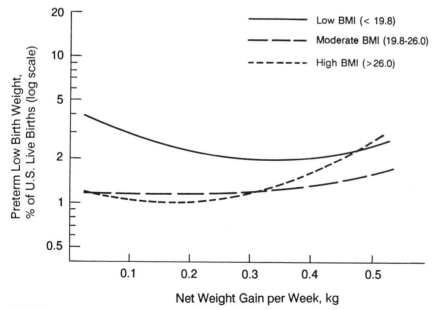

FIGURE 8-11 Preterm low birth weight of live-born singleton infants by net maternal weight gain per week and prepregnancy BMI of white non-Hispanic married mothers in the United States in 1980. From Kleinman (1990).

weight gain according to each of the three weight gain measures. As with full-term LBW, the effect of low weight gain on the relative odds of preterm LBW for women in the high BMI group was weak and insignificant, regardless of the weight gain measure used. For women in the low and moderate BMI groups, there were significant associations between low total or net weight gain and the relative odds of preterm LBW. But the odds ratios were close to, and not significantly different from, 1 when the analysis was based on the more appropriate measure of net gain per week.

One important methodologic caveat should be kept in mind in interpreting studies linking gestational weight gain to gestational duration. As discussed earlier in the section on fetal growth, errors in estimation of gestational age (particularly when based on menstrual dates) may well lead to misclassification of some growth-retarded infants as preterm. Since gestational weight gain has been shown to have an impact on fetal growth and the risk of IUGR, evidence of effects on gestational duration based on menstrual dates should be interpreted with caution. Nevertheless, some data do suggest a possible effect of low weight gain on reducing gestational duration and increasing the risk of preterm delivery. Further research in this area using validated gestational age measurements (e.g., based on early ultrasound examination) should receive high priority, given the well-known importance of preterm delivery on infant mortality and infant and child morbidity and performance.

TABLE 8-2   Preterm Low-Birth-Weight Odds Ratios for Low Maternal Weight Gain,[a] by Prepregnancy Body Mass Index (BMI)[b,c]

Weight Gain Measure	Odds Ratios (95% Confidence Intervals), by Prepregnancy BMI		
	Low (<19.8)	Moderate	High (>26.0)
Total weight gain, ≤10 vs >10 kg (≤22 vs >22 lb)	4.0 (2.7, 6.0)	2.8 (2.0, 4.0)	1.6 (0.8, 3.2)
Net weight gain, ≤6.8 vs >6.8 kg (≤15 vs >15 lb)	1.9 (1.2, 2.8)	1.8 (1.4, 2.6)	1.1 (0.6, 2.2)
Net weight gain per week ≤0.17 vs >0.17 kg/wk (≤0.375 vs >0.375 lb/wk)	1.2 (0.8, 1.9)	1.0 (0.7, 1.5)	1.0 (0.5, 1.9)

[a] Odds of preterm low birth weight (<2,500 g and <37 weeks of gestation) for mothers with low weight gain (below overall 25th percentile) compared with those of other mothers. Based on live births in single deliveries to white, non-Hispanic married mothers. Adjusted for maternal age, parity, height, cigarette smoking, and education.

[b] BMI expressed in metric units.

[c] From Kleinman (1990).

Spontaneous Abortion (Miscarriage)

There is a general paucity of data concerning the effects of gestational weight gain on the risk of spontaneous abortion, i.e., first- and early-second-trimester spontaneous abortions (later-second-trimester spontaneous abortions merge with preterm deliveries and probably share many of their etiologic determinants). Unfortunately, epidemiologic studies of early miscarriages are quite difficult, since these pregnancy losses may not be recognized or, if recognized, may not come to the attention of a physician or other health care worker.

Few data relate early miscarriage to maternal nutrition. A hospital-based study in New York City showed no association between chromosomally normal spontaneous abortion and prepregnancy BMI (Stein, 1989). Risch et al. (1988) found that neither height, weight, nor the presence or absence of obesity (all presumably at the time of the interview) was associated with the woman's risk of a previous spontaneous abortion.

In an early study of the effects of the Dutch famine, Smith (1947) noted an increased rate of "abortion and miscarriage" among Rotterdam women who conceived during the famine, but it is not clear whether the reported figures include induced abortions. Smith commented, "There is no reason to assume [the data] are accurate or that conclusions can be drawn from them," p. 603.

The only direct data linking gestational weight gain and spontaneous abortion came from a study in Bangladesh (Pebley et al., 1985). Conception from June to October—a lean period of arduous work and reduced diet—was associated with pregnancy loss primarily in the third trimester and, to a lesser extent, before and during the second trimester. Independent effects were reported both for reductions in prepregnancy weight as well as gestational weight gain, both of which were reduced during the lean period.

Congenital Anomalies

The subcommittee found no studies directly linking gestational weight gain to the risk either of congenital anomalies in general or of specific malformations. Such a link would not be expected, given the negligible weight changes that occur during the very early gestational period of embryonic morphogenesis.

MATERNAL OUTCOMES

Maternal Mortality

In most developed countries, maternal mortality during pregnancy, childbirth, or the puerperium is extremely rare—generally less than 10 per

100,000. The most common causes are pregnancy-induced hypertension (PIH), pulmonary embolism, ectopic pregnancy, and hemorrhage (ante- and postpartum) (NCHS, 1987). In the United States, rates are three to four times higher for black women than for white women (Buehler et al., 1986). This has been attributed to poor prenatal care among black women (Sachs et al., 1987), although the causal relationship between prenatal care and the risk of maternal death remains uncertain. Nutritional differences and many other explanations for the higher rates are possible. Neither gestational weight gain nor other nutritional factors have been investigated directly for this association.

Complications of Pregnancy, Labor, and Delivery

Large weight gains, especially in the second and third trimesters, have long been associated with an increased risk of PIH and preeclamptic tox- emia (including proteinuria and generalized edema) in primiparous women (Naeye, 1981b; Shepard et al., 1986; Thomson and Billewicz, 1957; Tomp- kins et al., 1955). Recognition of this association reinforced the earlier obstetric practice of limiting weight gain, which appears to have originated with an observed reduction in eclampsia that was temporally associated with food shortages in Germany during World War I (Anonymous, 1917; NRC, 1970). But the determination of causality in this association is highly problematic, since the edema and increased body water accompany- ing preeclampsia will, of course, be manifested by an increased maternal weight, irrespective of any change in maternal lean or fat mass. The typical pattern is a sudden increase in weight between visits in the third trimester.

The subcommittee was unable to locate any evidence linking increases in maternal lean or muscle mass early in pregnancy to subsequent PIH or preeclampsia. In fact, an expert committee of the World Health Organiza- tion concluded that it is difficult, based on the available evidence, to define the precise role of nutrition in toxemia (WHO, 1965). The severe energy restriction that occurred during the Dutch famine was associated with a significant reduction in systolic blood pressure near the time of delivery (Ribeiro et al., 1982). Although this might represent some reduction in the risk of PIH or preeclampsia, it could also be a mechanism for lowering uterine blood flow and thereby for impairing fetal growth. Tompkins et al. (1955) did note a higher risk of toxemia in women with low prepregnancy weights for height who had low weight gains during the second trimester. In a review of the published evidence, Chesley (1976) found that, despite the weight gain associated with preeclampsia, most women who develop the condition have total weight gains that are below average. Thus, the causal relationship between gestational weight gain and PIH/preeclampsia remains unclear. Low early gains may be a marker, or even a determinant, of subsequent gestational hypertensive disorders, but firmer inferences must await the results of future research.

As previously discussed, large gestational weight gains are associated with an increased risk of high birth weight and a corresponding increase in risk for dysfunctional labor, midforceps delivery, and cesarean delivery (Boyd et al., 1983; Koff and Potter, 1939; Modanlou et al., 1980). Moreover, there is some evidence that these consequences of fetopelvic disproportion are exacerbated in women with short stature or small pelvic size (Frame et al., 1985; Hughes et al., 1987). Cesarean delivery rates have skyrocketed over the last 15 to 20 years (Placek and Taffel, 1980; Placek et al., 1983), but the remarkable increase has been accompanied by rather modest increases in the rates of high birth weight (see Chapter 3). Thus, even if larger gestational weight gains are partly responsible for the trend toward slightly larger infants, their contribution to complications of labor and delivery must be quite small.

Varma (1984) examined the direct relationship between gestational weight gain and pregnancy complications. Although he reports a significantly higher rate of forceps and cesarean deliveries among women with fetal weight gains ≥16 kg (35.2 lb), and especially ≥21 kg (46.2 lb), these results are unadjusted for potentially confounding differences among women with different weight gains. Using a more sophisticated multivariate approach, however, Shepard et al. (1986) confirmed that women with large weight gains (>35% of their prepregnancy weight) had higher rates of cesarean deliveries and other operative deliveries (forceps and vacuum extraction), as well as a prolonged second stage of labor.

Lactation Performance

There is a general perception that fat deposition during pregnancy is required for optimal lactation performance. Although several studies have examined the relationship between milk production and maternal nutrition during lactation, few have related lactation performance to gestational weight gain.

In one longitudinal study of well-nourished women in the United States, gestational weight gain was not related to milk quantity or quality (Butte et al., 1984). Fat mobilization was not a prerequisite to adequate milk production, as indicated by the inverse relationship between the amount of energy mobilized from maternal stores and dietary energy intake.

Other studies on humans do not support the hypothesis that fat deposited during pregnancy is necessarily mobilized later during lactation. In one study of Swedish women, the mean gestational weight gain (13.8 kg, or ~30 lb) included substantial quantities of fat (5.8 kg, or ~13 lb) (Sadurskis et al., 1988). During the first 2 months of lactation, total body fat did not change; milk production and composition were normal. Energy costs of lactation were met by increased energy intake, not by body fat mobilization.

By contrast, investigators from The Gambia have inferred that fat deposition during pregnancy is of crucial importance for lactation performance. In one Gambian study, milk output at 3 months post partum was negatively correlated with the change in skinfold thicknesses from 6 to 12 weeks post partum (Paul et al., 1979). In women who were replenishing their fat stores during the dry (harvest) season, milk output was low. Although the investigators interpreted this observation to indicate competition between replenishment of maternal body fat and milk production, the data are also consistent with mobilization of maternal fat for milk production. Subsequent, conflicting results indicated higher milk production rates during the dry season compared with those during the wet (farming) season (Prentice and Whitehead, 1987). One study conducted in East Java, Indonesia, demonstrated that energy supplementation in the last trimester of pregnancy did not increase milk output among women with habitually low energy intakes (van Steenbergen et al., 1989).

The limited evidence from studies on the relationship between gestational weight gain and lactation performance in humans can be supplemented with findings from animal studies. Extrapolation of data on reproduction from nonprimate animal models to humans can be hazardous, since marked differences in the energy costs of gestation and lactation exist between primates and other mammals. Nonetheless, the evidence from animal studies indicates that *gestational* nutrition is less important than *postpartum* nutrition for lactation (Jenness, 1986; Kliewer and Rasmussen, 1987; Lodge, 1969; O'Grady et al., 1973; Sadurskis, 1988). This evidence thus supports the notion that gestational weight gain in humans has little impact on subsequent milk quantity or quality.

Postpartum Obesity

It is often alleged that women in developing countries become progressively malnourished (experience *maternal depletion*) and have correspondingly worse outcomes with successive pregnancies (Jelliffe, 1966). In contrast, many investigators report a net increase in body weight among women in industrialized countries during the interconceptional period that may persist and even increase with successive pregnancies.

Studies by Stander and Pastore (1940), Beazley and Swinhoe (1979), and Samra et al. (1988) did not control for the expected weight increase that normally occurs with age. In several population-based cross-sectional studies (Forster et al., 1986; Heliövaara and Aromaa, 1981; McKeown and Record, 1957; Newcombe, 1982; Noppa and Bengtsson, 1980), stratification or multivariate statistical approaches have been used to adjust for the confounding effect of age and, in some cases, for interpregnancy interval, socioeconomic status, and other potential confounders. But cross-sectional studies are prone to cohort effects; i.e., there has been a trend over time toward higher total body weights at any given age and parity. A recent longitudinal study in The Netherlands (Rookus et al., 1987) reported a slightly (but nonsignificantly) higher increase in BMI at 9 months post partum in 49 pregnant women compared with that in 400 nonpregnant controls followed for the same period. Similarly, in a cross-sectional study (Cederlöf and Kaij, 1970) comparing parous monozygotic twins with their childless co-twins, and in longitudinal studies of repeated pregnancies in Scotland (Billewicz and Thomson, 1970) and the United States (Greene et al., 1988), an independent effect of parity on body weight was confirmed. Overall, the evidence suggests an average weight retention of approximately 1 kg (2.2 lb) per birth.

The studies in Scotland and the United States are the only ones found by the subcommittee that attempt to relate the magnitude of the parity effect to the amount of weight gained in the preceding pregnancies. Billewicz and Thomson (1970) reported that weight increases (adjusted for age and cohort effects) above 2.5 kg (5.5 lb) between the first and second pregnancies were associated with high weight gains (average 10 to 12 kg, or 22 to 26 lb) after 20 weeks of gestation during the first pregnancy. Greene et al. (1988) reported an analysis of 7,116 women who had at least two singleton births in the 1959-1965 Collaborative Perinatal Project. There was a monotonic trend toward increasing (adjusted) interpregnancy retention of weight with increasing gestational weight gains in the earlier pregnancy. For the minority of women who had very high gestational weight gains, the increases were substantial: 5 kg (10.9 lb) for women gaining 16.4 to 18.2 kg (36 to 40 lb) and 8.0 kg (17.7 lb) for those gaining more than 18.2 kg. (The mean weight gain among the study women was 9.5 kg, or 20.8 lb.) These data should be interpreted with caution, however, since the pregnancies studied occurred nearly four decades ago, when gestational weight gains were considerably lower than those observed more recently (see Chapter 3). Women gaining ≥16.4 kg (36 lb) represented only 8% of those studied; that percentage would be far higher today. The fact that the study population was skewed toward black, urban, and poor women and was restricted to the 7,116 women with at least two singleton births during the study period (out of the 58,760 total study population) also limits the generalizability of the findings.

In summary, the evidence suggests that women with average gestational weight gains retain about 1 kg (2.2 lb) above and beyond their expected weight increase with age. The 1-kg figure is based largely on data from older studies, however, and may underestimate weight retention associated with the higher gestational weight gains seen in recent years. Women with very large weight gains appear to be at risk for considerably larger postpartum weight increases. For women who are well- or over-nourished prior to pregnancy, these large increases may contribute to the development of obesity and its adverse health sequelae. Since a given weight increase will have a greater impact on relative weight and, hence, obesity in short women, large weight gains may be particularly undesirable in such women. Further studies are required to document the effects of high gestational weight gain on subsequent maternal obesity.

SUMMARY

A large body of evidence indicates that gestational weight gain is a determinant of fetal growth, although the magnitude of the causal impact is somewhat less than that usually reported because of the failure of previous studies to adjust total weight gain for fetal weight. Even after such adjustment, however, lower net weight gains are associated with an increased risk of IUGR and increased perinatal mortality (probably mediated by effects on IUGR), whereas higher weight gains are associated with high birth weight and, secondarily, prolonged labor, shoulder dystocia, cesarean delivery, and birth trauma and asphyxia. There is convincing evidence that the effect of maternal weight gain on fetal growth is modified by pregnancy weight for height. Published data do not suggest an effect modification by age or ethnic background.

Data concerning the effects of maternal weight gain on gestational duration are suggestive but less conclusive, particularly in light of the difficulties in determining gestational age with accuracy. Further research is clearly indicated in this area, because even small reductions in risk for preterm deliveries, especially those that occur very early in gestation, would have a favorable impact on perinatal and later mortality and on infant and child morbidity and performance.

There is little evidence to suggest an important association between gestational weight gain and spontaneous abortion (miscarriage), congenital anomalies, maternal mortality, or lactation performance. There does appear to be a statistical association with PIH and preeclampsia, but it is difficult to interpret this association because of directionality (increased body water leads to increased weight gain) and the absence of data relating PIH to early gestational changes in maternal fat or lean body mass.

Pregnancy, in general, and gestational weight gain, in particular, are associated with retained maternal weight post partum. Women with extremely high weight gains during pregnancy may be at increased risk of subsequent obesity.

CLINICAL IMPLICATIONS

- Recommendations for gestational weight gain must be based on an adequate appreciation of potential benefits and risks for fetal growth, perinatal mortality, complications of labor and delivery, and birth trauma and asphyxia.
- Desirable weight gains are highest in thin women and lowest in obese, overweight, and short women (see Table 1-1 in Chapter 1).
- Young adolescent and black mothers should be encouraged to strive for weight gains toward the upper range desirable for adult white mothers with similar prepregnancy weights for height and heights.

REFERENCES

Abrams, B.F., and R.K. Laros, Jr. 1986. Prepregnancy weight, weight gain, and birth weight. Am. J. Obstet. Gynecol. 154:503-509.

Abrams, B., V. Newman, T. Key, and J. Parker. 1989. Maternal weight gain and preterm delivery. Obstet. Gynecol. 74:577-583.

Acker, D.B., B.P. Sachs, and E.A. Friedman. 1985. Risk factors for shoulder dystocia. Obstet. Gynecol. 66:762-768.

Anonymous. 1917. Eclampsia rare on war diet in Germany. J. Am. Med. Assoc. 68:732.

Arnold, C.C., C.A. Hobbs, R.H. Usher, and M.S. Kramer. 1988. What's wrong with the concept of "very low birth weight" (VLBW)? Pediatr. Res. 23:288A.

Arora, N.K., V.K. Paul, and M. Singh. 1987. Morbidity and mortality in term infants with intrauterine growth retardation. J. Trop. Pediatr. 33:186-189.

Babson, S.G. 1970. Growth of low-birth-weight infants. J. Pediatr. 77:11-18.

Babson, S.G., and D.S. Phillips. 1973. Growth and development of twins dissimilar in size at birth. N. Engl. J. Med. 289:937-940.

Beazley, J.M., and R.J. Swinhoe. 1979. Body weight in parous women: is there any alteration between successive pregnancies? Acta Obstet. Gynecol. Scand. 58:45-47.

Berkowitz, G.S. 1981. An epidemiologic study of preterm delivery. Am. J. Epidemiol. 113:81-92.

Billewicz, W.Z., and A.M. Thomson. 1970. Body weight in parous women. Br. J. Prev. Soc. Med. 24:97-104.

Boyd, M.E., R.H. Usher, and F.H. McLean. 1983. Fetal macrosomia: prediction, risks, proposed management. Obstet. Gynecol. 61:715-722.

Briend, A. 1985. Do maternal energy reserves limit fetal growth? Lancet 1:38-40.

Brown, J.E., K.W. Berdan, P. Splett, M. Robinson, and L.J. Harris. 1986. Prenatal weight gains related to the birth of healthy-sized infants to low-income women. J. Am. Diet. Assoc. 86:1679-1683.

Buehler, J.W., A.M. Kaunitz, C.J.R. Hogue, J.M. Hughes, J.C. Smith, and R.W. Rochat. 1986. Maternal mortality in women aged 35 years or older: United States. J. Am. Med. Assoc. 255:53-57.

Butte, N.F., C. Garza, J.E. Stuff, E.O. Smith, and B.L. Nichols. 1984. Effect of maternal diet and body composition on lactational performance. Am. J. Clin. Nutr. 39:296-306.

Campbell, D.M., and I. MacGillivray. 1975. The effect of a low calorie diet or a thiazide diuretic on the incidence of pre-eclampsia and on birth-weight. Br. J. Obstet. Gynaecol. 82:572-577.

Campbell-Brown, M., and I.R. McFadyen. 1985. Maternal energy reserves and birthweight. Lancet 1:574-575.

Cederlöf, R., and L. Kaij. 1970. The effect of childbearing on body-weight. Acta Psychiatr. Scand., Suppl. 219:47-49.

Chesley, L.C. 1976. Blood pressure, edema and proteinuria in pregnancy. 1. Historical developments. Prog. Clin. Biol. Res. 7:19-66.

Duenhoelter, J.H., J.M. Jimenez, and G. Baumann. 1975. Pregnancy performance of patients under fifteen years of age. Obstet. Gynecol. 46:49-52.

Duffus, G.M., I. MacGillivray, and K.J. Dennis. 1971. The relationship between baby weight and changes in maternal weight, total body water, plasma volume, electrolytes and proteins, and urinary oestriol excretion. J. Obstet. Gynaecol. Br. Commonw. 78:97-104.

Ellenberg, J.H., and K.B. Nelson. 1979. Birth weight and gestational age in children with cerebral palsy or seizure disorders. Am. J. Dis. Child. 133:1044-1048.

Erhardt, C.L., G.B. Joshi, F.G. Nelson, B.H. Kroll, and L. Weiner. 1964. Influence of weight and gestation on perinatal and neonatal mortality by ethnic group. Am. J. Public Health 54:1841-1855.

Fancourt, R., S. Campbell, D. Harvey, and A.P. Norman. 1976. Follow-up study of small-for-date babies. Br. Med. J. 1:1435-1437.

Fitzhardinge, P.M., and S. Inwood. 1989. Long-term growth in small-for-date children. Acta Paediatr. Scand., Suppl. 349:27-33.

Fitzhardinge, P.M., and E.M. Steven. 1972. The small-for-date infant. I. Later growth patterns. Pediatrics 49:671-681.

Forster, J.L., E. Bloom, G. Sorensen, R.W. Jeffery, and R.J. Prineas. 1986. Reproductive history and body mass index in black and white women. Prev. Med. 15:685-691.

Frame, S., J. Moore, A. Peters, and D. Hall. 1985. Maternal height and shoe size as predictors of pelvic disproportion: an assessment. Br. J. Obstet. Gynaecol. 92:1239-1245.

Frentzen, B.H., D.L. Dimperio, and A.C. Cruz. 1988. Maternal weight gain: effect on infant birth weight among overweight and average-weight low-income women. Am. J. Obstet. Gynecol. 159:1114-1117.

Frisancho, A.R., J.E. Klayman, and J. Matos. 1977. Influence of maternal nutritional status on prenatal growth in a Peruvian urban population. Am. J. Phys. Anthropol. 46:265-274.

Frisancho, A.R., J. Matos, W.R. Leonard, and L.A. Yaroch. 1985. Developmental and nutritional determinants of pregnancy outcome among teenagers. Am. J. Phys. Anthropol. 66:247-261.

Greene, G.W., H. Smiciklas-Wright, T.O. Scholl, and R.J. Karp. 1988. Postpartum weight change: how much of the weight gained in pregnancy will be lost after delivery? Obstet. Gynecol. 71:701-707.

Gross, S., C. Librach, and A. Cecutti. 1989. Maternal weight loss associated with hyperemesis gravidarum: a predictor of fetal outcome. Am. J. Obstet. Gynecol. 160:906-909.

Guaschino, S., A. Spinillo, E. Stola, P.C. Pesando, G.P. Gancia, and G. Rondini. 1986. The significance of ponderal index as a prognostic factor in a low-birth-weight population. Biol. Res. Preg. Perinatol. 7:121-127.

Haas, J.D., H. Balcazar, and L. Caulfield. 1987. Variation in early neonatal mortality for different types of fetal growth retardation. Am. J. Phys. Anthropol. 73:467-473.

Haiek, L., and S.A. Lederman. 1989. The relationship between maternal weight for height and term birth weight in teens and adult women. J. Adol. Health Care 10:16-22.

Harrison, G.G., J.N. Udall, and G. Morrow III. 1980. Maternal obesity, weight gain in pregnancy, and infant birth weight. Am. J. Obstet. Gynecol. 136:411-412.

Harvey, D., J. Prince, J. Bunton, C. Parkinson, and S. Campbell. 1982. Abilities of children who were small-for-gestational-age babies. Pediatrics 69:296-300.

Hediger, M.L., T.O. Scholl, D.H. Belsky, I.G. Ances, and R.W. Salmon. 1989. Patterns of weight gain in adolescent pregnancy: effects on birth weight and preterm delivery. Obstet. Gynecol. 74:6-12.

Heliövaara, M., and A. Aromaa. 1981. Parity and obesity. J. Epidemiol. Community Health 35:197-199.

Herrera, M.G., J.O. Mora, B. de Paredes, and M. Wagner. 1980. Maternal weight/height and the effect of food supplementation during pregnancy and lactation. Pp. 252-263 in H. Aebi and R. Whitehead, eds. Maternal Nutrition during Pregnancy and Lactation. Hans Huber, Bern.

Hill, R.M., W.M. Verniaud, R.L. Deter, L.M. Tennyson, G.M. Rettig, T.E. Zion, A.L. Vorderman, P.G. Helms, L.B. McCulley, and L.L. Hill. 1984. The effect of intrauterine malnutrition on the term infant: a 14-year progressive study. Acta Paediatr. Scand. 73:482-487.

Hingson, R., J.J. Alpert, N. Day, E. Dooling, H. Kayne, S. Morelock, E. Oppenheimer, and B. Zuckerman. 1982. Effects of maternal drinking and marijuana use on fetal growth and development. Pediatrics 70:539-546.

Hoffman, H.J., and L.S. Bakketeig. 1984. Heterogeneity of intrauterine growth retardation and recurrence risks. Semin. Perinatol. 8:15-24.

Hoffman, H.J., F.E. Lundin, Jr., L.S. Bakketeig, and E.E. Harley. 1977. Classification of births by weight and gestational age for future studies of prematurity. Pp. 297-333 in D.M. Reed and F.J. Stanley, eds. The Epidemiology of Prematurity. Urban & Schwarzenberg, Baltimore.

Hogue, C.J.R., J.W. Buehler, L.T. Strauss, and J.C. Smith. 1987. Overview of the National Infant Mortality Surveillance (NIMS) Project—design, methods, results. Public Health Rep. 102:126-138.

Horon, I.L., D.M. Strobino, and H.M. MacDonald. 1983. Birth weights among infants born to adolescent and young adult women. Am. J. Obstet. Gynecol. 146:444-449.

Hughes, A.B., D.A. Jenkins, R.G. Newcombe, and J.F. Pearson. 1987. Symphysis-fundus height, maternal height, labor pattern, and mode of delivery. Am. J. Obstet. Gynecol. 156:644-648.

Hytten, F.E., and A.M. Thomson. 1976. Weight gain in pregnancy. Pp. 179-187 in M.D. Lindheimer, A.I. Katz, and F.P. Zuspan, eds. Hypertension in Pregnancy. John Wiley & Sons, New York.

Jelliffe, D.B. 1966. The Assessment of the Nutritional Status of the Community. WHO Monograph Series No. 53. World Health Organization, Geneva. 271 pp.

Jenness, R. 1986. Lactational performance of various mammalian species. J. Dairy Sci. 69:869-885.

Kaminski, M., and E. Papiernik. 1974. Multifactorial study of the risk of prematurity at 32 weeks of gestation. II. A comparison between an empirical prediction and a discriminant analysis. J. Perinat. Med. 2:37-44.

Kleinman, J.C. 1990. Maternal Weight Gain During Pregnancy: Determinants and Consequences. NCHS Working Paper Series No. 33. National Center for Health Statistics, Public Health Service, U.S. Department of Health and Human Services, Hyattsville, Md. 24 pp.

Kleinman, J.C., and S.S. Kessel. 1987. Racial differences in low birth weight: trends and risk factors. N. Engl. J. Med. 317:749-753.

Kliewer, R.L., and K.M. Rasmussen. 1987. Malnutrition during the reproductive cycle: effects on galactopoietic hormones and lactational performance in the rat. Am. J. Clin. Nutr. 46:926-935.

Koff, A.K., and E.L. Potter. 1939. The complications associated with excessive development of the human fetus. Am. J. Obstet. Gynecol. 38:412-423.

Koops, B.L., L.J. Morgan, and F.C. Battaglia. 1982. Neonatal mortality risk in relation to birth weight and gestational age: update. J. Pediatr. 101:969-977.

Kramer, M.S. 1987. Determinants of low birth weight: methodological assessment and meta-analysis. Bull. W.H.O. 65:663-737.

Kramer, M.S., F.H. McLean, M. Olivier, D.M. Willis, and R.H. Usher. 1989. Body proportionality and head and length 'sparing' in growth-retarded neonates: a critical reappraisal. Pediatrics 84:717-723.

Langhoff-Roos, J., G. Lindmark, and M. Gebre-Medhin. 1987. Maternal fat stores and fat accretion during pregnancy in relation to infant birthweight. Br. J. Obstet. Gynaecol. 94:1170-1177.

Lawton, F.G., G.C. Mason, K.A. Kelly, I.N. Ramsay, and G.A. Morewood. 1988. Poor maternal weight gain between 28 and 32 weeks gestation may predict small-for-gestational-age infants. Br. J. Obstet. Gynaecol. 95:884-887.

Lazar, R. 1981. General commentary. Pp. 181-186 in J. Dobbing, ed. Maternal Nutrition in Pregnancy: Eating for Two? Academic Press, London.

Lechtig, A., J.P. Habicht, H. Delgado, R.E. Klein, C. Yarbrough, and R. Martorell. 1975. Effect of food supplementation during pregnancy on birthweight. Pediatrics 56:508-520.

Lodge, G.A. 1969. The effects of pattern of feed distribution during the reproductive cycle on the performance of sows. Anim. Prod. 11:133-143.

Low, J.A., R.S. Galbraith, D. Muir, H. Killen, B. Pater, and J. Karchmar. 1982. Intrauterine growth retardation: a study of long-term morbidity. Am. J. Obstet. Gynecol. 142:670-677.

Lubchenco, L.O., D.T. Searls, and J.V. Brazie. 1972. Neonatal mortality rate: relationship to birth weight and gestational age. J. Pediatr. 81:814-822.

Luke, B., C. Dickinson, and R.H. Petrie. 1981. Intrauterine growth: correlations of maternal nutritional status and rate of gestational weight gain. Eur. J. Obstet., Gynecol. Reprod. Biol. 12:113-121.

Maso, M.J., E.J. Gong, M.S. Jacobson, D.S. Bross, and F.P. Heald. 1988. Anthropometric predictors of low birth weight outcome in teenage pregnancy. J. Adol. Health Care 9:188-193.

McCormick, M.C. 1985. The contribution of low birth weight to infant mortality and childhood morbidity. N. Engl. J. Med. 312:82-90.

McKeown, T., and R.G. Record. 1957. The influence of reproduction on body weight in women. J. Endocrinol. 15:393-409.

Metropolitan Life Insurance Company. 1959. New weight standards for men and women. Stat. Bull. Metrop. Life Insur. Co. 40:1-4.

Miller, H.C., and T.A. Merritt. 1979. Fetal Growth in Humans. Year Book Medical Publishers, Chicago. 180 pp.

Mitchell, M.C., and E. Lerner. 1987. Factors that influence the outcome of pregnancy in middle-class women. J. Am. Diet. Assoc. 87:731-735.

Mitchell, M.C., and E. Lerner. 1989. Weight gain and pregnancy outcome in underweight and normal weight women. J. Am. Diet. Assoc. 89:634-638.

Modanlou, H.D., W.L. Dorchester, A. Thorosian, and R.K. Freeman. 1980. Macrosomia—maternal, fetal, and neonatal implications. Obstet. Gynecol. 55:420-424.

Mora, J.O., B. de Paredes, M. Wagner, L. de Navarro, J. Suescum, N. Christiansen, and M.G. Herrera. 1979. Nutritional supplementation and the outcome of pregnancy. I. Birth weight. Am. J. Clin. Nutr. 32:455-462.

Naeye, R.L. 1979. Weight gain and the outcome of pregnancy. Am. J. Obstet. Gynecol. 135:3-9.

Naeye, R.L. 1981a. Maternal blood pressure and fetal growth. Am. J. Obstet. Gynecol. 141:780-787.

Naeye, R.L. 1981b. Maternal nutrition and pregnancy outcome. Pp. 89-111 in J. Dobbing, ed. Maternal Nutrition in Pregnancy: Eating for Two? Academic Press, London.

Naeye, R.L. 1981c. Nutritional/nonnutritional interactions that affect the outcome of pregnancy. Am. J. Clin. Nutr. 34:727-731.

Naeye, R.L. 1981d. Teenaged and pre-teenaged pregnancies: consequences of the fetal-maternal competition for nutrients. Pediatrics 67:146-150.

Naeye, R.L., and R.A. Chez. 1981. Effects of maternal acetonuria and low pregnancy weight gain on children's psychomotor development. Am. J. Obstet. Gynecol. 139:189-193.

NCHS (National Center for Health Statistics). 1987. Vital Statistics of the United States, 1983. Vol. 2—Mortality, Part A. DHHS Publ. No. (PHS) 87-1102. National Center for Health Statistics, Public Health Service, U.S. Department of Health and Human Services, Hyattsville, Md. 713 pp.

Neligan, G.A., I. Kolvin, D.McI. Scott, and R.F. Garside. 1976. Born Too Soon or Born Too Small: A Follow-up Study to Seven Years of Age. Clinics in Developmental Medicine, No. 61. Heineman, London. 101 pp.

Newcombe, R.G. 1982. Development of obesity in parous women. J. Epidemiol. Community Health 36:306-309.

Noppa, H., and C. Bengtsson. 1980. Obesity in relation to socioeconomic status: a population study of women in Göteborg, Sweden. J. Epidemiol. Community Health 34:139-142.

NRC (National Research Council). 1970. Maternal Nutrition and the Course of Pregnancy. Report of the Committee on Maternal Nutrition, Food and Nutrition Board. National Academy of Sciences, Washington, D.C. 241 pp.

O'Grady, J.F., F.W.H. Elsley, R.M. MacPherson, and I. McDonald. 1973. The response of lactating sows and their litters to different dietary energy allowances. 1. Milk yield and composition, reproductive performance of sows and growth rate of litters. Anim. Prod. 17:65-74.

Ounsted, M., and A. Scott. 1981. Associations between maternal weight, height, weight-for-height, weight-gain and birth weight. Pp. 113-129 in J. Dobbing, ed. Maternal Nutrition in Pregnancy: Eating for Two? Academic Press, London.

Ounsted, M., and M.E. Taylor. 1971. The postnatal growth of children who were small-for-dates or large-for-dates at birth. Dev. Med. Child Neurol. 13:421-434.

Ounsted, M., V. Moar, and W.A. Scott. 1981. Perinatal morbidity and mortality in small-for-date babies: the relative importance of some maternal factors. Early Hum. Dev. 5:367-375.

Ounsted, M.K., V.A. Moar, and A. Scott. 1984. Children of deviant birthweight at the age of seven years: health, handicap, size and developmental status. Early Hum. Dev. 9:323-340.

Ounsted, M., V.A. Moar, and A. Scott. 1988. Neurological development of small-for-gestational age babies during the first year of life. Early Hum. Dev. 16:163-172.

Papiernik, E., and M. Kaminski. 1974. Multifactorial study of the risk of prematurity at 32 weeks of gestation. I. A study of the frequency of 30 predictive characteristics. J. Perinat. Med. 2:30-36.

Paul, A.A., E.M. Muller, and R.G. Whitehead. 1979. The quantitative effects of maternal dietary energy intake on pregnancy and lactation in rural Gambian women. Trans. R. Soc. Trop. Med. Hyg. 73:686-692.

Pebley, A.R., S.L. Huffman, A.K.M.A. Chowdhury, and P.W. Stupp. 1985. Intra-uterine mortality and maternal nutritional status in rural Bangladesh. Popul. Stud. 39:425-440.

Picone, T.A., L.H. Allen, P.N. Olsen, and M.E. Ferris. 1982. Pregnancy outcome in North American women. II. Effects of diet, cigarette smoking, stress, and weight gain on placentas, and on neonatal physical and behavioral characteristics. Am. J. Clin. Nutr. 36:1214-1224.

Pipe, N.G.J., T. Smith, D. Halliday, C.J. Edmonds, C. Williams, and T.M. Coltart. 1979. Changes in fat, fat-free mass and body water in human normal pregnancy. Br. J. Obstet. Gynaecol. 86:929-940.

Placek, P.J., and S.M. Taffel. 1980. Trends in cesarean section rates for the United States, 1970-78. Public Health Rep. 95:540-548.

Placek, P.J., S. Taffel, and M. Moien. 1983. Cesarean section delivery rates: United States, 1981. Am. J. Public Health 73:861-862.

Prentice, A.M., and R.G. Whitehead. 1987. The energetics of human reproduction. Symp. Zool. Soc. London 57:275-304.

Prentice, A.M., R.G. Whitehead, M. Watkinson, W.H. Lamb, and T.J. Cole. 1983. Prenatal dietary supplementation of African women and birth-weight. Lancet 1:489-492.

Ribeiro, M.D., Z. Stein, M. Susser, P. Cohen, and R. Neugut. 1982. Prenatal starvation and maternal blood pressure near delivery. Am. J. Clin. Nutr. 35:535-541.

Risch, H.A., N.S. Weiss, E.A. Clarke, and A.B. Miller. 1988. Risk factors for spontaneous abortion and its recurrence. Am. J. Epidemiol. 128:420-430.

Rookus, M.A., P. Rokebrand, J. Burema, and P. Deurenberg. 1987. The effect of pregnancy on the body mass index 9 months postpartum in 49 women. Int. J. Obesity 11:609-618.

Rosso, P. 1985. A new chart to monitor weight gain during pregnancy. Am. J. Clin. Nutr. 41:644-652.

Rubin, R.A., C. Rosenblatt, and B. Balow. 1973. Psychological and educational sequelae of prematurity. Pediatrics 52:352-363.

Sachs, B.P., D.A.J. Brown, S.G. Driscoll, E. Schulman, D. Acker, B.J. Ransil, and J.F. Jewett. 1987. Maternal mortality in Massachusetts: trends and prevention. N. Engl. J. Med. 316:667-672.

Sadurskis, A. 1988. Energy Costs of Pregnant and Lactating Females in Relation to Nutritional Status and Energy Intake. Studies in Humans and Rats. Dissertation, Department of Medical Nutrition, Karolinska Institute, Stockholm, Sweden. 60 pp.

Sadurskis, A., N. Kabir, J. Wager, and E. Forsum. 1988. Energy metabolism, body composition, and milk production in healthy Swedish women during lactation. Am. J. Clin. Nutr. 48:44-49.

Samra, J.S., L.C.H. Tang, and M.S. Obhrai. 1988. Changes in body weight between consecutive pregnancies. Lancet 2:1420-1421.

Sandmire, H.F., and T.J. O'Halloin. 1988. Shoulder dystocia: its incidence and associated risk factors. Int. J. Gynaecol. Obstet. 26:65-73.

Scholl, T.O., E. Decker, R.J. Karp, G. Greene, and M. De Sales. 1984. Early adolescent pregnancy: a comparative study of pregnancy outcome in young adolescents and mature women. J. Adol. Health Care 5:167-171.

Scholl, T.O., R.W. Salmon, L.K. Miller, P. Vasilenko III, C.H. Furey, and M. Christine. 1988. Weight gain during adolescent pregnancy: associated maternal characteristics and effects on birth weight. J. Adol. Health Care 9:286-290.

Scholl, T.O., M.L. Hediger, R.W. Salmon, D.H. Belsky, and I.G. Ances. 1989. Influence of prepregnant body mass and weight gain for gestation on spontaneous preterm delivery and duration of gestation during adolescent pregnancy. Am. J. Hum. Biol. 1:657-664.

Seidman, D.S., P. Ever-Hadani, and R. Gale. 1989. The effect of maternal weight gain in pregnancy on birth weight. Obstet. Gynecol. 74:240-246.

Shapiro, S., M.C. McCormick, B.H. Starfield, J.P. Krischer, and D. Bross. 1980. Relevance of correlates of infant deaths for significant morbidity at 1 year of age. Am. J. Obstet. Gynecol. 136:363-373.

Shepard, M.J., K.G. Hellenbrand, and M.B. Bracken. 1986. Proportional weight gain and complications of pregnancy, labor, and delivery in healthy women of normal prepregnant stature. Am. J. Obstet. Gynecol. 155:947-954.

Singer, J.E., M. Westphal, and K. Niswander. 1968. Relationship of weight gain during pregnancy to birth weight and infant growth and development in the first year of life: a report from the Collaborative Study of Cerebral Palsy. Obstet. Gynecol. 31:417-423.

Smith, C.A. 1947. The effect of wartime starvation in Holland upon pregnancy and its product. Am. J. Obstet. Gynecol. 53:599-608.

Stander, H.J., and J.B. Pastore. 1940. Weight changes during pregnancy and puerperium. Am. J. Obstet. Gynecol. 39:928-937.

Stein, A. 1989. Maternal pre-pregnant nutritional status and the risk for spontaneous abortion. Master's Essay. Columbia University School of Public Health, New York.

Stein, Z., M. Susser, G. Saenger, and F. Marolla. 1975. Famine and Human Development: The Dutch Hunger Winter of 1944-1945. Oxford University Press, New York. 284 pp.

Taffel, S.M. 1986. Maternal Weight Gain and the Outcome of Pregnancy: United States, 1980. Vital and Health Statistics, Series 21, No. 44. DHHS Publ. No. (PHS) 86-1922. National Center for Health Statistics, Public Health Service, U.S. Department of Health and Human Services, Hyattsville, Md. 25 pp.

Taffel, S.M., and K.G. Keppel. 1986. Advice about weight gain during pregnancy and actual weight gain. Am. J. Public Health 76:1396-1399.

Tavris, D.R., and J.A. Read. 1982. Effect of maternal weight gain on fetal, infant, and childhood death and on cognitive development. Obstet. Gynecol. 60:689-694.

Thomson, A.M., and W.Z. Billewicz. 1957. Clinical significance of weight trends during pregnancy. Br. Med. J. 1:243-247.

Thomson, A.M., F.E. Hytten, and W.Z. Billewicz. 1967. The epidemiology of oedema during pregnancy. J. Obstet. Gynaecol. Br. Commonw. 74:1-10.

Tompkins, W.T., and D.G. Wiehl. 1951. Nutritional deficiencies as a causal factor in toxemia and premature labor. Am. J. Obstet. Gynecol. 62:898-919.

Tompkins, W.T., D.G. Wiehl, and R.M. Mitchell. 1955. The underweight patient as an increased obstetric hazard. Am. J. Obstet. Gynecol. 69:114-123.

Udall, J.N., G.G. Harrison, Y. Vaucher, P.D. Walson, and G. Morrow III. 1978. Interaction of maternal and neonatal obesity. Pediatrics 62:17-21.

Usher, R.H. 1970. Clinical and therapeutic aspects of fetal malnutrition. Pediatr. Clin. North Am. 17:169-183.

van den Berg, B.J., and F.W. Oechsli. 1984. Prematurity. Pp. 69-85 in M.B. Bracken, ed. Perinatal Epidemiology. Oxford University Press, New York.

van Steenbergen, W.M., J.A. Kusin, S. Kardjati, and C. de With. 1989. Energy supplementation in the last trimester of pregnancy in East Java, Indonesia: effect on breast-milk output. Am. J. Clin. Nutr. 50:274-279.

Varma, T.R. 1984. Maternal weight and weight gain in pregnancy and obstetric outcome. Int. J. Gynaecol. Obstet. 22:161-166.

Viegas, O.A.C., P.H. Scott, T.J. Cole, P. Eaton, P.G. Needham, and B.A. Wharton. 1982. Dietary protein energy supplementation of pregnant Asian mothers at Sorrento, Birmingham. II. Selective during third trimester only. Br. Med. J. 285:592-595.

Viegas, O.A.C., T.J. Cole, and B.A. Wharton. 1987. Impaired fat deposition in pregnancy: an indicator for nutritional intervention. Am. J. Clin. Nutr. 45:23-28.

Villar, J., V. Smeriglio, R. Martorell, C.H. Brown, and R.E. Klein. 1984. Heterogeneous growth and mental development of intrauterine growth-retarded infants during the first 3 years of life. Pediatrics 74:783-791.

Walther, F.J. 1988. Growth and development of term disproportionate small-for-gestational age infants at the age of 7 years. Early Hum. Dev. 18:1-11.

Walther, F.J., and L.H.J. Ramaekers. 1982. Growth in early childhood of newborns affected by disproportionate intrauterine growth retardation. Acta Paediatr. Scand. 71:651-656.

Westwood, M., M.S. Kramer, D. Munz, J.M. Lovett, and G.V. Watters. 1983. Growth and development of full-term nonasphyxiated small-for-gestational-age newborns: follow-up through adolescence. Pediatrics 71:376-382.

WHO (World Health Organization). 1965. Nutrition in Pregnancy and Lactation. Report of a WHO Expert Committee. Technical Report Series No. 302. World Health Organization, Geneva. 54 pp.

Winikoff, B., and C.H. Debrovner. 1981. Anthropometric determinants of birth weight. Obstet. Gynecol. 58:678-684.

Yerushalmy, J., B.J. van den Berg, C.L. Erhardt, and H. Jacobziner. 1965. Birth weight and gestation as indices of "immaturity". Am. J. Dis. Child. 109:43-57.

Ylitalo, V., P. Kero, and R. Erkkola. 1988. Neurological outcome of twins dissimilar in size at birth. Early Hum. Dev. 17:245-255.

9

Weight Gain in Twin Pregnancies

Twin pregnancies are excluded from most pregnancy studies. Although some reports give infant weights for large numbers of twin births, few provide data on maternal weight gain, body composition changes, or postpartum weight loss. A better understanding of twin pregnancies could be of major public health importance. In the United States in 1986, less than 2% of all births were twin births, but 16% of the low-birth-weight infants were twins (NCHS, 1988); infant mortality is also correspondingly higher in twin births. Figure 9-1 illustrates the continuing high incidence of low birth weight and very low birth weight among twins.

Weight gain in a twin pregnancy is expected to exceed weight gain in a single-fetus pregnancy because of greater increases in both maternal tissues and intrauterine weight. Selection of twin pregnancies to identify the appropriate weight gain or the normal or optimal course poses a number of problems, in addition to those encountered in studying singleton pregnancies, specifically:

• More mothers of twins may have taken action to restrict their weight gain, especially if they do not know until late in gestation that they are pregnant with twins.

• Many twin infants have low birth weights, even at full-term.

• Outcomes may differ for mixed-sex twin pairs in comparison with those for same-sex pairs.

• Many twin deliveries are preterm.

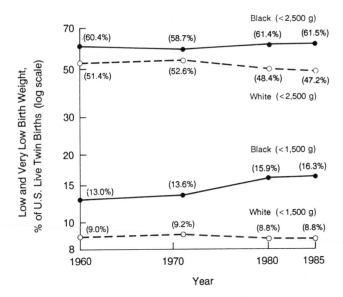

FIGURE 9-1 Trends in low and very low birth weight of live-born twins in the United States from 1960 through 1985. Based on unpublished data from the National Vital Statistics System, computed by the Division of Analysis from data compiled by the Division of Vital Statistics, National Center for Health Statistics.

• Elective cesarean delivery and labor induction before 40 weeks of gestation are more common for women carrying twins.

• Certain complications (e.g., preeclampsia and anemia) are more common for women carrying twins.

• Outcomes may differ for monozygotic and dizygotic twins.

Standards for identifying a normal twin pregnancy have not yet been established. Some studies indicate that approximately one-third of twin births occur before 37 weeks of gestation (Ho and Wu, 1975) and that the mean gestational age at delivery is near 37 weeks (see Tables 9-1A and 9-1B). Longer gestations, with the resultant higher birth weights and lower mortalities, might be achievable if more could be learned about the physiology and progress of optimal twin pregnancies. Although the birth weights of twins start to fall below the weights of similar-aged infants at about 30 weeks of gestation, it is arguable whether this difference should be accepted as inevitable.

If twins have not yet been identified during prenatal care, high maternal weight gain (especially early in pregnancy) may lead to self-imposed food restriction or may stimulate warnings from the health care provider for the woman to curb her food intake. If twins are expected, concern about hypertension (more frequent in women with twin pregnancies) may also

TABLE 9-1A   Mean Birth Weights of Twins of Both Genders Combined

Location of Study and Reference	Number of Twin Pairs	Stage of Gestation at Birth, wk	Mean Birth Weights, g ± SD[a] Twin 1	Twin 2	Both Twins
New Haven, Conn., USA Yarkoni et al., 1987	35	37.5	2,673 ± 582	2,614 ± 490	NR[b]
Chicago, Ill., USA Keith et al., 1980	488	NR	2,388 ± 742	2,314 ± 766	NR
Sweden Grennert et al., 1978	153	NR	2,540[c]	2,470[c]	NR
Holland Hofman, 1984	239	37.4	NR	NR	2,388 ± 576
Finland Lammintausta and Erkkola, 1979	10	36.8	2,720 ± 310[d]	2,743 ± 332[d]	
Africa Farrell, 1964	1,000	NR	2,385[c]	2,349[c]	2,367[c]

[a] SD = Standard deviation.
[b] NR = Not reported.
[c] Standard deviation was not reported.
[d] Standard deviation was derived from the reported data.

TABLE 9-1B   Mean Birth Weight of Twins, by Gender and Zygosity When Known

Reference and Location of Study	Birth Weight ± SD[a] by Gender and Zygosity Males Dizygotic	Monozygotic	Females Dizygotic	Monozygotic
Corney et al., 1981 Oxford, United Kingdom	2,728 ± 516, N[b] = 160	2,595 ± 684, N = 36	2,601 ± 490, N = 144	2,385 ± 607, N = 18
Aberdeen, United Kingdom	2,542 ± 591, N = 110	2,439 ± 528, N = 56	2,557 ± 516, N = 112	2,428 ± 463, N = 48
Pilic et al., 1985 Belgrad, Yugoslavia	2,455 ± 704,[c] N = 360		2,316 ± 651,[c] N = 360	

[a] SD = Standard deviation.
[b] N = sample size.
[c] Zygosity not specified.

result in some degree of dietary control. Current data do not address these issues and their possible contribution to observed outcomes. In the following sections, data on pregnancy outcome are reviewed along with information on maternal factors that might influence pregnancy outcome.

MORTALITY

The high mortality rates of twins appear to be influenced by the preponderance of low-weight, early births. In England and Wales in 1983, twins represented 2% of all births but 9% of perinatal deaths (Botting et al., 1987). Declining twin mortality rates over time have been documented in several studies (De Muylder et al., 1982; van der Pol et al., 1982). A decrease in the proportion of low-birth-weight twins would have a very large effect on mortality. However, since preterm delivery leads to a substantial proportion of the lower mean birth weight of twins, effective interventions may be dependent on improved understanding of the factors that contribute to early labor.

BIRTH WEIGHT

Table 9-1A and 9-1B include data on twin birth weights from several studies, more than half of which were conducted outside of the United States. In twin pregnancies, as in singleton pregnancies, birth weight is lower in female infants, infants born to primiparous women (van der Pol et al., 1982), and infants of smokers (Luke, 1987), as well as in the second twin. The data indicate that twin mean birth weight is as much as 700 g lower than the singleton birth weight and that gestation is about 2 to 3 weeks shorter. As in singleton pregnancies, it has also been shown that light-for-date twins have lower weight placentas than those of appropriate-for-date twins (Tayama et al., 1983).

GESTATION LENGTH AND LOW BIRTH WEIGHT

The mean gestation length for twins is between 37 and 38 weeks (Tables 9-1A and 9-1B). Preterm delivery rates of 42.2% have been reported in Canada (De Muylder et al., 1982). Low-birth-weight rates were higher in live-born white twins in the United States during a similar period, specifically, 51.4% in 1960 declining to 47.2% in 1985 (J. Kleinman, National Center for Health Statistics, personal communication, 1989). Iffy et al. (1983) examined twin and single fetuses that were aborted 8.5 to 21 weeks after the last menstrual period and concluded that twin fetuses may be about 6 days younger than would ordinarily be estimated from the date of the last menstrual period. This conclusion would be consistent with the smaller head size noted in twins throughout gestation, but means that they are even younger at delivery than their generally early delivery date indicates.

MATERNAL FACTORS

Physical Characteristics and Weight Gain

In one observational study, Konwinski et al. (1974) noted that none of the five women weighing over 65 kg (143 lb) before pregnancy delivered at or before 37 weeks of gestation, whereas 15 of the 22 women weighing less than 65 kg (143 lb) delivered early. No such relationship was found between length of gestation and insufficient pregnancy weight gain (categorized as <6 kg, or 13 lb, at 28 weeks, <7 kg, or 15 lb, at 32 weeks; and <8 kg, or ~18 lb, at 36 weeks of gestation). However, a statistically significant increase in preterm delivery *was* observed in those twin gestations in which the mother lost 1 kg or more between weeks 32 and 36 of gestation. More recently, Luke (1987) has related low early weight gain to preterm delivery of twins.

In an observational, prospective study of 132 twin pregnancies, Houlton et al. (1981) have shown that obese mothers have a reduced risk for one or both twins to be growth retarded. They also identified a maternal height of less than 156 cm (~61 in.) and a weight loss or stable weight over three consecutive prenatal visits as factors that were predictive of twins at risk for growth retardation.

Weight gains in twin pregnancies have been reported in a few studies. In Finland, Lammintausta and Erkkola (1979) observed that maternal weight gain through 30 to 33 weeks of gestation was 11.4 ± 1.6 kg (25 ± 3.5 lb; mean ± standard deviation). If weight gain had continued at the same rate until 37 weeks of gestation, from 13 to 14 kg (29 to 31 lb) would have been gained. Schneider et al. (1978) distinguished weight gain by zygosity in a prospective study of 86 twin pregnancies. By week 36 of gestation, mothers of monozygotic twins had gained 12.25 kg ± 4.27SD (27.0 ± 9.4 lb) and mothers of dizygotic twins had gained 13.86 ± 4.18 kg (30.5 ± 9.2 lb) (not significantly different). An earlier study in France also showed higher weight gains at 28 weeks of gestation by mothers of dizygotic twins (Konwinski et al., 1974) (see Table 9-2).

Using data from earlier studies, Campbell (1986) reported a mean weight gain of 14.6 kg (32.1 lb) at 36 weeks of gestation in twin pregnancies and a mean gain of 11.1 kg (24.4 lb) in the same period in singleton pregnancies (standard deviation and number of participants were not given; Table 9-3). The reported difference in weight gain barely accounted for the difference that would be expected from the weight of the additional fetus

TABLE 9-2   Weight Gain in Women Bearing Monozygotic or Dizygotic Twins

Reference and Study Population Size	Length of Gestation, wk	Mean Maternal Weight Gain ± SD,[a] kg, by Type of Twin Pregnancy	
		Monozygotic	Dizygotic
Schneider et al., 1978;	28	8.89 ± 3.43[b]	10.18 ± 3.13[b]
monozygotic: N = 40;	32	10.95 ± 3.84[b]	10.95 ± 3.46[b]
dizygotic: N = 46	36	12.25 ± 4.27[b]	13.86 ± 4.18[b]
Konwinski et al., 1974 (population size not reported)	28	7.3 ± 1.7[c]	8.3 ± 1.5[c]

[a] SD = Standard deviation.
[b] Standard deviation was erroneously reported as standard error.
[c] It was not stated whether this variance represented standard deviation or standard error.

TABLE 9-3   Weight Gain in Twin and Singleton Pregnancies[a]

Period of Gestation, wk	Weight Gain, kg/wk, by Type of Pregnancy[b]	
	Single	Twin
13–20	0.42	0.60
20–30	0.47	0.54
30–36	0.40	0.64
0–36	11.1 kg total gain	14.6 kg total gain

[a] From Campbell (1986) with permission.
[b] Standard deviations not given.

and placenta and thus does not indicate additional weight increases in the body of the twin-bearing mother.

Three studies, two of which were reported as abstracts, have provided more current data. Luke (1987) found a rate of weight gain in twin pregnancies of nonsmokers (Table 9-4) that was higher than the rate reported by Campbell (1986; Table 9-3), but the rate for smokers was not. The data in Table 9-4 indicate that a lower rate of early weight gain may contribute to early delivery in both smokers and nonsmokers. Their data also show that smokers have lower-weight infants at term (2,478 g) than do nonsmokers (2,692 g).

Brown and Schloesser (1989) studied the birth records of nearly 2,000 twins born in Kansas from 1980 to 1986. They found that birth weight increased with increasing maternal weight gain (not controlled for length

TABLE 9-4   Weight Gain During Twin Gestations in
Smokers and Nonsmokers[a]

| Period of Gestation, wk | Weight Gain, kg/wk, by Maternal Smoking Status[b] | |
	Nonsmokers	Smokers
0 to 30	0.72	0.60
30 to birth, preterm	0.57	0.50
30 to birth, at full term	0.88	0.65
0 to 38	13 kg total gain	10.5 kg total gain

[a] Based on Luke (1987).
[b] Standard deviations not given.

of gestation). The rate of low birth weight ranged from a high of 32.3%
in underweight women to 20.0% in very obese women, based on maternal
prepregnancy weight for height. The lowest perinatal mortality occurred in
the 3,000- to 3,500-g birth-weight group. For this group, maternal weight
gain was 20.1 kg (44.2 lb) for underweight women, 18.6 kg (40.9 lb) for
normal-weight women, and 13.3 kg (29.2 lb) for very obese women.

A retrospective medical records study of 217 twin pregnancies of
women over age 18 delivering in Seattle, Washington, indicated that unrestricted weight gain (from prepregnancy to within 1 week of delivery) was
18.5 kg (40.6 lb) (Pederson et al., 1989). The prepregnancy weight averaged
63.2 kg (139.6 lb). Weight gain averaged 20 kg (44 lb) for those mothers
who gave birth at term to two live-born infants weighing at least 2,500 g
and with 5-minute Apgar scores of at least 7, termed "optimal outcome."
Mothers with a "less than optimal outcome" had gained 16.8 kg (37 lb).
(For the entire group, the mean birth weight was 2,602 ± 586.6 g and the
mean gestational age was 36.9 ± 3.2 weeks.)

Data from the 1980 National Natality Survey for 124 white, non-
Hispanic, married mothers carrying twins are shown in Table 9-5. On
average, mothers of twins gained approximately 2 to 4 kg (4 to 9 lb) more
than did mothers of single infants. Adjustment for increased placental
weight in twin pregnancies changes these figures only slightly. The data in
Table 9-5 provide evidence that mothers of twins in the United States gain
more per week than do those who have single births.

In general, the study results are consistent in that they show a relationship of weight gain to birth weight and low-birth-weight rates in twin as
well as in singleton pregnancies. A relationship of weight gain to duration
is less uniformly reported. Weight gains in twin pregnancies with good
birth weight outcomes are substantially higher than they are in singleton
pregnancies, averaging about 22 kg (44 lb).

TABLE 9-5   Comparison of Full-Term Total Weight Gain and Net Gain per Week for Women Delivering Single and Twin Births, by Body Mass Index (BMI)[a]

| | Maternal Weight Gain, kg, by Type of Birth (and Sample Size) | | | |
| | Single | | Twin | |
BMI Category	Total Weight Gain, kg	Net Weight Gain per Week, kg[b]	Total Weight Gain, kg	Net Weight Gain per Week, kg[b]
Low (<19.8)	13.6	0.27	18.2	0.37
	(N = 1,027)		(N = 31)	
Moderate (19.8–26.0)	13.8	0.26	17.7	0.37
	(N = 2,393)		(N = 62)	
High (>26.0)	12.4	0.21	14.1	0.25
	(N = 526)		(N = 31)	

[a] Unpublished data based on the 1980 National Natality Survey.
[b] Net weight gain per week is calculated by subtracting the weight of the baby from the total gestational weight gain before computing the weekly gain.

Body Composition

It is not clear from body composition studies of twin pregnancies whether the additional maternal weight gain is composed of maternal fat or lean tissue. Internal contradictions in reported studies (Campbell, 1983, 1986; Campbell and MacGillivray, 1977) suggest that they are unreliable and do not warrant discussion. Further study is clearly needed.

Physiologic Adaptations

Romney et al. (1955) found that uterine circulation in one twin gestation was double the average value observed in a set of five singleton pregnancies. It is of interest that this twin pregnancy was a full-term pregnancy—the two infants weighed 3.3 and 3.6 kg. Adequate uterine circulation may be critical to maintaining the growth of the twins late in pregnancy.

In another study, calcium balance remained positive in a woman pregnant with twins, largely because of a marked reduction in urinary calcium excretion (Duggin et al., 1974). Several studies demonstrated that levels of many of the major pregnancy hormones are higher in twin pregnancies than they are in singleton pregnancies (e.g., Knight et al., 1981; MacGillivray, 1978; Tayama et al., 1983). These hormones could contribute to augmenting pregnancy adjustments, increasing weight gain (Schneider et al., 1978), and altering maternal body composition.

SUMMARY

The literature suggests that in twin pregnancies weight gain is higher than the weight accounted for by the mass of the additional conceptus. Data on the association of twin weight with mortality indicate that birth weights that are similar to those of singleton births, and that are much higher than the usual birth weights of twins, are associated with minimum perinatal mortality. As in singleton pregnancies, twin birth weight appears to be related to maternal weight gain and inversely related to maternal smoking. Evidence suggests that maternal weight gain in a twin pregnancy is related to both the length of gestation and the percentage of infants born with a low birth weight.

Since information on body composition is incomplete and unreliable, it is not possible to draw conclusions about the components of the additional weight gain. Limited information suggests that physiologic and metabolic adaptations are greater during twin pregnancies than they are in singleton pregnancies. This information is consistent with observations on weight gain but is insufficient to provide a definitive statement about which changes are necessary for a successful twin pregnancy.

CLINICAL IMPLICATIONS

Total weight gain of 16 to 20.5 kg (35 to 45 lb) is consistent with a favorable outcome of a full-term twin pregnancy. This suggests that a woman who is pregnant with twins should aim for a weekly weight gain of approximately 0.75 kg (1.5 lb) during the second and third trimesters of pregnancy.

REFERENCES

Botting, B.J., I.M. Davies, and A.J. MacFarlane. 1987. Recent trends in the incidence of multiple births and associated mortality. Arch. Dis. Child. 62:941-950.

Brown, J.E., and P. Schloesser. 1989. Prepregnancy weight status, prenatal weight gain, birth weight, and perinatal mortality relationships in term, twin pregnancies. FASEB J. 3:A648.

Campbell, D.M. 1983. Dietary restriction in obesity and its effect on neonatal outcome. Pp. 243-250 in D.M. Campbell and M.D.G. Gillmer, eds. Nutrition in Pregnancy: Proceedings of the Tenth Study Group in the Royal College of Obstetricians and Gynaecologists, September, 1982. The Royal College of Obstetricians and Gynaecologists, London.

Campbell, D.M. 1986. Maternal adaptation in twin pregnancy. Semin. Perinatol. 10:14-18.

Campbell, D.M., and I. MacGillivray. 1977. Maternal physiological responses and birthweight in singleton and twin pregnancies by parity. Eur. J. Obstet., Gynecol. Reprod. Biol. 7:17-24.

Corney, G., D. Seedburgh, B. Thompson, D.M. Campbell, I. MacGillivray, and D. Timlin. 1981. Multiple and singleton pregnancy: differences between mothers as well as offspring. Prog. Clin. Biol. Res. 69A:107-114.

De Muylder, X., J.M. Moutquin, M.F. Desgranges, B. Leduc, and F. Lazaro-Lopez. 1982. Obstetrical profile of twin pregnancies: a retrospective review of 11 years (1969-1979) at Hôspital Notre-Dame, Montréal, Canada. Acta. Genet. Med. Gemellol. 31:149-155.

Duggin, G.G., N.E. Dale, R.C. Lyneham, R.A. Evans, and D.J. Tiller. 1974. Calcium balance in pregnancy. Lancet 2:926-927.

Farrell, A.G.W. 1964. Twin pregnancy: a study of 1,000 cases. S. Afr. J. Obstet. Gynaecol. 2:35-41.

Grennert, L., P.H. Persson, and G. Gennser. 1978. Intrauterine growth of twins judged by BPD measurements. Acta Obstet. Gynecol. Scand., Suppl. 78:28-32.

Ho, S.K., and P.Y.K. Wu. 1975. Perinatal factors and neonatal morbidity in twin pregnancy. Am. J. Obstet. Gynecol. 122:979-987.

Hofman, M.A. 1984. Energy metabolism and relative brain size in human neonates from single and multiple gestations: an allometric study. Biol. Neonate 45:157-164.

Houlton, M.C.C., M. Marivate, and R.H. Philpott. 1981. The prediction of fetal growth retardation in twin pregnancy. Br. J. Obstet. Gynecol. 88:264-273.

Iffy, L., M.A. Lavenhar, A. Jakobovits, and H.A. Kaminetzky. 1983. The rate of early intrauterine growth in twin gestation. Am. J. Obstet. Gynecol. 146:970-972.

Keith, L., R. Ellis, G.S. Berger, and R. Depp. 1980. The Northwestern University Multihospital Twin Study. I. A description of 588 twin pregnancies and associated pregnancy loss, 1971 to 1975. Am. J. Obstet. Gynecol. 138:781-789.

Knight, G.J., E.M. Kloza, D.E. Smith, and J.E. Haddow. 1981. Efficiency of human placental lactogen and alpha-fetoprotein measurement in twin pregnancy detection. Am. J. Obstet. Gynecol. 141:585-586.

Konwinski, T., C. Gerard, A.M. Hult, and E. Papiernik-Berkhauer. 1974. Maternal pregestational weight and multiple pregnancy duration. Acta Genet. Med. Gemollol., Suppl. 22:44-47.

Lammintausta, R., and R. Erkkola. 1979. Effect of long-term salbutamol treatment on renin-aldosterone system in twin pregnancy. Acta Obstet. Gynecol. Scand. 58:447-451.

Luke, B. 1987. Twin births: influence of maternal weight on intrauterine growth and prematurity. Fed. Proc., Fed. Am. Soc. Exp. Biol. 46:1015.

MacGillivray, I. 1978. Twin pregnancies. Obstet. Gynecol. Annu. 7:135-151.

NCHS (National Center for Health Statistics). 1988. Vital Statistics of the United States, 1986. Vol. I—Natality. DHHS Publ. No. (PHS) 88-1123. National Center for Health Statistics, Public Health Service, U.S. Department of Health and Human Services, Hyattsville, Md. 454 pp.

Pederson, A.L., B. Worthington-Roberts, and D.E. Hickok. 1989. Weight gain patterns during twin gestation. J. Am. Diet. Assoc. 89:642-646.

Pilic, Z., V. Sulovic, S. Markovic, R. Radosevic, and V. Kesic. 1985. Genetic factors and fetal growth sex constitution and birthweight in twins. Int. J. Gynaecol. Obstet. 23:421-425.

Romney, S.L., D.E. Reid, J. Metcalfe, and C.S. Burwell. 1955. Oxygen utilization by the human fetus in utero. Am. J. Obstet. Gynecol. 70:791-799.

Schneider, L., M. Rigaud, J.L. Tabaste, P. Chebroux, B. Lacour, and J. Baudet. 1978. HPL measurements: relationships with maternal weight gain in twin pregnancy. Prog. Clin. Biol. Res. 24C:123-128.

Tayama, C., S. Ichimaru, M. Ito, M. Nakayama, M. Maeyama, and I. Miyakawa. 1983. Unconjugated estradiol, estriol and total estriol in maternal peripheral vein, cord vein, and cord artery serum at delivery in pregnancies with intrauterine growth retardation. Endocrinol. Jpn. 30:155-162.

van der Pol, J.G., O.P. Bleker, and P.E. Treffers. 1982. Clinical bedrest in twin pregnancies. Eur. J. Obstet., Gynecol. Reprod. Biol. 14:75-80.

Yarkoni, S., E.A. Reece, T. Holford, T.Z. O'Connor, and J.C. Hobbins. 1987. Estimated fetal weight in the evaluation of growth in twin gestations: a prospective longitudinal study. Obstet. Gynecol. 69:636-639.

10

Causality and Opportunities for Intervention

One of the major issues under consideration by this subcommittee is the relationship between gestational weight gain and a variety of maternal and child health outcomes. In particular, its interest focuses on gestational weight gain as an etiologic *determinant*, i.e., a cause, of these maternal and child outcomes. An understanding of cause is often a prerequisite for effecting change (improving maternal and child health). As mentioned in Chapters 2 and 4, however, low gestational weight gain might also be of potential value as a noncausal *marker* of risk for adverse pregnancy outcome.

A change in pregnancy outcome therefore depends on the ability to alter causal determinants. Since clinicians and public health practitioners cannot directly affect gestational weight gain (without surgically removing or adding tissue to the pregnant woman), factors that can be modified must be considered. The two major modifiable factors are energy intake and expenditure (as they have an impact on energy balance). But these can be modified only indirectly, such as by offering nutritional advice or supplementation, either in the context of regular prenatal care or as part of a special program. It may also be possible to change maternal attitudes that have an impact on energy intake, either by apprising the community of recent research findings and expert opinion or through more formal avenues of health education.

In identifying modifiable factors and the likely impact of such modifications on maternal and child health, the entire causal pathway depicted in Figure 2-3 must be considered, beginning with attitudes, counseling, and

222

supplementation and working through actual increases or decreases in energy intake; subsequent changes in gestational weight gain; the short-term maternal and fetal/child outcomes of pregnancy; and finally, longer-term maternal and child health. In the following section, these causal links are discussed in greater detail.

THE CAUSAL PATHS

Most of the evidence examined by the subcommittee concerns the possible causal relationship between gestational weight gain and a variety of short-term health outcomes for the mother (mortality, complications of pregnancy, lactation performance, and postpartum obesity) and the fetus and infant (mortality, fetal growth, gestational duration, spontaneous abortion, and congenital anomalies). As discussed in Chapter 2 and as shown in Figure 2-3, however, these limited causal paths require both proximal and distal extensions. They need to be extended proximally because neither clinical and public health interventions nor changes in maternal attitudes have a direct impact on gestational weight gain. Consideration must be given, at least briefly, to causal paths from maternal attitudes, nutritional counseling, and energy supplementation to energy intake, and from energy intake to gestational weight gain. The paths must be extended distally to examine the relationship between the short-term outcomes enumerated above and the longer-term maternal and child health outcomes that may be of greater importance. For the mother, the main long-term outcome of interest is obesity. For the child, such outcomes include all aspects of survival, morbidity, growth, and performance that could be affected by changes in fetal growth or gestational duration.

Very few reports directly link the proximal factors to the important long-term health outcomes at the end of the causal pathway. Exceptions include publications by Naeye and Chez (1981), Singer et al. (1968), and Tavris and Read (1982), which link childhood cognitive development to maternal weight gain. Moreover, there is no strong evidence that long-term outcomes are affected directly, i.e., independently of shorter-term outcomes. In the remainder of this chapter, therefore, discussion is limited to examination of the evidence involving each of the individual causal links. Although most of the evidence and most of the deliberations of the subcommittee focus on links between gestational weight gain and maternal and child outcomes, the entire causal pathway summarized in Figure 2-3 needs to be kept in mind when formulating recommendations and contemplating possible clinical or public health interventions.

In examining the evidence for causality in these individual links, the subcommittee based its inferences on standard epidemiologic criteria. These criteria include the strength, biologic gradient (dose-response effect), lack of bias, statistical significance, specificity, consistency, and biologic plausibility and coherence of the association between exposure (the putative cause) and outcome (DHEW, 1964; Hill 1965; Susser 1973, 1988).

THE EVIDENCE

Do Nutritional Counseling, Energy Supplementation, and Maternal Attitudes Affect Energy Intake?

Remarkably few studies have been conducted to assess the efficacy of nutritional counseling (without supplementation) on energy intake by pregnant women either within or outside the context of regular prenatal care. In early studies carried out at the Montreal Diet Dispensary, for example, counseling was combined with some degree of energy supplementation, and inappropriate comparisons were made between women who either were referred for or requested those nutrition services and those who did not (Higgins, 1976; Primrose and Higgins, 1971). Thus, the rather large increases in net energy intake (and birth weight) attributed to use of the nutrition services are likely to be overestimates. Rush (1981) attempted to pair-match Montreal Diet Dispensary participants and nonparticipants according to potential confounding factors. The increases in energy intake and birth weight were more modest than those reported by Higgins (1976) and Primrose and Higgins (1971), but they were still in the expected direction. Higgins et al. (1989) found an increase in infant birth weight among mothers who participated in the program in the second but not the first of two pregnancies, but they provided no data on differences in energy intake.

The Special Supplemental Food Program for Women, Infants, and Children (WIC) in the United States also includes a mixture of nutritional counseling and supplementation. Pregnant women are given vouchers that can be used to obtain highly nutritious foods; however, there is no guarantee that the women will consume these foods and not share them with others. Several evaluations of WIC, including the largest and most recent one by Rush et al. (1988), indicate that WIC participants increase their energy intake and have higher gestational weight gains as a result of participation in the program (Edozien et al., 1979; Endres et al., 1981; Metcoff et al., 1985; Rush et al., 1988). The net increase in energy intake is modest, however, probably on the order of 100 to 150 kcal/day.

Supplementation trials indicate that women who are given energy supplements during pregnancy increase their total energy intakes (Lechtig et al., 1975; Mora et al., 1979; Prentice et al., 1983; Rush et al., 1980), but in most studies, the magnitude of the increased intake ranged from 100 to 250 kcal/day—less than the energy content of the supplement provided. Larger increments have been achieved in certain undernourished populations in developing countries, e.g., in The Gambia (Prentice et al., 1983). The subcommittee found no formal research to determine the effect of maternal attitudes on energy intake. These attitudes change slowly in response to many factors, including the reporting (and mass media dissemination) of new research findings, recommendations by national and international bodies or individual experts, health education (including that provided at schools and public prenatal classes), practices of health care providers, and word of mouth. Such factors are difficult to measure objectively. Moreover, concurrent controls are often impossible to obtain, since entire countries tend to be exposed to the messages simultaneously. Before-and-after comparisons may therefore be the only feasible way to assess the influence of these factors on energy intake. Unfortunately, small changes in energy intake are also difficult to measure (see Chapter 7). Thus, any attempt to assess changes in energy intake as a consequence of (i.e., caused by) changes in maternal attitudes would be difficult, to say the least.

Nonetheless, as discussed in Chapter 3, authorities have increased their recommended energy intakes and target weight gains for pregnant women over the past 30 to 40 years, and these changes have been accompanied by corresponding increases in gestational weight gain. It is difficult to ascribe recent weight gain changes to anything other than increased energy intake during pregnancy (see discussion below). Although increased energy intake may be attributable, in part, to individual nutritional counseling by obstetricians, nurse-midwives, dietitians, and other health care professionals, it seems reasonable to infer that gradual changes in public awareness and maternal attitudes have also played a role.

Does Energy Intake Affect Gestational Weight Gain?

Everyday experience and carefully controlled experimental studies (Sims et al., 1968) have demonstrated that people who consume excess energy gain weight. There is no reason to believe that pregnant women are an exception to this general rule. Many of the clinical and epidemiologic studies linking energy intake to gestational weight gain have found rather modest, and often nonsignificant, correlations between the two, in part because most women with high energy intakes also have high energy expenditures and, in part, because of the difficulty of accurately measuring the change in energy intake. Problems in measurement of energy intake have probably led to underestimates of the true correlation between maternal energy intake and gestational weight gain.

The clearest evidence favoring the link between energy intake and gestational weight gain comes from studies of human famine and from supplementation trials. It is clear from the Dutch famine study that reduced energy intake leads to reduced gestational weight gain (Stein et al., 1975; Susser and Stein, 1982). It is equally clear from supplementation trials in both developed (Rush et al., 1980) and developing (Mora et al., 1979) countries that increased energy intake leads to larger maternal weight gains.

Does Gestational Weight Gain Affect Short-Term Maternal/Child Health?

Virtually all epidemiologic studies with adequate sample sizes have demonstrated an association between gestational weight gain and fetal growth. Many supplementation trials and observational studies have been based on rigorous epidemiologic methods to minimize most sources of bias; however, reverse causality (temporal precedence) has not received adequate attention. For example, the amount of weight that a woman gains during a pregnancy is influenced not only by the deposition of fat, protein, and glycogen stores potentially available for provision of nutrients to the fetus but also by large increases in body water. It is well known that expanded plasma volume and modest degrees of dependent edema are associated with favorable pregnancy outcomes (Campbell and MacGillivray, 1975; Duffus et al., 1971; Hytten and Thomson, 1976; Naeye, 1981a,b; Thomson et al., 1967); but in the absence of data establishing that increases in body water precede increases in fetal growth rate, they may just as likely be an effect, rather than a cause, of a well-functioning fetoplacental unit. A specific example of reverse causality is provided by the evidence that twin births are associated with higher *net* maternal weight gains. Thus, it seems clear that the fetus and placenta can affect maternal weight gain apart from the weight they contribute.

Furthermore, the amount of weight gained during pregnancy is influenced by the weights of the fetus, placenta, and amniotic fluid. Nonetheless, studies that examined net (i.e., maternal) weight gain have shown smaller, but consistent, effects on fetal growth (see Chapter 8).

The strongest evidence that gestational weight gain can affect fetal growth is provided by supplementation trials (Lechtig et al., 1975; Mora et al., 1979, Prentice et al., 1983; Rush et al., 1980) and studies of human famine (Stein et al., 1975; Susser and Stein, 1982). In both of these settings, changes in energy intake result in changes in both gestational weight gain and gestational age-adjusted birth weight. Both nutritional and nonnutritional (i.e., expansion of body water) factors may be involved in producing the effect of gestational weight gain on fetal growth, as suggested by the trial of Campbell and MacGillivray (1975) that included use of energy restriction and diuretics. The causal link is further strengthened by coincidental temporal trends over the last 20 to 30 years: increasing gestational weight gains and mean birth weights and decreasing rates of intrauterine growth retardation.

However, the magnitude of the causal effect size (e.g., increase in birth weight) is modest. The data indicate, for example, that in women with a normal prepregnancy weight for height, birth weight increases 20 g, on average, for a change of 1 kg in gestational weight gain (Kramer, 1987). Thus, a 5-kg (11-lb) difference in gestational weight gain is associated with an average difference in birth weight of only 100 g. The actual change in birth weight for an individual woman who increases or decreases her gestational weight gain by this amount is likely to vary considerably around this average. Moreover, the 20-g/kg effect is probably an overestimate, since the analyses in most studies are based on total rather than on net weight gain (see Chapter 4). When based on net weight gain, the effect appears to be reduced by one-third to about 13 g of birth weight per 1 kg (2.2 lb) of gestational weight gain (Kramer et al., 1989).

Given this modest effect size and the large variability in weight gains associated with optimal fetal growth, even within groups with similar prepregnancy weights for height, knowledge of an individual mother's weight gain does not substantially enhance her (or her physician's) ability to predict the growth of her fetus. Nor is the evidence bearing on this causal link particularly useful in the diagnostic setting. The low birth weight of an infant born to a mother who gained only 5 kg (11 lb) cannot, therefore, be confidently attributed to her low gestational weight gain, nor can the high birth weight of a baby whose mother gained 25 kg (55 lb) be attributed to the high gestational weight gain. Thus, despite the strong evidence that gestational weight gain *can* affect fetal growth, the chance that it *will* (or *did*) in an individual case may be far from clear (Kramer, 1988; Lane, 1984).

With regard to the effects of gestational weight gain on gestational duration, the evidence for causality is considerably weaker than that for fetal growth. Once again, reverse causality is a key issue and one that has not been adequately considered in most epidemiologic studies, especially those in which gestational weight gain has been based on total weight gain, rather than on early weight gain or rate of weight gain. Obviously, a pregnancy that ends prematurely will be associated with a smaller total weight gain, because the mother will have had less total time in which to gain weight.

Birth weight can be measured without appreciable random or systematic error. By contrast, as mentioned above, gestational age is difficult to estimate and errors in such estimates, particularly at the extremes of maturity (Kramer et al., 1988), are likely to lead to misclassification of some growth-retarded babies as preterm and preterm babies as growth retarded.

Nonetheless, evidence from many of the better epidemiologic studies does suggest that a low rate of gestational weight gain can increase the risk of preterm delivery (Abrams et al., 1989; Berkowitz, 1981; Hediger et al., 1989; Miller and Merritt, 1979; Scholl et al., 1989; van den Berg and Oechsli,

1984). The evidence is not unanimous, however (Kleinman, 1990), and there is no clear biologic mechanism whereby changes in gestational weight gain would lead to earlier or later labor and delivery. Furthermore, there has been no clear trend toward increasing gestational duration paralleling the increase in gestational weight gain in the United States during the past two or three decades. For all these reasons, the subcommittee finds that the evidence for an important causal impact on gestational duration is inconclusive.

There are fewer data concerning the links between gestational weight gain and the other short-term maternal and child outcomes shown in Figure 2-3. Data from the Collaborative Perinatal Project (Naeye, 1979) and the 1980 National Fetal Mortality Survey (Taffel, 1986) indicate an increased perinatal mortality rate among infants born to women with low gestational weight gains, especially those with low prepregnancy weights for height. The evidence does not suggest that gestational weight gain affects congenital anomalies, spontaneous abortion, maternal mortality, or the volume or composition of human milk during lactation.

Evidence from the large body of literature concerning the effects of gestational weight gain on fetal growth indicates that large gestational weight gains do increase the risk of high-birth-weight infants (Ounsted and Scott, 1981; Scholl et al., 1988; Udall et al., 1978), which can lead to fetopelvic disproportion and, secondarily, to increased risks of midforceps delivery, cesarean delivery, shoulder dystocia, meconium aspiration, clavicular fracture, brachial plexus injury, and neonatal asphyxia (Acker et al., 1985; Boyd et al., 1983; Koff and Potter, 1939; Modanlou et al., 1980; Sandmire and O'Halloin, 1988). But the magnitude of the effect of gestational weight gain on these outcomes appears to be small. In particular, very little of the recent marked increase in the rate at which cesarean deliveries are performed can be attributed to larger maternal weight gains. Finally, published evidence indicates that women who have large weight gains during pregnancy tend to remain somewhat heavier in the immediate postpartum period (Billewicz and Thomson, 1970; Greene et al., 1988).

Do Short-Term Maternal and Child Health Effects Lead to Longer-Term Effects?

Most of the questions about the long-term effects of gestational weight gain on maternal or child health concern postpartum maternal obesity and the survival, morbidity, growth, and performance of the offspring. Some maternal weight added during pregnancy may be retained permanently, particularly if weight is retained following each of several pregnancies (see Chapter 8). Further research in this area is clearly required. Obesity has well-documented adverse health consequences, including hypertension, non-insulin-dependent diabetes mellitus, gallbladder disease, osteoarthritis, and increased overall mortality (Hoffmans et al., 1988; Mann, 1974a,b; NIH, 1985; Van Itallie, 1979). Therefore, any tendency toward excessive fat retention must be regarded as undesirable. Fortunately, most women retain only an average of approximately 1 kg (2.2 lb) per pregnancy, although this figure might underestimate weight retentions associated with the large weight gains observed in recent years.

Most of the issues regarding the effects on the child focus on the prognostic implications of intrauterine growth retardation (IUGR) or high birth weight. There is fairly convincing evidence that IUGR infants have increased morbidity in the newborn period, including increased risks of polycythemia, hypoglycemia, hypocalcemia, and birth asphyxia (Arora et al., 1987; Kramer et al., 1989; Ounsted et al., 1988; Usher, 1970). The evidence also indicates that IUGR leads to small but persistent effects in stature, brain growth, and neurocognitive performance (as reviewed by Teberg et al., 1988), although control for confounding postnatal influences has not always been adequate in previous studies. In addition, a small but definite risk of fetal and infant mortality seems to be attributable to IUGR (Arora et al., 1987; Haas et al., 1987; Koops et al., 1982; Kramer et al., 1989; Usher, 1970). High-birth-weight infants, on the other hand, tend to be taller and heavier throughout childhood and have an increased risk of obesity (Binkin et al., 1988; Fisch et al., 1975; Kramer et al., 1985; Ounsted et al., 1982).

If there is confirmation of several recent studies suggesting that increased maternal weight gain can increase gestational duration and that women with low weight gain are at increased risk for preterm delivery, the promotion of gestational weight gain might have important long-term benefits for child health. Preterm infants, especially those born before 34 weeks of gestation, are at greatly increased risk for perinatal and infant mortality, as well as rather severe and persistent pulmonary and neurocognitive sequelae. The causal impact of preterm birth on these adverse outcomes is extremely well established and of large magnitude. Thus, even if insufficient gestational weight gain increases the risk of preterm birth only to a small degree, the negative effects on child health may be large. These considerations once again underline the need for further research on the link between maternal weight gain and gestational duration.

IMPLICATIONS

The evidence suggests that an across-the-board increase in gestational weight gain among U.S. women would have both beneficial and adverse effects on maternal and child health. Fetal and infant mortality would be reduced, as would the incidence of IUGR (and its short-term and longer-term sequelae). Such an increase in weight gain would also result in an increased risk of maternal obesity (and its secondary health sequelae) for women with very large weight gains and an increased incidence of high-birth-weight infants, which has some undeniable consequences both for mothers and infants.

A formal decision analysis, in which probabilities and utilities (values) are assigned to each potential outcome, might assist in balancing these risks and benefits. Essential components of such an analysis include the probability of each beneficial and adverse outcome occurring with and without nutritional counseling, energy supplementation, or changes in maternal attitudes and the value that mothers, children, and society place on each of those outcomes. Even then, it is important to consider who would be helped and who would be harmed, as well as whose values should be considered. For example, if increased energy intakes lead to an elevated risk of maternal obesity but better overall outcomes in the infants, how should risks to the mother be balanced against benefits to the child? And who will make the decision?

The analysis could be refined by taking into account the fact that the risks and benefits are likely to differ according to the mother's prepregnancy weight for height, existing energy intake, and other factors that affect the outcomes under consideration. It may well be possible to maximize benefits and minimize risks by focusing educational efforts, individual nutritional counseling, and energy supplementation on women who are undernourished or who have other risk factors. Increased energy intakes by such women can be expected to have a substantial impact on intrauterine growth and its longer-term child health sequelae without incurring the appreciable risks of maternal obesity and high birth weight.

Finally, even if the overall benefits of increased energy intake exceed the risks, and even if the above technical and philosophical objections can be overcome, society will need to consider the costs of these interventions. Cost-benefit and cost-effectiveness analytic techniques could be used to decide whether the net benefit is worth the expense, or whether the required resources can be more productively channeled in other directions. Public media campaigns, individual nutritional counseling, and energy supplementation all require financial resources. Even if those resources were kept within the maternal and child health sector, the benefit:cost ratio for the various interventions should be compared with that for public health and clinical interventions to convince mothers to stop smoking during pregnancy and with that for family planning and contraceptive services (particularly for adolescents). Although such a balancing of benefits, risks, and costs should play an important role in public health policy in this domain, these considerations extend considerably beyond the subcommittee's mandate.

REFERENCES

Abrams, B., V. Newman, T. Key, and J. Parker. 1989. Maternal weight gain and preterm delivery. Obstet. Gynecol. 74:577-583.

Acker, D.B., B.P. Sachs, and E.A. Friedman. 1985. Risk factors for shoulder dystocia. Obstet. Gynecol. 66:762-768.

Arora, N.K., V.K. Paul, and M. Singh. 1987. Morbidity and mortality in term infants with intrauterine growth retardation. J. Trop. Pediatr. 33:186-189.

Berkowitz, G.S. 1981. An epidemiologic study of preterm delivery. Am. J. Epidemiol. 113:81-92.

Billewicz, W.Z., and A.M. Thomson. 1970. Body weight in parous women. Br. J. Prev. Soc. Med. 24:97-104.

Binkin, N.J., R. Yip, L. Fleshood, and F.L. Trowbridge. 1988. Birth weight and childhood growth. Pediatrics 82:828-834.

Boyd, M.E., R.H. Usher, and F.H. McLean. 1983. Fetal macrosomia: prediction, risks, proposed management. Obstet. Gynecol. 61:715-722.

Campbell, D.M., and I. MacGillivray. 1975. The effect of a low calorie diet or a thiazide diuretic on the incidence of pre-eclampsia and on birth-weight. Br. J. Obstet. Gynaecol. 82:572-577.

DHEW (Department of Health, Education, and Welfare). 1964. Smoking and Health: Report of the Advisory Committee to the Surgeon General of the Public Health Service. PHS Publ. No. 1103. Public Health Service, U.S. Department of Health, Education, and Welfare. U.S. Government Printing Office, Washington, D.C. 387 pp.

Duffus, G.M., I. MacGillivray, and K.J. Dennis. 1971. The relationship between baby weight and changes in maternal weight, total body water, plasma volume, electrolytes and proteins, and urinary oestriol excretion. J. Obstet. Gynaecol. Br. Commonw. 78:97-104.

Edozien, J.C., B.R. Switzer, and R.B. Bryan. 1979. Medical evaluation of the Special Supplemental Food Program for Women, Infants, and Children. Am. J. Clin. Nutr. 32:677-692.

Endres, J.M., M. Sawicki, and J.A. Casper. 1981. Dietary assessment of pregnant women in a supplemental food program. J. Am. Diet. Assoc. 79:121-126.

Fisch, R.O., M.K. Bilek, and R. Ulstrom. 1975. Obesity and leanness at birth and their relationship to body habitus in later childhood. Pediatrics 56:521-528.

Greene, G.W., H. Smiciklas-Wright, T.O. Scholl, and R.J. Karp. 1988. Postpartum weight change: how much of the weight gained in pregnancy will be lost after delivery. Obstet. Gynecol. 71:701-707.

Haas, J.D., H. Balcazar, and L. Caulfield. 1987. Variation in early neonatal mortality for different types of fetal growth retardation. Am. J. Phys. Anthropol. 73:467-473.

Hediger, M.L., T.O. Scholl, D.H. Belsky, I.G. Ances, and R.W. Salmon. 1989. Patterns of weight gain in adolescent pregnancy: effects on birth weight and preterm delivery. Obstet. Gynecol. 74:6-12.

Higgins, A.C. 1976. Nutritional status and the outcome of pregnancy. J. Can. Diet. Assoc. 37:17-35.

Higgins, A.C., J.E. Moxley, P.B. Pencharz, D. Mikolainis, and S. Dubois. 1989. Impact of the Higgins Nutrition Intervention Program on birth weight: a within-mother analysis. J. Am. Diet. Assoc. 89:1097-1103.

Hill, A.B. 1965. The environment and disease: association or causation? Proc. R. Soc. Med. 58:295-300.

Hoffmans, M.D., D. Kromhout, and C. de Lezenne Coulander. 1988. The impact of body mass index of 78,612 18-year old Dutch men on 32-year mortality from all causes. J. Clin. Epidemiol. 41:749-756.

Hytten, F.E., and A.M. Thomson. 1976. Weight gain in pregnancy. Pp. 179-187 in M.D. Lindheimer, A.I. Katz, and F.P. Zuspan, eds. Hypertension in Pregnancy. John Wiley & Sons, New York.

Kleinman, J.C. 1990. Maternal Weight Gain During Pregnancy: Determinants and Consequences. NCHS Working Paper Series No. 33. National Center for Health Statistics, Public Health Service, U.S. Department of Health and Human Services, Hyattsville, Md. 24 pp.

Koff, A.K., and E.L. Potter. 1939. The complications associated with excessive development of the human fetus. Am. J. Obstet. Gynecol. 38:412-423.

Koops, B.L., L.J. Morgan, and F.C. Battaglia. 1982. Neonatal mortality risk in relation to birth weight and gestational age: update. J. Pediatr. 101:969-977.

Kramer, M.S. 1987. Determinants of low birth weight: methodological assessment and meta-analysis. Bull. W.H.O. 65:663-737.

Kramer, M.S. 1988. Causality. Pp. 255-269 in Clinical Epidemiology and Biostatistics: A Primer for Clinical Investigators and Decision-Makers. Springer-Verlag, Berlin.

Kramer, M.S., R.G. Barr, D.G. Leduc, C. Boisjoly, and I.B. Pless. 1985. Infant determinants of childhood weight and adiposity. J. Pediatr. 107:104-107.

Kramer, M.S., F.H. McLean, M.E. Boyd, and R.H. Usher. 1988. The validity of gestational age estimation by menstrual dating in term, preterm, and postterm gestations. J. Am. Med. Assoc. 260:3306-3308.

Kramer, M.S., F.H. McLean, M. Olivier, D.M. Willis, and R.H. Usher. 1989. Body proportionality and head and length 'sparing' in growth-retarded neonates: a critical reappraisal. Pediatrics 84:717-723.

Lane, D.A. 1984. A probabilist's view of causality assessment. Drug Inf. J. 18:323-330.

Lechtig, A., J.P. Habicht, H. Delgado, R.E. Klein, C. Yarbrough, and R. Martorell. 1975. Effect of food supplementation during pregnancy on birthweight. Pediatrics 56:508-520.

Mann, G.V. 1974a. The influence of obesity on health (first of two parts). N. Engl. J. Med. 291:178-185.

Mann, G.V. 1974b. The influence of obesity on health (second of two parts). N. Engl. J. Med. 291:226-232.

Metcoff, J., P. Costiloe, W.M. Crosby, S. Dutta, H.H. Sandstead, D. Milne, C.E. Bodwell, and S.H. Majors. 1985. Effect of food supplementation (WIC) during pregnancy on birth weight. Am. J. Clin. Nutr. 41:933-947.

Miller, H.C., and T.A. Merritt. 1979. Fetal Growth in Humans. Year Book Medical Publishers, Chicago. 180 pp.

Modanlou, H.D., W.L. Dorchester, A. Thorosian, and R.K. Freeman. 1980. Macrosomia—maternal, fetal, and neonatal implications. Obstet. Gynecol. 55:420-424.

Mora, J.O., B. de Paredes, M. Wagner, L. de Navarro, J. Suescum, N. Christiansen, and M.G. Herrera. 1979. Nutritional supplementation and the outcome of pregnancy. I. Birth weight. Am. J. Clin. Nutr. 32:455-462.

Naeye, R.L. 1979. Weight gain and the outcome of pregnancy. Am. J. Obstet. Gynecol. 135:3-9.

Naeye, R.L. 1981a. Maternal blood pressure and fetal growth. Am. J. Obstet. Gynecol. 141:780-787.

Naeye, R.L. 1981b. Nutritional/nonnutritional interactions that affect the outcome of pregnancy. Am. J. Clin. Nutr. 34:727-731.

Naeye, R.L., and R.A. Chez. 1981. Effects of maternal acetonuria and low pregnancy weight gain on children's psychomotor development. Am. J. Obstet. Gynecol. 139:189-193.

NIH (National Institutes of Health). 1985. Health implications of obesity: National Institutes of Health Consensus Development Conference Statement. Ann. Intern. Med. 103:1073-1077.

Ounsted, M., and A. Scott. 1981. Associations between maternal weight, height, weight-for-height, weight-gain and birth weight. Pp. 113-129 in J. Dobbing, ed. Maternal Nutrition in Pregnancy: Eating for Two? Academic Press, London.

Ounsted, M., V. Moar, and A. Scott. 1982. Growth in the first four years. II. Diversity within groups of small-for-date and large-for-date babies. Early Hum. Dev. 7:29-39.

Ounsted, M., V.A. Moar, and A. Scott. 1988. Neurological development of small-for-gestational age babies during the first year of life. Early Hum. Dev. 16:163-172.

Prentice, A.M., R.G. Whitehead, M. Watkinson, W.H. Lamb, and T.J. Cole. 1983. Prenatal dietary supplementation of African women and birth-weight. Lancet 1:489-492.

Primrose, T., and A. Higgins. 1971. A study in human antepartum nutrition. J. Reprod. Med. 7:257-264.

Rush, D. 1981. Nutritional services during pregnancy and birthweight: a retrospective matched pair analysis. Can. Med. Assoc. J. 125:567-576.

Rush, D., Z. Stein, and M. Susser. 1980. A randomized controlled trial of prenatal nutritional supplementation in New York City. Pediatrics 65:683-697.

Rush, D., N.L. Sloan, J. Leighton, J.M. Alvir, D.G. Horvitz, W.B. Seaver, G.C. Garbowski, S.S. Johnson, R.A. Kulka, M. Holt, J.W. Devore, J.T. Lynch, M.B. Woodside, and D.S. Shanklin. 1988. The National WIC Evaluation: evaluation of the Special Supplemental Food Program for Women, Infants, and Children. V. Longitudinal study of pregnant women. Am. J. Clin. Nutr. 48:439-483.

Sandmire, H.F., and T.J. O'Halloin. 1988. Shoulder dystocia: its incidence and associated risk factors. Int. J. Gynaecol. Obstet. 26:65-73.

Scholl, T.O., M.L. Hediger, I.G. Ances, and C.E. Cronk. 1988. Growth during early teenage pregnancies. Lancet 1:701-702.

Scholl, T.O., M.L. Hediger, R.W. Salmon, D.H. Belsky, and I.G. Ances. 1989. Influence of prepregnant body mass and weight gain for gestation on spontaneous preterm delivery and duration of gestation during adolescent pregnancy. Am. J. Hum. Biol. 1:657-664.

Sims, E.A.H., R.F. Goldman, C.M. Gluck, E.S. Horton, P.C. Kelleher, and D.W. Rowe. 1968. Experimental obesity in man. Trans. Assoc. Am. Physicians 81:153-170.

Singer, J.E., M. Westphal, and K. Niswander. 1968. Relationship of weight gain during pregnancy to birth weight and infant growth and development in the first year of life: a report from the Collaborative Study of Cerebral Palsy. Obstet. Gynecol. 31:417-423.

Stein, Z., M. Susser, G. Saenger, and F. Marolla. 1975. Famine and Human Development: The Dutch Hunger Winter of 1944-1945. Oxford University Press, New York. 284 pp.

Susser, M. 1973. Causal Thinking in the Health Sciences: Concepts and Strategies of Epidemiology. Oxford University Press, New York. 181 pp.

Susser, M. 1988. Falsification, verification and causal inference in epidemiology: reconsiderations in the light of Sir Karl Popper's philosophy. Pp. 33-57 in K.J. Rothman, ed. Causal Inference. Epidemiology Resources, Chestnut Hill, Mass.

Susser, M., and Z. Stein. 1982. Third variable analysis: application to causal sequences among nutrient intake, maternal weight, birthweight, placental weight, and gestation. Stat. Med. 1:105-120.

Taffel, S.M. 1986. Maternal Weight Gain and the Outcome of Pregnancy: United States, 1980. Vital and Health Statistics, Series 21, No. 44. DHHS Publ. No. (PHS) 86-1922. National Center for Health Statistics, Public Health Service, U.S. Department of Health and Human Services, Hyattsville, Md. 25 pp.

Tavris, D.R., and J.A. Read. 1982. Effect of maternal weight gain on fetal, infant, and childhood death and on cognitive development. Obstet. Gynecol. 60:689-694.

Teberg, A.J., F.J. Walther, and I.C. Pena. 1988. Mortality, morbidity, and outcome of the small-for-gestational age infant. Semin. Perinatol. 12:84-94.

Thomson, A.M., F.E. Hytten, and W.Z. Billewicz. 1967. The epidemiology of oedema during pregnancy. J. Obstet. Gynaecol. Br. Commonw. 74:1-10.

Udall, J.N., G.G. Harrison, Y. Vaucher, P.D. Walson, and G. Morrow III. 1978. Interaction of maternal and neonatal obesity. Pediatrics 62:17-21.

Usher, R.H. 1970. Clinical and therapeutic aspects of fetal malnutrition. Pediatr. Clin. North Am. 17:169-183.

van den Berg, B.J., and F.W. Oechsli. 1984. Prematurity. Pp. 69-85 in M.B. Bracken, ed. Perinatal Epidemiology. Oxford University Press, New York.

Van Itallie, T.B. 1979. Obesity: adverse effects on health and longevity. Am. J. Clin. Nutr. 32:2723-2733.

PART II

DIETARY INTAKE AND
NUTRIENT SUPPLEMENTS

11

Introduction

In addition to increased energy requirements during pregnancy, a topic covered in Part I of this volume, it has long been recognized that pregnancy also increases a woman's need for protein, vitamins, and minerals. Some reports suggest that the usual dietary intake of certain nutrients is inadequate to meet the needs of pregnant women, and many suggest that supplemental intake of one or more nutrients might be desirable. Recently, health care providers have asked for guidance in counseling pregnant women about the use of nutrient supplements with regard to their safety, efficacy, and appropriate dosage if used.

In the past, several reports issued by expert Food and Nutrition Board (FNB) committees on maternal nutrition have given detailed consideration to certain vitamins, minerals, and protein. One of these reports contained an overview of laboratory indices of a broad spectrum of nutrients (NRC, 1978); another covered certain practices, such as pica (the ingestion of nonfood substances such as laundry starch) and vegetarianism, that may influence nutritional status during pregnancy (NRC, 1982). Four reports recommended 30 to 60 mg of supplemental iron per day (NRC, 1970, 1980, 1981, 1982), and two recommended supplemental folic acid (NRC, 1970, 1980) during pregnancy as a means of reducing the risk of anemia. No FNB reports have recommended the routine use of multivitamin-mineral supplements.

PREVIOUS RECOMMENDATIONS FROM
PROFESSIONAL ORGANIZATIONS

Professional organizations concerned with maternal and child health have made recommendations pertaining to nutrient intake and supplement use during pregnancy. For example, a special task force of the American Dietetic Association released the following statement regarding vitamin and mineral supplementation. Although this statement was targeted toward the general population, it specifically mentions pregnant women:

> Healthy children and adults should obtain adequate nutrient intakes from dietary sources. Meeting nutrient needs by choosing a variety of foods in moderation, rather than by supplementation, reduces the potential risk for both nutrient deficiencies and nutrient excesses. Individual recommendations regarding supplements and diets should come from physicians and registered dietitians. Supplement usage may be indicated in some circumstances including: Women who are pregnant or breastfeeding need more of certain nutrients, especially iron, folic acid and calcium (ADA, 1987, p. 1342).

A virtually identical statement was released by the American Institute of Nutrition jointly with the American Society for Clinical Nutrition (Callaway et al., 1987).

In its publication *Standards for Obstetric-Gynecologic Services*, the American College of Obstetricians and Gynecologists (ACOG) included the following statement:

> Protein, iron, folic acid, and certain other vitamins and minerals are required in greater amounts during pregnancy. If these needs are not met by increased dietary intake, a vitamin/mineral supplement equal to the recommended dietary allowances (RDA) for pregnant women should be given (ACOG, 1985, p. 20).

In a separate publication the same year, the Task Force on Adolescent Pregnancy (1985) addressed nutritional needs of pregnant adolescents in somewhat more detail, providing specific suggestions to consume protein-rich foods with a goal of achieving a daily protein intake of 76 to 78 g. Regarding iron, it stated: "Pregnancy requires 30-60 mg of iron per day. Since dietary sources of iron are limited, and diet alone cannot supply the needed iron, a supplement is recommended in appropriate amounts to meet the increased need" (Task Force on Adolescent Pregnancy, 1985, p. 28). It also recommended a calcium intake of 1.2 to 1.6 g daily and stated: "If the teen's normal diet includes large amounts of milk and dairy products, supplemental calcium will be unnecessary" (Task Force on Adolescent Pregnancy, 1985, p. 29). Further relevant recommendations include the following: "During all pregnancies, a supplement of folic acid—not to exceed 1 mg per day—is recommended" (p. 29) and "Because certain vitamins may cause fetal malformations, general recommendations for a vitamin supplement would be unwise" (p. 29).

The American Academy of Pediatrics (AAP) and ACOG jointly published *Guidelines for Perinatal Care* (AAP/ACOG, 1988), which includes slightly different recommendations: folic acid supplementation of at least 400 μg/day and, for adolescents, calcium and phosphorus supplementation or additional milk (more than 1 quart daily). With regard to other vitamins and minerals:

> The increased amounts of other vitamins and minerals recommended during pregnancy . . . can usually be obtained through dietary intake, and the routine use of a multivitamin supplement is not necessary. If there are doubts about the adequacy of a patient's diet, however, a vitamin and mineral supplement that provides the recommended dietary allowances can be given safely. It is important to avoid excessive vitamin and mineral intakes (ie, more than twice the recommended dietary allowances) during pregnancy because both fat-soluble and water-soluble vitamins may have toxic effects (AAP/ACOG, 1988, p. 196).

The recommendations made by these professional groups were strongly influenced by earlier FNB reports, including the 1980 (ninth) edition of *Recommended Dietary Allowances* (NRC, 1980). The recently published tenth edition of the RDAs (NRC, 1989) includes a number of revised recommendations for nutrient intake. For example, the 1989 RDA for folate (often called folacin or folic acid) intake during pregnancy is 400 μg, compared with 800 μg in 1980. The 1989 RDAs for pregnant women appear in Table 11-1.

Directions on the labels of certain prenatal vitamin-mineral supplements may lead to intakes well in excess of the 1989 RDAs. This is not readily apparent to either the user or the physician issuing the prescription, since label information is expressed in terms of the Food and Drug Administration's U.S. Recommended Daily Allowances (U.S. RDA)—not the RDAs, which are substantially different for several nutrients (see Table 11-1): 100% of the U.S. RDA may be more or less than the RDA. The safety of vitamin-mineral supplementation deserves close examination, as does the possibility of benefit to mother or infant.

USAGE PATTERNS

Prenatal vitamin-mineral supplementation has been widespread in the United States for many years. Approximately 92% of 7,825 married mothers* in the 1980 National Natality Survey reported taking vitamin supplements during pregnancy (K. Keppel, National Center for Health Statistics, personal communication, 1988), as did nearly 88% of the 116

---

*Unmarried women were not interviewed in the 1980 National Natality Survey. For more information about the survey, see Chapter 5.

TABLE 11-1   Recommended Dietary Allowances (RDAs) and Estimated Safe and Adequate Daily Dietary Intakes (ESADDIs) Compared with U.S. Recommended Daily Allowances (U.S. RDAs) for Nonpregnant and Pregnant Women

Nutrient	RDA or ESADDI for Pregnant Adult Women[a]	U.S. RDA[b] Adults and Children over 3 Years Old[c]	U.S. RDA[b] Pregnant or Lactating Women[d]
	RDA:		
Protein	60 g	65 g	65 g
Vitamin A	800 mg RE[e]	5,000 IU	8,000 IU
Vitamin D	10 μg[f]	400 IU	400 IU
Vitamin E	10 mg of α-TE[g]	30 IU	30 IU
Vitamin K	65 μg	—[h]	—
Vitamin C	70 mg	60 mg	60 mg
Thiamin	1.5 mg	1.5 mg	1.7 mg
Riboflavin	1.6 mg	1.7 mg	2.0 mg
Niacin	17 mg NE[i]	20 mg	20 mg
Vitamin B_6	2.2 mg	2.0 mg	2.5 mg
Folacin	400 μg	400 μg	800 μg
Vitamin B_{12}	2.2 μg	6 μg	8 μg
Calcium	1,200 mg	1,000 mg	1,300 mg
Phosphorus	1,200 mg	1,000 mg	1,300 mg
Magnesium	300 mg	400 mg	450 mg
Iron	30 mg	18 mg	18 mg
Zinc	15 mg	15 mg	15 mg
Iodine	175 μg	150 μg	150 μg
Selenium	65 μg	—	—
	ESADDI:		
Biotin	30–100 μg	300 μg	300 μg
Pantothenic acid	4–7 mg	10 mg	10 mg
Copper	1.5–3.0 mg	2 mg	2 mg
Manganese	2.0–5.0 mg	—	—
Fluoride	1.5–4.0 mg	—	—
Chromium	50–200 μg	—	—
Molybdenum	75–250 μg	—	—

[a] From NRC, 1989.

[b] From National Nutrition Consortium, 1975.

[c] Used in the labeling of most foods, e.g., ready-to-eat cereals, and vitamin and mineral supplements for adults.

[d] Used in the labeling of vitamin-mineral supplements designed for pregnant and lactating women.

[e] 1 RE (retinol equivalent) = 1 μg of retinol, 6 μg of β-carotene, or 12 μg of other provitamin A carotenoids; whereas 1 IU is usually equated to 0.3 μg of retinol and to 0.6 μg of β-carotene. By calculation, 8,000 IU of vitamin A from vitamin supplements or cereal fortified with retinol equals 2,400 RE.

[f] 1 μg of vitamin D (cholecalciferol) = 40 IU.

[g] 1 α-TE (tocopherol equivalent) = 1 mg of RRR-α-tocopherol = 1.49 IU RRR-α-tocopherol = 0.74 IU of all-*rac*-α-tocopherol (the synthetic form).

[h] — = Not established.

[i] 1 NE (niacin equivalent) is equal to 1 mg of niacin or 60 mg of dietary tryptophan.

pregnant women in the U.S. Department of Agriculture's (USDA's) Continuing Survey of Food Intake by Individuals (S. Krebs-Smith, Food and Nutrition Service, personal communication, 1988).

Vitamin-mineral supplementation early in pregnancy, before prenatal care, may be of particular interest because of associations (both positive and negative) between supplement use and teratogenesis. Although supplement usage rates by women in the first few weeks of gestation have not been reported, they may parallel those reported for nonpregnant, nonlactating women in the childbearing years, which vary substantially by ethnic background, education, and income (Block et al., 1988; Koplan et al., 1986). The less advantaged groups have lower supplement usage rates. For example, 55% of all women in their childbearing years reported taking a vitamin or mineral supplement regularly or occasionally (USDA, 1987b) compared with 48% of low-income women who were not participating in the Food Stamp Program and 39% of those who were (USDA, 1987a). Analysis of data collected in the first (1971-1975) National Health and Nutrition Examination Survey indicates that among females between 25 and 34 years of age, 26.4% of the whites and 15.5% of the blacks reported regular use of vitamin and mineral supplements (Block et al., 1988).

SCOPE OF REPORT

The Subcommittee on Dietary Intake and Nutrient Supplements During Pregnancy was asked to review recent studies of dietary intake, supplement usage, laboratory indices reflecting nutrient intake, and nutrient requirements as a basis for developing conclusions and recommendations pertaining to the use of nutrient supplements during pregnancy. The sponsor, the Bureau of Maternal and Child Health and Resources Development of the U.S. Department of Health and Human Services, also asked the subcommittee to give special attention to calcium, iron, zinc, folate, and protein—most of which have been the subject of an increasing amount of research because of their suspected influence on the short- and long-term health status of mothers or their infants.

The subcommittee considered the following questions as they pertain to pregnancy:

- For which nutrients is it reasonable to expect that food alone will provide adequate intake?
- For which nutrients, if any, is supplementary intake from pharmaceutical preparations desirable?
- If supplementation is recommended or practiced, what level is appropriate?
- Is there danger of toxicity from use of any nutrient supplements?

• Do interactions among nutrients and between drugs and nutrients substantially change the pregnant woman's ability to achieve satisfactory nutritional status?

• Should recommendations differ for adolescents, for women aged 35 and over, and for women of different ethnic backgrounds?

These are questions faced by pregnant women as well as by the practitioners and the health and nutrition programs that serve them.

New findings relative to nutrient-nutrient interactions may be relevant in providing nutritional advice to pregnant women, both from the standpoint of desirable types of food combinations and when considering the use of supplemental nutrients. In addition, the subcommittee considered the use of such substances as street drugs, alcohol, and tobacco, which may have far-reaching consequences on the developing fetus and the family unit. It recognized the need to determine the nutritional implications of different forms of substance abuse and to develop realistic approaches to modifying food intake, recommending supplement use, or delivering nutrition services—without losing sight of the importance of taking steps to modify the harmful practice. The subcommittee also searched for evidence relating differences in body size, genetic makeup, age, recent life circumstances (e.g., living in a refugee settlement), and customary eating practices to the need for supplementation. However, the lack of scientific data limited the extent to which the subcommittee was able to address these issues.

UNDERLYING ASSUMPTIONS

During the course of its deliberations, the subcommittee agreed that the following concepts were important in guiding its work:

• Supplementation is justified only when there is evidence that dietary intake of the nutrient is likely to be sufficiently low to produce adverse effects on maternal or fetal health or on pregnancy outcomes.

• Laboratory indices of nutrient deficiencies developed for nonpregnant women are frequently inappropriate for women who are pregnant. Standards for pregnant women are often unavailable. This is an additional reason why optimal maternal and fetal health should be a major criterion on which to judge the need for supplementation.

• Supplementation is an intervention, for which both safety and efficacy are of concern.

• It is important to review the effects of nutrient supplements during organogenesis, which occurs very early in pregnancy.

• The practical issue of the patient's willingness to take supplements must be considered when making recommendations for supplementation.

ORGANIZATION OF THE REPORT

Chapter 12 presents useful background information pertaining to the assessment of prenatal nutrient needs. Chapter 13 presents an analysis of evidence about the dietary intake of pregnant women. These two chapters provide a framework for the next six chapters (Chapters 14 through 19), which address specific nutrients of possible concern during pregnancy. In Chapter 20, the subcommittee presents data on interactions among food, nutrients, and certain nonnutritive substances (e.g., cigarettes, coffee or caffeine, alcohol, marijuana, and cocaine) used during pregnancy and examines how these interactions may influence recommendations for supplementation. Periconceptional nutrition and the evidence for and against the use of multivitamins in the prevention of neural tube defects are discussed in Chapter 21. Chapter 1 contains the subcommittee's conclusions and recommendations.

REFERENCES

AAP/ACOG (American Academy of Pediatrics/American College of Obstetricians and Gynecologists). 1988. Guidelines for Perinatal Care, 2nd ed. American Academy of Pediatrics, Elk Grove, Ill. 356 pp.
ACOG (American College of Obstetricians and Gynecologists). 1985. Standards for Obstetric-Gynecologic Services, 6th ed. The American College of Obstetricians and Gynecologists, Washington, D.C. 109 pp.
ADA (American Dietetic Association). 1987. Recommendations concerning supplement usage: ADA statement. J. Am. Diet. Assoc. 87:1342-1343.
Block, G., C. Cox, J. Madans, G.B. Schreiber, L. Licitra, and N. Melia. 1988. Vitamin supplement use, by demographic characteristics. Am. J. Epidemiol. 127:297-309.
Callaway, C.W., K.W. McNutt, R.S. Rivlin, A.C. Ross, H.H. Sanstead, and A.P. Simopoulos. 1987. Statement on vitamin and mineral supplements. J. Nutr. 117:1649.
Koplan, J.P., J.L. Annest, P.M. Layde, and G.L. Rubin. 1986. Nutrient intake and supplementation in the United States (NHANES II). Am. J. Public Health 76:287-289.
National Nutrition Consortium. 1975. Nutrition Labeling: How it Can Work for You. National Nutrition Consortium, Bethesda, Md. 134 pp.
NRC (National Research Council). 1970. Maternal Nutrition and the Course of Pregnancy. Report of the Committee on Maternal Nutrition, Food and Nutrition Board. National Academy of Sciences, Washington, D.C. 241 pp.
NRC (National Research Council). 1978. Laboratory Indices of Nutritional Status in Pregnancy. Report of the Committee on Nutrition of the Mother and Preschool Child, Food and Nutrition Board. National Academy of Sciences, Washington, D.C. 195 pp.
NRC (National Research Council). 1980. Recommended Dietary Allowances, 9th ed. Report of the Committee on Dietary Allowances, Food and Nutrition Board, Division of Biological Sciences, Assembly of Life Sciences. National Academy Press, Washington, D.C. 185 pp.
NRC (National Research Council). 1981. Nutrition Services in Perinatal Care. Report of the Committee on Nutrition of the Mother and Preschool Child, Food and Nutrition Board, Assembly of Life Sciences. National Academy Press, Washington, D.C. 72 pp.
NRC (National Research Council). 1982. Alternative Dietary Practices and Nutritional Abuses in Pregnancy: Proceedings of a Workshop. Report of the Committee on Nutrition of the Mother and Preschool Child, Food and Nutrition Board, Commission on Life Sciences. National Academy Press, Washington, D.C. 211 pp.

NRC (National Research Council). 1989. Recommended Dietary Allowances, 10th ed. Report of the Subcommittee on the Tenth Edition of the RDAs, Food and Nutrition Board, Commission on Life Sciences. National Academy Press, Washington, D.C. 284 pp.

Task Force on Adolescent Pregnancy. 1985. Adolescent Perinatal Health: A Guidebook for Services. The American College of Obstetricians and Gynecologists, Washington, D.C. 40 pp.

USDA (U.S. Department of Agriculture). 1987a. Nationwide Food Consumption Survey. Continuing Survey of Food Intakes by Individuals. Low-Income Women 19-50 Years and Their Children 1-5 Years, 1 Day, 1986. Report No. 86-2. Nutrition Monitoring Division, Human Nutrition Information Service, U.S. Department of Agriculture, Hyattsville, Md. 166 pp.

USDA (U.S. Department of Agriculture). 1987b. Nationwide Food Consumption Survey. Continuing Survey of Food Intakes by Individuals. Women 19-50 Years and Their Children 1-5 Years, 1 Day, 1986. Report No. 86-1. Nutrition Monitoring Division, Human Nutrition Information Service, U.S. Department of Agriculture, Hyattsville, Md. 98 pp.

12

Assessment of
Nutrient Needs

In considering nutrient supplementation for pregnant women, the subcommittee reviewed nutrient requirements and evidence regarding whether those requirements can be and are ordinarily met by dietary means. Among the lines of evidence reviewed were overt (clinical) signs of deficiency, results of laboratory and functional tests, and dietary intake data. Special attention was given to physiologic changes during pregnancy—changes that make it particularly difficult to assess the nutrient requirements and nutritional status of pregnant women.

NUTRIENT HOMEOSTASIS

Unless the usual dietary intake of a nutrient is severely deficient, the body is able to maintain relatively constant tissue levels of most nutrients, even in the face of the wide variations in intake that occur from meal to meal and day to day. The same homeostatic mechanisms also afford some protection against longer-term, chronic marginal deficits or excesses in the intakes of specific nutrients.

Four major types of homeostatic responses can help to maintain tissue levels when dietary intakes are low: use of body stores (applicable to most vitamins and minerals), an increased absorption of the nutrient (e.g., calcium, iron, zinc, magnesium, copper, and carotene), reduced excretion in urine (e.g., of sodium and calcium), and a slowing down of nutrient utilization or turnover (e.g., of protein). These responses are described in more detail for individual nutrients in Chapters 14 to 19.

Physiologic changes that occur in pregnancy stimulate some of these homeostatic responses, regardless of the nutritional status of the mother, thereby increasing the supply of nutrients to help meet increased demands. Most notably, there is more efficient absorption of several minerals, such as calcium (Heaney and Skillman, 1971) and iron (Svanberg et al., 1976a,b), and urinary excretion of some nutrients, e.g., riboflavin, is reduced (Sauberlich, 1978). However, the utilization and turnover rate of most nutrients are probably increased during pregnancy, although there are few quantitative data concerning this issue. To some extent, it is considered normal for tissue stores of nutrients—especially vitamins and minerals—to be drawn upon during pregnancy. Thus, a drop in tissue levels may be of concern only if such levels were initially low and become depleted during pregnancy, or if there is evidence that stores are not repleted at a later date.

ASSESSMENT OF NUTRITIONAL STATUS

Nutrient deficiency or excess in an individual progresses in a continuum from the initial signs to severe tissue pathology. One of the difficulties in assessing nutrient status, especially in the early stages of deficiency or excess, is the lack of precision and sensitivity in most methods. In addition, most changes in nutritional status can be observed only if the homeostatic mechanisms described above are unable to modulate body nutrient levels. The likelihood that the homeostatic mechanisms will be inadequate increases in proportion to the severity and duration of the specific nutrient deficiency.

A variety of methods have been developed for use in the assessment of nutrient status. Conceptually, they fall into two categories: *static measurements*, which include determination of nutrient levels in blood or tissues, and *functional measurements*, which include a wide range of tests to determine the adequacy of nutritional status to support the functions of subcellular constituents, cells, tissues, organs, biologic systems, or the whole body. The advantages and limitations of static as compared with functional measurements have been reviewed by Solomons and Allen (1983).

In the assessment of nutritional status during pregnancy, static measurements include determination of overt signs of clinical deficiency, which are extremely rare in pregnant women in the United States and Canada; estimates of tissue stores; and determination of levels of nutrients or metabolites in maternal and infant blood and in other body tissues and fluids. Functional measurements include determination of activity of nutrient-dependent enzymes or amounts of hormones, nutrient-dependent metabolic or structural changes, rates at which maternal and infant anthropometric measurements change, and indicators of the course and outcome of pregnancy, including maternal and infant health, gestational duration, birth weight, and infant neurobehavioral development.

In nonpregnant, nonlactating women, a number of static measurements and the first two types of functional measurements have been found to give useful information about nutrient status, especially with regard to vitamins and iron. However, blood levels of some nutrients are maintained within a narrow range, e.g., the calcium level is controlled by hormones and the magnesium level by renal reabsorption. This prevents them from being useful in assessment of nutrient status, even in the nonpregnant state. Assessment of the nutritional status of pregnant women is complicated by altered nutrient needs in conjunction with shifts in plasma volume, hormone-induced changes in metabolism, and changes in renal function and resulting urinary excretion, as described in the Food and Nutrition Board's report *Laboratory Indices of Nutritional Status in Pregnancy*(NRC, 1978). Nutrient concentrations in blood or plasma during pregnancy are decreased by hemodilution, but they may be increased, decreased, or unaffected by the concentration of carrier proteins. Placental transfer of nutrients varies from nutrient to nutrient. The impact of these factors changes over the course of pregnancy, so that a laboratory value that is normal during week 12 of gestation may be abnormal at week 34. Furthermore, the pattern of change differs for each nutrient. Nutrient status parameters usually revert to normal after delivery, suggesting that these changes reflect physiologic adjustments to pregnancy rather than a state of deficiency (NRC, 1978).

These complexities in the assessment and interpretation of the nutritional status of pregnant women explain in part the relative sparseness of such data and the difficulties faced by the subcommittee in evaluating the need for nutrient supplements. Changes in static measurements, such as blood levels of nutrients, very likely result from the physiologic changes of pregnancy rather than from a nutrient deficiency. For this reason, the subcommittee gave more weight to evidence showing that usual nutrient intakes were inadequate to support optimal function than to evidence of decreases in static levels of nutrients. For example, low serum zinc levels might be regarded as normal during pregnancy, but if linked to low dietary zinc intake and adverse pregnancy outcomes, this would provide a strong argument for recommending supplementation with this nutrient.

ASSESSMENT OF NUTRIENT NEEDS

Nutrient needs can be defined as the amount of each nutrient required in the diet to support optimal metabolism; functions of cells, tissues, and organs; and the maintenance of adequate tissue stores. Four principal methods have been used to estimate nutrient requirements: evidence from epidemiologic studies relating intake to outcome, the factorial approach, balance studies, and nutrient turnover.

Epidemiologic approaches include observational and experimental studies, each of which is useful in investigating possible determinants of health outcomes. Observational studies, which comprise cohort, case-control, and cross-sectional investigations, have been used to assess associations between estimates of usual nutrient intake and measures of biologic outcome such as anemia or infant birth weight. The cross-sectional approach has proven to be an important method for evaluating nutrients (such as iron) for which deficiency states are identifiable and relatively common. For example, population-based data comparing iron intake with iron status in nonpregnant women in the United States were used as supporting evidence that the Recommended Dietary Allowance (RDA) for iron could safely be lowered (NRC, 1989). Cohort investigations have been conducted to assess pregnancy outcomes for women with low, intermediate, and high hemoglobin concentrations during early and midgestation (Murphy et al., 1986). Case-control studies, in which a sample of affected individuals (cases) is compared with a group of individuals who are free of the disorder (controls), present a particularly useful approach for studying rare pregnancy outcomes, such as neural tube defects. Finally, experimental studies, specifically, randomized controlled clinical trials, provide a powerful method for determining the safety and efficacy of nutrient supplements in preventing pregnancy complications and improving outcomes.

In the *factorial approach,* the total nutrient requirement is calculated by summing the estimated amounts required by category of need. During pregnancy, these needs include increased requirements for maternal tissue expansion or metabolism; placental growth; and growth, nutrient storage, and metabolism in the fetus. An additional amount is added to the estimated sum of nutrient requirements for these purposes to allow for endogenous secretion and incomplete maternal intestinal absorption. This approach has been used to estimate the maternal requirements for protein; some minerals such as iron, calcium, and zinc; and vitamins A and C.

Balance studies are conducted to estimate nutrient requirements based on measurements of all dietary intake and physiologic loss of the nutrient and its metabolites. During pregnancy, a nutrient requirement is considered to be that amount necessary to replace obligatory maternal nutrient losses and to allow for normal growth of fetal and maternal tissues and for accretion of nutrient stores. This approach has been used to estimate requirements for protein and some minerals during pregnancy.

Measurements of *nutrient turnover* (utilization and replacement) can provide additional information about the dynamics of nutrient metabolism. This relatively new approach has been used to quantify the rate at which some nutrients are transferred from the mother to the fetus and the rate of nutrient turnover in both the mother and fetus.

Because each of these approaches has its limitations, there is sometimes a lack of agreement, on both theoretical and experimental grounds, regarding nutrient requirements. Observational epidemiologic studies are useful for establishing the relationship between nutrient intake and adequacy in population groups—not in individuals. Unless other potentially important factors are controlled effectively, the results of epidemiologic studies can be misleading. The factorial approach requires assumptions that are not always testable, and it neglects the dynamic nature of metabolism. Balance studies are technically tedious and difficult for many reasons; their usefulness is limited by the body's ability to maintain balance over a wide range of intakes (Mertz, 1987). Turnover measurements have provided valuable insights into metabolism, but for most nutrients, the models for estimating requirements from such measurements have yet to be developed. Nonetheless, these multiple approaches serve to bracket general estimates of nutrient requirements.

ASSESSMENT OF DIETARY ADEQUACY

Dietary assessment serves as the foundation for appropriate nutrition counseling and intervention. It enables investigators and clinicians to identify both poor and desirable food habits and dietary patterns, and thus is fundamental in determining the risk of inadequate intakes of specific nutrients, possibilities for dietary improvement, and the potential need for supplementation of individual pregnant women. Food intake data can be collected by a variety of methods, both quantitative (where the goal is to collect accurate information on the usual total daily intake of specific nutrients) and qualitative (such as an assessment of food groups or food patterns). Useful reviews of dietary assessment methods include those by Block (1982) and Todd et al. (1983). However, few studies have been conducted to validate methods for use with pregnant women (Abramson et al., 1963; Hunt et al., 1983; Krebs-Smith and Clark, 1989; Suitor et al., 1989), and there is a need for research to develop and validate practical methods of assessing dietary intake for use in routine prenatal care.

Quantitative intake data are useful in several areas, e.g., in nutrition research, in the evaluation of effects of interventions, and in surveys; however, even the most accurate methods for obtaining information on nutrient intakes are imprecise (Medlin and Skinner, 1988; Quandt, 1986), or they may alter food intake.

Methods for collecting quantitative data include 24-hour recalls and food records. In the recall method, the individual is asked to recall the types and amounts of the foods and beverages consumed during the previous day. This is a relatively inexpensive and practical quantitative method for collecting data about 1 day's intake, but its accuracy is limited by such factors as memory, lack of knowledge about the ingredients used in foods, and an inability to describe portion sizes correctly (Beaton et al., 1979). In the food record method, the subjects record the type and amount of items consumed, preferably immediately after eating. One of the problems with this method is that individuals must be cooperative and able to record detailed information, resulting in a bias toward better-quality data on women who are concerned about their diet and who are well educated (Sampson, 1985).

Estimation of intake over 1 day is very unlikely to represent a person's usual nutrient consumption (Garn et al., 1976) because of the wide variation in day-to-day food and nutrient intake. A single day's intake can be used to estimate the nutrient intake of a group of individuals, but this is not the usual intent in clinical practice. For such nutrients as energy and protein, which are consumed relatively consistently from day to day (Beaton et al., 1979), assessment of average intake over 3 days is sufficient to estimate usual intake by an individual. Unfortunately, many days would have to be sampled to obtain an accurate estimate of the usual intake of nutrients such as vitamins A and C, for which intake is highly variable (Beaton et al., 1983).

For these reasons, a pregnant woman's risk of dietary inadequacy may be assessed more efficiently and practically by a food frequency or diet history questionnaire. In these approaches, the woman is asked (either orally or in written form) for the usual frequency with which specific foods are consumed over time. Both methods are useful for detecting poor dietary patterns and low intake of specific food groups; food frequency questionnaires have also provided a practical means of collecting data on relationships between dietary patterns and either nutrition or health outcomes (see the review by Sampson, 1985). Examples of interview forms used for this purpose have been published (Sampson, 1985; Williams, 1989). The accuracy of the nutrient estimates may improve somewhat if the questionnaire includes portion size (Block and Hartman, 1989), but the addition of such questions would increase the time required to complete the form and may make the approach less practical in the clinical setting.

If food intake information is collected carefully by the diet recall or diet record method, it can be used to calculate the intake of specific nutrients. This is done most efficiently by using one of the many diet analysis programs available for either personal or mainframe computers (Frank and Pelican, 1986). Responses to food frequency questionnaires and diet histories are often evaluated by comparing the usual number of servings of foods in specific food groups to a recommended number of servings (see Williams, 1989, for examples), but there are also computer programs for estimating usual daily nutrient intake (NCI, 1988; Willett et al., 1985). The best method to use in a particular clinic depends on the purposes of the data collection and practical considerations within the clinic. Practical methods for collecting dietary data from pregnant women, often tailored to specific ethnic groups, are available from the state departments of health, from the Supplemental Food Program for Women, Infants, and Children, the American Dietetic Association, and the American College of Obstetricians and Gynecologists.

In general, the dietary assessment methods outlined above serve to identify nutritionally unsound dietary practices. However, additional questions can be asked, as appropriate, to determine whether the pregnant woman has special problems that may affect her dietary adequacy. The following are examples of problems that may be identified by questioning and reviewing the woman's medical/obstetric chart.

- Low income and inadequate access to food.
- Avoidance of certain types of food because of intolerance or aversion, e.g., avoidance of milk because of lactose intolerance or because of fad diets or cultural practices involving food taboos (Cassidy, 1982).
- Adherence to completely vegetarian diets. (The diets of lacto-ovovegetarians are more likely to be nutritionally adequate.)
- Consumption of substantial amounts of alcohol or use of tobacco or illicit drugs (see Chapter 20).
- A life-style that is unlikely to support adequate acquisition, preparation, or consumption of food, e.g., that of a busy professional person as well as that of a poor woman living without a partner.
- Diet restriction in an attempt to control weight.
- The practice of pica (consumption of nonfood substances such as laundry starch).
- Unhappiness with being pregnant.

Clinical information that may signify a risk of nutritional problems includes:

- Substantial under- or overweight
- Early teenage pregnancy
- Multiple gestation (e.g., twins or triplets)
- Anemia

To the extent possible, the subcommittee recommends that poor dietary practices be improved by appropriate interventions. These may include general nutrition education, individualized diet counseling, and referral to food assistance programs or to programs (e.g., the Expanded Food and Nutrition Education Program) that promote improved food acquisition or preparation practices. If, in the judgment of the clinician, such interventions are likely to be or have been unsuccessful, then recommendation of a multivitamin-mineral supplement may be the only practical strategy to improve nutrient intake. Later chapters distinguish between nutrients that warrant careful attention and those for which intake is likely to be adequate to meet the increased demands of pregnancy.

RECOMMENDED DIETARY ALLOWANCES

There is considerable variation in nutrient requirements among individuals within a population. In recognition of this problem, and after considering data on both nutrient requirements and their variability by using the four approaches described above, the Food and Nutrition Board set RDAs at a level high enough to meet the requirements of nearly all healthy individuals in the U.S. population (NRC, 1989). Energy recommendations are the only exception, since intake of energy above requirements causes obesity. The extent of the data base on which the RDAs are based varies from nutrient to nutrient, but the needs of most pregnant women will be met, by definition, even when their nutrient intakes fall somewhat below the RDAs.

The subcommittee concluded that a nutrient intake that is lower than the RDA for pregnancy, by itself, is an insufficient basis for recommending supplementation. Given the difficulties of assessing usual nutrient intake and nutritional status during pregnancy, the subcommittee concluded that a decision to recommend routine supplementation should be based on evidence that usual intakes are inadequate to support optimal maternal and fetal health and function.

Although the subcommittee did not rely on the RDAs as the sole basis on which to judge the adequacy of usual dietary intakes of nutrients, it did use the RDAs for several other purposes. In Chapter 13, for example, the average nutrient intakes of pregnant women are compared with the RDAs. If the average intake of a nutrient exceeds the RDAs, the subcommittee is less concerned about the need for supplements. A similar approach was used in the report *Nutrition Monitoring in the United States* (LSRO, 1989). When the subcommittee recommended supplements, the RDAs were considered in suggesting the amount of supplement to be provided.

FACTORS INFLUENCING NUTRIENT REQUIREMENTS AND THE NEED FOR SUPPLEMENTATION

Factors that may increase nutrient needs above the ordinary demands of pregnancy are poor nutritional status, young maternal age, a multiple pregnancy, closely spaced births, a continued high level of physical activity, certain disease states (e.g., malabsorption), and use of such substances as cigarettes, alcohol, some legal drugs (e.g., antibiotics and phenytoin), and illegal drugs. For women whose nutrient needs are increased by one or more of these factors, an increased supply of selected nutrients may be indicated. Ordinarily, this is most effectively accomplished with food, because an increased need for specific vitamins and minerals is often accompanied by an increased need for energy and for other nutrients not provided in multivitamin-mineral supplements.

Attempts have been made to categorize pregnant women as being at low, moderate, or high risk of nutrient inadequacy. Methods for making such assignments have included comparison of food or dietary patterns and nutrient intake with various standards or using such criteria as young maternal age, multiple gestation, closely spaced births, and substance abuse to identify high-risk women. Results of laboratory tests have also been used for this purpose, but this is not a practical approach for most nutrients.

Unfortunately, there are no validated guidelines on how to use information based on such criteria to assign women to a specific risk category, because there has been no determination of the relative risk that the mother or fetus will have one or more deficiencies if the mother meets such criteria. Nor has it been established which individual women in a category are likely to benefit from extra nutrients through food or supplements or which women are likely to be harmed if there is no intervention. Whether or not a level of dietary or supplementary intake of a nutrient reduces the risk of pregnancy complications and adverse pregnancy outcomes can be determined most convincingly when there are data on many women from carefully controlled, randomized studies. Such studies are rare because of their high cost, difficulty in recruiting subjects, and ethical considerations.

Thus, the decision to provide special dietary intervention or nutrient supplementation must be made on an individual basis, using the best judgment of the health professional. The information provided in later chapters is intended to assist in such judgments.

NUTRIENT-NUTRIENT INTERACTIONS

Supplements pose a much greater potential problem of nutrient-nutrient interactions than does the typical U.S. diet. An excess of one nutrient in a supplement may interact with another nutrient in the supplement or in food—thereby affecting absorption or utilization adversely or, less often, beneficially. Numerous such interactions have been identified. The effects result from competitive biologic interactions (Hill and Matrone, 1970) and a variety of other mechanisms.

Interactions may occur at any stage in the digestion, absorption, transport, metabolism, utilization, or excretion of nutrients. Among the micronutrients, there are interactions among trace elements, between vitamins and trace elements, and between vitamins. For example, iron inhibits the absorption of zinc (Hambidge et al., 1987), and zinc inhibits the absorption of copper (Festa et al., 1985). Major minerals such as calcium, phosphorus, and magnesium also participate in important interactions among themselves and with other nutrients. For example, calcium interferes with the absorption of both iron and zinc (Seligman et al., 1983), and protein increases urinary calcium losses (Allen et al., 1979) and vitamin B_6 requirements (NRC, 1989).

Subsequent chapters include further discussions of nutrient-nutrient interactions and highlight reasons why the routine use of supplements should be viewed with caution. It is important to avoid a situation in which supplementation with one nutrient increases the need for another, so that yet one more nutrient must be added to the supplement.

NUTRIENT TOXICITIES

The use of high levels (e.g., >10 times the RDA) of supplements, which are often self-prescribed, by a substantial portion of the general public has led to concern about nutrient toxicities. Women in the childbearing years are among the frequent users of vitamin-mineral supplements. The vulnerability of the fetus to nutrient toxicity is an additional concern. An extensive review of this topic is found in an earlier Food and Nutrition Board report (Pitkin, 1982). Unique features of the maternal-fetal relationship make it difficult to predict the extent to which an excess of a nutrient will cross the placenta, accumulate, and harm the fetus. Nutrients that potentially can exert toxic effects include iron; zinc; selenium; and vitamins A, B_6, C, and D. Even when there is no conclusive evidence that teratogenicity or signs of toxicity result from excessive intake of a specific nutrient, Pitkin (1982) argued that potential for harm, in the absence of any clear benefits, is a sound reason for caution in the use of supplements.

According to the subcommittee, pharmacologic (high) doses of nutrients should be prescribed during pregnancy only when there is solid evidence of a beneficial effect, as in the treatment of vitamin dependency states.

SUMMARY

In the laboratory and in routine clinical practice, there are serious limitations in diagnosing states of nutritional deficiency and in determining who may benefit from supplementation. Given that biochemical changes in pregnancy are often poorly understood, correction and prevention of functional impairments caused by nutrient deficiency are the most important criteria on which to judge the need for, and benefits of, nutrient supplementation. Subsequent chapters of this report provide information relative to making decisions regarding the desirability of supplementation.

CLINICAL IMPLICATIONS

• The usefulness of laboratory tests for assessment of nutritional status in pregnant women is limited by changes in blood levels of nutrients or in nutrient-dependent enzymes or reactions, which most likely reflect normal physiologic changes that occur in pregnancy rather than a state of nutrient deficiency.

• Dietary assessment is recommended for all pregnant women in the United States. It is important to have information on the usual dietary intake of individual women before recommendations can be made about their need for specific nutrient supplements.

• The most practical method of evaluating the adequacy of usual food intake patterns is to use some type of food frequency questionnaire.

• In addition to questions about food intake, it is important to ask pregnant women whether they have special problems that may affect their dietary adequacy and to consider clinical information that may signify additional nutritional risk.

• To the extent possible, the approach should be to remedy poor dietary practices by appropriate interventions. Supplements may fail to supply all the nutrients needed, and they raise concerns about the adverse effects of nutrient-nutrient interactions and toxicities. If recommendations to change dietary intake are judged likely to be unsuccessful or insufficient, then recommendation of a nutrient supplement may be indicated.

• If nutrient supplements are recommended to pregnant women for any reason, the subcommittee urges clinicians to provide counseling at the same time in the proper use of supplements to prevent overdosing.

REFERENCES

Abramson, J.H., C. Slome, and C. Kosovsky. 1963. Food frequency interview as an epidemiological tool. Am. J. Public Health 53:1093-1101.

Allen, L.H., E.A. Oddoye, and S. Margen. 1979. Protein-induced hypercalciuria: a longer term study. Am. J. Clin. Nutr. 32:741-749.

Beaton, G.H., J. Milner, P. Corey, V. McGuire, M. Cousins, E. Stewart, M. de Ramos, D. Hewitt, P.V. Grambsch, N. Kassim, and J.A. Little. 1979. Sources of variance in 24-hour dietary recall data: implications for nutrition study design and interpretation. Am. J. Clin. Nutr. 32:2546-2559.

Beaton, G.H., J. Milner, V. McGuire, T.E. Feather, and J.A. Little. 1983. Source of variance in 24-hour dietary recall data: implications for nutrition study design and interpretation. Carbohydrate sources, vitamins, and minerals. Am. J. Clin. Nutr. 37:986-995.

Block, G. 1982. A review of validations of dietary assessment methods. Am. J. Epidemiol. 115:492-505.

Block, G., and A.M. Hartman. 1989. Issues in reproducibility and validity of dietary studies. Am. J. Clin. Nutr. 50:1133-1138.

Cassidy, C.M. 1982. Subcultural prenatal diets of Americans. Pp. 25-60 in Alternative Dietary Practices and Nutritional Abuses in Pregnancy: Proceedings of a Workshop. Report of the Committee on Nutrition of the Mother and Preschool Child, Food and Nutrition Board, Commission on Life Sciences. National Academy Press, Washington, D.C.

Festa, M.D., H.L. Anderson, R.P. Dowdy, and M.R. Ellersieck. 1985. Effect of zinc intake on copper excretion and retention in men. Am. J. Clin. Nutr. 41:285-292.

Frank, G.C., and S. Pelican. 1986. Guidelines for selecting a dietary analysis system. J. Am. Diet. Assoc. 86:72-75.

Garn, S.M., F.A. Larkin, and P.E. Cole. 1976. The problem with one-day dietary intakes. Ecol. Food Nutr. 5:245-247.

Hambidge, K.M., N.F. Krebs, L. Sibley, and J. English. 1987. Acute effects of iron therapy on zinc status during pregnancy. Obstet. Gynecol. 4:593-596.

Heaney, R.P., and T.G. Skillman. 1971. Calcium metabolism in normal human pregnancy. J. Clin. Endocrinol. Metab. 33:661-670.

Hill, C.H., and G. Matrone. 1970. Chemical parameters in the study of in vivo and in vitro interactions of transition elements. Fed. Proc., Fed. Am. Soc. Exp. Biol. 29:1474-1481.

Hunt, I.F., N.J. Murphy, A.E. Cleaver, N. Laine, and C.A. Clark. 1983. Protective foods recall as a tool for dietary assessment in the evaluation of public health programs for pregnant Hispanics. Ecol. Food Nutr. 12:235-245.

Krebs-Smith, S.M., and L.D. Clark. 1989. Validation of a nutrient adequacy score for use with women and children. J. Am. Diet. Assoc. 89:775-780,783.

LSRO (Life Sciences Research Office). 1989. Nutrition Monitoring in the United States: An Update Report on Nutrition Monitoring. Prepared for the U.S. Department of Agriculture and the U.S. Department of Health and Human Services. DHHS Publ. No. (PHS) 89-1225. U.S. Government Printing Office, Washington, D.C. (various pagings).

Medlin, C., and J.D. Skinner. 1988. Individual dietary intake methodology: a 50-year review of progress. J. Am. Diet. Assoc. 88:1250-1257.

Mertz, W. 1987. Use and misuse of balance studies. J. Nutr. 117:1811-1813.

Murphy, J.F., J. O'Riordan, R.G. Newcombe, E.C. Coles, and J.F. Pearson. 1986. Relation of haemoglobin levels in first and second trimesters to outcome of pregnancy. Lancet 1:992-995.

NCI (National Cancer Institute). 1988. Health Habits and History Questionnaire: Diet History and Other Risk Factors. Personal Computer System Packet. Division of Cancer Prevention and Control, National Cancer Institute, National Institutes of Health, Public Health Service, U.S. Department of Health and Human Services, Bethesdsa, Md. (various pagings).

NRC (National Research Council). 1978. Laboratory Indices of Nutritional Status in Pregnancy. Report of the Committee on Nutrition of the Mother and Preschool Child, Food and Nutrition Board. National Academy of Sciences, Washington, D.C. 195 pp.

NRC (National Research Council). 1989. Recommended Dietary Allowances, 10th ed. Report of the Subcommittee on the Tenth Edition of the RDAs, Food and Nutrition Board, Commission on Life Sciences. National Academy Press, Washington, D.C. 284 pp.

Pitkin, R.M. 1982. Megadose nutrients during pregnancy. Pp. 203-211 in Alternative Dietary Practices and Nutritional Abuses in Pregnancy: Proceedings of a Workshop. Report of the Committee on Nutrition of the Mother and Preschool Child, Food and Nutrition Board, Commission on Life Sciences. National Academy Press, Washington, D.C.

Quandt, S.A. 1986. Nutritional anthropology: individual focus. Pp. 3-20 in S.A. Quandt and C. Ritenbaugh, eds. Training Manual in Nutritional Anthropology. Special Publication No. 20. American Anthropological Association, Washington, D.C.

Sampson, L. 1985. Food frequency questionnaires as a research instrument. Clin. Nutr. 4:171-178.

Sauberlich, H.E. 1978. Vitamin indices. Pp. 109-156 in Laboratory Indices of Nutritional Status in Pregnancy. Report of the Committee on Nutrition of the Mother and Preschool Child, Food and Nutrition Board. National Academy of Sciences, Washington, D.C.

Seligman, P.A., J.H. Caskey, J.L. Frazier, R.M. Zucker, E.R. Podell, and R.H. Allen. 1983. Measurements of iron absorption from prenatal multivitamin-mineral supplements. Obstet. Gynecol. 61:356-362.

Solomons, N.W., and L.H. Allen. 1983. The functional assessment of nutritional status: principles, practice and potential. Nutr. Rev. 41:33-50.

Suitor, C.J.W., J. Gardner, and W.C. Willett. 1989. A comparison of food frequency and diet recall methods in studies of nutrient intake of low-income pregnant women. J. Am. Diet. Assoc. 89:1786-1794.

Svanberg, B., B. Arvidsson, A. Norrby, G. Rybo, and L. Sölvell. 1976a. Absorption of supplemental iron during pregnancy—a longitudinal study with repeated bone-marrow studies and absorption measurements. Acta Obstet. Gynecol. Scand., Suppl. 48:87-108.

Svanberg, B., B. Arvidsson, E. Björn-Rasmussen, L. Hallberg, L. Rossander, and B. Swolin. 1976b. Dietary iron absorption in pregnancy—a longitudinal study with repeated measurements of non-haeme iron absorption from whole diet. Acta Obstet. Gynecol. Scand., Suppl. 48:43-68.

Todd, K.S., M. Hudes, and D.H. Calloway. 1983. Food intake measurement: problems and approaches. Am. J. Clin. Nutr. 37:139-146.

Willett, W.C., L. Sampson, M.J. Stampfer, B. Rosner, C. Bain, J. Witschi, C.H. Hennekens, and F.E. Speizer. 1985. Reproducibility and validity of a semiquantitative food frequency questionnaire. Am. J. Epidemiol. 122:51-65.

Williams, S.R. 1989. Nutrition assessment and guidance in prenatal care. Pp. 141-171 in B. Worthington-Roberts and S.R. Williams, eds. Nutrition in Pregnancy and Lactation, 4th ed. Times Mirror/Mosby, St. Louis.

13

Dietary Intake During Pregnancy

Since nutrient supplementation of healthy pregnant women is necessary only when the usual intake of nutrients from the diet is insufficient to meet physiologic requirements (see Chapter 12), in this chapter the subcommittee reviews data on the usual dietary intake of nutrients by pregnant women and identifies nutrients that are frequently consumed below the recommended levels. The subcommittee noted that if a population group were to consume, on average, less of a nutrient than the Recommended Dietary Allowance (RDA) (NRC, 1989), this would not necessarily imply that they are *deficient* in that nutrient. It may, however, mean that some individuals within the group are at risk of deficiency.

AVAILABLE DIETARY DATA

The following review of data on nutrient intakes during pregnancy is restricted to women residing in the United States. Lack of data prevented the inclusion of some essential nutrients, and certain others were excluded (e.g., phosphorus) because adequacy of intake has been well established. Limited data on the nutrients omitted from Table 13-1 are provided in Chapters 15, 17, and 18. All reports published since 1978 were selected if they included data for energy and at least four nutrients. That year was selected as a cutoff point because older data are unlikely to be representative of current nutrient intakes for several reasons. For example, advice to restrict weight gain during pregnancy by reducing food intake is given less frequently than it was in the past. Furthermore, estimates of the nutrient composition of foods have been revised. Thus, nutrient data bases have changed accordingly over time and have become more complete. There have also been changes in the types of foods available to and consumed by the U.S. public, and in the 1980s, the food intake of increasing numbers of pregnant women was affected by their participation in the Special Supplemental Food Program for Women, Infants, and Children (WIC) (see Chapter 3, Figure 3-5).

Table 13-1 summarizes the references from which data were abstracted; provides the year of each report; and notes the population groups studied, the stage of pregnancy at which intake was measured, the dietary data collection method, and the number of days that intake was measured.

LIMITATIONS OF THE DATA

Neither the National Health and Nutrition Examination Surveys (NHANES), the Nationwide Food Consumption Surveys (NFCS), nor the Continuing Survey of Food Intake by Individuals (CSFII) serves as a source of representative dietary data for pregnant women in the United States. Since the number of pregnant women included in the surveys is small, e.g., 116 of 2,910 women in the first wave of CSFII in 1985 (USDA, 1985), valid comparisons cannot be made across age, ethnic, or socioeconomic groups. However, results from one analysis of CSFII data on pregnant women are included in Table 13-2.

Low-income women were heavily represented in the recent dietary intake studies (at least 8 of the 11 studies) of pregnant women included in Table 13-2. That is, many studies were conducted with WIC participants, whose family income is less than 185% of the national poverty level. This factor, combined with the small sample size of most studies, introduces some uncertainty regarding the extent to which the data can be generalized to the ethnic and age groups specified in Tables 13-1 and 13-2.

Differences between studies make it difficult to compare their results. Although most investigators used a 24-hour diet recall method to obtain the dietary data, the accuracy of the food intake information must have varied with the level of training of the interviewers, the use of food models, the time available for the interview, characteristics of the subjects such as their education level and economic status, and the sensitivity and knowledge of interviewers concerning cultural food patterns. In the studies in which women were asked to record or to record and weigh their intake, it is likely that some women changed their food intake because of the need to keep a record. Different investigators used different nutrient data bases, which vary in completeness and accuracy (Dwyer and Suitor, 1984). This is especially likely to affect estimates of the intakes of such nutrients as folacin, vitamin B_6, and zinc.

TABLE 13-1 Population Groups and Methods Used in Dietary Intake Studies of Pregnant Women

Population Group and Reference	Age Group	WIC[a] Participation	Number in Sample	Gestational Period	Data Collection Method	Duration of Study, days
Mixed ethnic groups:						
Hartford, Conn., 33% white, 33% black, 33% Hispanic; Picone et al., 1982	Mixed	Unspecified	144	Mixed	24-h recall	1
Second National WIC Evaluation, 56% white, 21% Hispanic, 20% black for entire study group, of which three separate samples were studied; Rush et al., 1988	Mixed	No No Yes	530 530 2,762	Trimester 1 Trimester 3 Trimester 3	24-h recall 24-h recall 24-h recall	1 1 1
Nationwide sample from CSFII,[b] 89% white, 10% black; S. Murphy and B. Abrams, unpublished data, University of California at Berkeley, 1989	Mixed	Unspecified	144	Mixed	24-h recall	1
Massachusetts, 59% white, 21% black, 20% Hispanic; Suitor et al., 1989	Mixed	56% Yes, 44% No	95	Mixed	24-h recall	3
Location and ethnic background unspecified; Endres et al., 1987	>35 yr Adolescents	Yes Yes	63 526	25 wk of gestation >23 wk of gestation	24-h recall 24-h recall	1
Location unspecified, 88% white, 12% black; Endres et al., 1985	Adults Adolescents	Yes Yes	204 91	24 wk of gestation 20 wk of gestation	24-h recall 24-h recall	1 1
Sacramento, Calif., 56% white, 16% black, 23% Hispanic; Loris et al., 1985	Adolescents	Unspecified	54	Trimesters 2 and 3	24-h recall	1

Whites:

Blacksburg, Va.; Taper et al., 1985	Young adult	Unspecified	8–11	18–26 wk of gestation	Duplicate weighed portions	14

Blacks:

Low-income blacks in St. Louis, Mo.; Brennan et al., 1983a	Unspecified	Unspecified	22	Trimester 3	Duplicate weighed portions	1

Hispanics:

Low-income Mexican-American women in Los Angeles; Hunt et al., 1983	Unspecified	Unspecified	106	20 wk of gestation	24-h recall	14
	Unspecified	Unspecified	78	36 wk of gestation	24-h recall	14

American Indians:

Navajo Indians; Butte et al., 1981	16–23 yr	70% Yes, 30% No	22	40 wk of gestation	24-h recall	1

[a] WIC = Supplemental Food Program for Women, Infants, and Children.
[b] CSFII = Continuing Survey of Food Intake by Individuals.

TABLE 13-2 Reported Average Nutrient Intakes by Pregnant Women in Comparison with 1989 Recommended Dietary Allowances[a]

Study Description and Reference	Energy, kcal	Protein, g	Vitamins A, µg of RE[b]	D, µg	E, mg	Folate, µg	Thiamin, mg	Riboflavin, mg	B6, mg	B12, µg	Niacin, mg	C, mg	Minerals Iron, mg	Zinc, mg	Calcium, mg	Magnesium, mg
Recommended Dietary Allowances (RDA), NRC, 1989	2,500	60	800	10	10	400	1.5	1.6	2.2	2.2	17	70	30	15	1,200	300
Mixed ethnic backgrounds and ages:																
Picone et al., 1982	1,972	86	1,043	NR[c]	NR	NR	1.2	2.0	NR	NR	20	106	12.0	NR	1,002	NR
Rush et al., 1988	2,001	81	1,133	NR	NR	NR	1.5	2.0	1.6	5.7	20	120	14.5	NR	918	254
Non-WIC,[d] trimesters 1 and 2	1,905	76	1,200	NR	NR	NR	1.4	2.0	1.6	5.4	19	112	14.1	NR	871	244
Non-WIC, trimester 3	2,016	81	1,400	NR	NR	NR	1.7	2.4	1.9	6.6	22	144	17.2	NR	1,004	269
WIC, trimester 3	1,736	68	1,021	NR	8.4	232	1.2	1.7	1.4	4.9	17	92	11.4	9.5	828	232
S. Murphy and B. Abrams, unpublished data, 1989	NR	NR	NR	NR	NR	NR	NR	NR	2.1	NR	NR	134	16.5	12.0	1,195	NR
Suitor et al., 1989	2,226	91	1,311	NR	NR	NR	NR	NR	NR	NR	NR	NR	NR	NR	NR	NR

Mixed ethnic backgrounds, adults only: Endres et al., 1985	**1,903**	75	1,250	**5.2**	12	**252**	1.6	2.3	**1.1**	NR	19	120	**15.8**	NR	929	NR
Mixed ethnic backgrounds, adults over 35 years of age: Endres et al., 1987	**1,512**	70	1,163	**4.4**	**7.6**	**183**	**1.4**	2.3	**0.8**	2.6	18	122	**14.1**	**6.0**	**800**	**187**
Mixed ethnic backgrounds, adolescents: Loris et al., 1985	2,822	110	1,440	NR	NR	NR	1.9	3.2	NR	NR	22	133	**16.6**	NR	1,670	NR
Endres et al., 1985	**1,927**	77	1,169	**5.3**	**9.5**	**243**	1.5	2.3	**1.0**	NR	19	99	**15.1**	NR	**943**	NR
Endres et al., 1987	**1,876**	74	972	**4.6**	**7.5**	**231**	1.5	2.2	**0.9**	4.8	19	123	**13.8**	**6.4**	**796**	**191**
Whites: Taper et al., 1985	**2,065**	75	NR	NR	NR	NR	NR	NR	NR	NR	NR	NR	**12.8**	**10.8**	**1,024**	NR
Blacks: Brennan et al., 1983a Study 1	**1,873**	74	1,017	NR	NR	**175**	**1.2**	1.8	NR	NR	**15**	87	**11.0**	**8.7**	**790**	**200**
Study 2	**1,722**	68	1,110	NR	NR	**168**	**1.2**	1.8	NR	NR	17	**48**	**14.4**	**8.4**	**931**	**204**
Mexican-Americans: Hunt et al., 1983 20 wk of gestation	**1,646**	68	1,191	NR	**5.2**	**241**	**1.2**	1.7	**1.4**	NR	26	116	**11.2**	**9.7**	**956**	NR
36 wk of gestation	**1,910**	75	1,299	NR	**6.2**	**293**	**1.3**	2.0	**1.6**	NR	28	142	**12.7**	**11.1**	**1,110**	NR
Navajo Indians: Butte et al., 1981	**2,406**	82	**711**	**3.0**	**3.4**	144	1.5	1.6	**1.5**	4.6	19	112	16.2	**11.4**	668	**230**

[a] Values in bold type are less than the 1989 RDA.
[b] RE = Retinol equivalent.
[c] NR = Not reported.
[d] WIC = Supplemental Food Program for Women, Infants, and Children.

In 1988, approximately 523,000 pregnant women per month were participants in WIC (J. Hirshman, Food and Nutrition Service, personal communication, 1988). Several investigators (see Table 13-1) did not identify the proportion of their subjects who were enrolled in WIC or separate the dietary intake data of participants from those of nonparticipants. Nutrient intakes by women from lower socioeconomic groups may be increased by participation in this program, as described later in this chapter.

Information on the *effects* of pregnancy on food choices and patterns, diet quality, and nutrient intake in the United States is virtually nonexistent. Since 1978, no investigator in the United States has made a systematic study of intake before and throughout pregnancy in the same women. With two exceptions (Endres et al., 1985; S. Murphy and B. Abrams, University of California at Berkeley, personal communication, 1988), no comparisons were made between nonpregnant and pregnant women.

It is unclear whether or how appetite changes during pregnancy. Data on intakes during the first trimester are scarce because most women make no more than one prenatal visit during this time. (In 1985, 18.1% of the pregnant women in the United States received no prenatal care in the first trimester. For teenagers and black women, first-trimester prenatal care was even less common [IOM, 1988].) In the few early studies in which appetite was investigated, some women reported that their appetite was greater, whereas others reported no difference (see review by Taggart, 1961). Beal (1971) reported that appetite decreased in the first trimester, improved in the fifth month, and declined thereafter.

Nausea during early pregnancy was reported by about half of the pregnant women studied by Brandes (1967). It is not known how nausea and vomiting affect the daily amount and nutritional quality of food consumed, but these unpleasant conditions have been associated with *favorable* pregnancy outcomes (Brandes, 1967; Klebanoff et al., 1985; Tierson et al., 1986). The few attempts to investigate whether maternal diet contributes to nausea or vomiting have failed to find a relationship. The lack of evidence that vitamin B_6 supplements help relieve nausea is discussed in Chapter 18.

Food-related behaviors that change more often during pregnancy than at any other stage of life include cravings, aversions to specific foods, and pica (the ingestion of nonfood substances such as laundry starch) (NRC, 1982). In one study of married pregnant women of northern European background from middle- and upper-income groups in the United States, 76% reported a craving for at least one food item, and 85% reported aversion to at least one (Tierson et al., 1985). These cravings and aversions had predictable effects on the amounts of the specific foods consumed, but it was not possible to generalize about the overall nutritional impact because of the large number and variety of foods involved. In another study of a random sample of 463 women who had recently delivered babies, more

than 90% reported a craving for at least one food item during then ...
trimester of pregnancy, and more than 50% reported aversion to at least
one (Worthington-Roberts et al., 1989).

NUTRIENT INTAKES OF PREGNANT WOMEN

Nutrient intake data from studies of pregnant women during the 1980s
are summarized in Table 13-2. Average intakes reported to be lower than
the 1989 RDAs for pregnant women are set in boldface type. The RDAs for
protein, vitamins, and minerals provide a substantial margin of safety and
exceed the requirements of almost all individuals in a specific population
group. For example, approximately 50% of the population has an adequate
intake of a nutrient at $\geq 77\%$ of the RDA, and 97.5% has an adequate
intake at 100% of the RDA, assuming that the RDAs are 30% (about 2
standard deviations) higher than the mean requirement of the population.

The following generalizations can be made about the data presented
in Table 13-2:

• The nutrient intake by pregnant women in the United States has
been measured in relatively few studies during the last decade. Information
is particularly sparse on adult women of northern European descent.

• Reported mean daily energy intakes varied markedly, ranging from
approximately 1,500 to 2,800 kcal. The extent to which this reflects differences in data collection techniques (and consequently over- or underreporting of food intake) or differences in age, body size, or activity level is
not clear. Not surprisingly, with a few exceptions, mean nutrient intakes by
the groups tended to rise or fall with the reported energy intake.

• On average, intakes of protein, riboflavin, vitamin B_{12}, and niacin
exceeded the RDAs, and there was only one report of low vitamin C intake.
This exception (Brennan et al., 1983a,b) was for the chemically *analyzed*
vitamin C content of the foods consumed, which was substantially lower
than that calculated from food composition tables. Average thiamin intakes
were close to the RDA in all studies.

• Some nutrients were consumed consistently in amounts substantially less than the RDA. These include vitamins B_6, D, E, and folacin;
iron; zinc; and magnesium.

• Mean calcium intake was less than the RDA in all but one study, in
which high intakes of all nutrients were reported for a group of teenagers
(Loris et al., 1985), and very close to the RDA in another study (Suitor
et al., 1989). Calcium values shown in Table 13-2 were especially low for
nonparticipants in WIC (Rush et al., 1988), black women (Brennan et al.,
1983a), and Navajo women (Butte et al., 1981).

• In the few studies that included vitamin E, intake averaged about half of the RDA for women of Hispanic and Navajo origin but was somewhat higher for others. The few studies including vitamin D indicated that intake of that vitamin was approximately half the RDA.

• There was a wide range in mean nutrient intake across different samples of pregnant teenagers. One group of investigators (Endres et al., 1985, 1987) found that the quantity and quality of the diet consumed by pregnant adolescents was similar to that consumed by pregnant adults. In contrast, Loris et al. (1985) observed higher intakes of energy and most other nutrients among adolescents as well as a greater weight gain than is typical for adults. Adolescents receiving more nutrition education consumed greater amounts of energy—400 kcal/day on average more than did those with little nutrition education.

• Some of the food composition data bases lacked information on nutrients that may be present in the diets of pregnant women at levels that are substantially less than recommended. This may partially explain why many of the investigators did not present values for zinc; magnesium; copper; and vitamins B_6, B_{12}, D, and E.

• The mean daily consumption of iron from foods ranged from 10.3 to 16.6 mg. The highest iron intakes were reported for black and Navajo women. However, comparisons of adequacy of iron intake were not made based on the amount of available iron (see Chapter 14).

• Vitamin A intakes were reported in international units (IUs) or in milligrams, whereas the RDAs are given as micrograms of retinol equivalents (REs). The subcommittee converted intake data to micrograms of RE based on the assumption that 1 RE is equivalent to 5 IU of vitamin A obtained from the typical U.S. diet in the form of retinol (from animal products) and carotenoids (from plants) (Olson, 1987) and that 1 mg of retinol equals 3,333 IU. Mean intakes of this vitamin appeared to be close to the RDA, on average, but were low in pregnant Navajo women.

In summary, the data in Table 13-2 indicate that, on average, pregnant women in the studies cited probably met their RDA for protein, thiamin, riboflavin, niacin, and vitamins A, B_{12}, and C. They were less likely to have met their RDAs for vitamins B_6, D, E, and folacin; iron; calcium; zinc; and magnesium. Because the RDA for iron during pregnancy is more than twice as high as average intake, it cannot be met from dietary sources without the use of highly fortified foods or very careful food selection (see Chapter 14).

The fact that the average intake of eight nutrients by almost all groups studied was substantially below the RDAs for pregnant women should be interpreted with caution. The RDAs for all vitamins and minerals include a safety factor to cover the needs of even those healthy individuals whose metabolism is such that their requirements are especially high; thus, it is possible that the RDAs for these eight nutrients are quite generous for most women. The food intake methods used in these studies may have underestimated true consumption. In the case of vitamin D, synthesis in the skin during summer months can contribute substantially to vitamin D adequacy. Finally, the number of women studied is relatively small, and women with medium to high incomes were underrepresented.

These data should also be interpreted in light of the fact that even the well-balanced diets of healthy, nonpregnant adults provide low amounts of these same nutrients relative to the RDAs (King et al., 1978; Peterkin, 1986). In the 1985 CSFII, a sample of all women aged 19 to 50 consumed less than three-quarters of their 1980 RDAs for iron, magnesium, calcium, zinc, vitamin B_6, and folate (Peterkin, 1986). (Vitamin D intakes were not reported.) Nonetheless, of these nutrients, the *Report on Nutrition Monitoring in the United States* (LSRO, 1989) categorized only iron and calcium as food components that are recommended for high-priority monitoring status because they represent public health problems in the population.

ASSOCIATIONS OF MATERNAL CHARACTERISTICS WITH NUTRIENT INTAKE DURING PREGNANCY

Ethnic Background

There have been no studies of both dietary and sociodemographic factors in a large, random sample of pregnant women in the United States. In a national sample of 1,503 women between the ages of 19 and 50, 93.4 % of whom were not pregnant or lactating (USDA, 1985), the most notable ethnic difference was calcium intake, which was 464 mg/day for blacks compared with 656 mg/day for whites (Peterkin, 1986). The data in Table 13-2 suggest that this difference persists during pregnancy.

In the National WIC Evaluation (Rush et al., 1988), in which all of the subjects were from low-income households, a few notable differences in intake were ascribed to ethnic background after a variety of maternal characteristics had been controlled statistically. Before registration in WIC, blacks had much lower intakes (703 mg/day) of calcium than did white non-Hispanics (1,045 mg/day), whereas Hispanic women consumed intermediate amounts (862 mg/day). Suitor et al. (1990) reported similar trends in calcium intake by ethnic groups among low-income pregnant women in Massachusetts. This situation may be explained in part by the much higher prevalence of lactose intolerance among blacks and Hispanics, sometimes resulting in their subsequent avoidance of milk. Data from one study (Villar et al., 1988) indicated that lactose intolerance abates during pregnancy, but this is unlikely to change dietary patterns substantially. Rush et al. (1988)

reported that enrollment in WIC was associated with 170- and 150-mg/day increases in calcium intake by blacks and Hispanics, respectively; however, average intakes remained low, especially for blacks. Lactose intolerance may not prevent blacks and Hispanics from consuming at least some of the dairy products supplied by WIC. It is also possible, however, that women *reported* a higher than actual consumption of the foods from the WIC package.

Socioeconomic and Demographic Factors

In the National WIC Evaluation (Rush et al., 1988), investigators examined associations between nutrient intake and factors such as income and occupation at the time of registration in the program. In this analysis, the relationships between specific socioeconomic or demographic factors and intake were controlled for all other maternal characteristics at registration that might confound interpretation of the results by differentially affecting intake. These included maternal ethnic background, age, parity, history of low birth weight or infant death, cigarette smoking, alcohol intake, participation in assistance programs, income, family size, and parental work status.

In these WIC-eligible, low-income women, employment was generally not associated with higher nutrient intakes and, in fact, was negatively related to calcium consumption. Wives of agricultural workers consumed substantially more energy, protein, and iron than did other women. The reasons for these associations were not established. On the other hand, Suitor et al. (1990) reported higher intakes of protein and zinc by employed rather than by unemployed low-income pregnant women. In the National WIC Evaluation, the number of people in the household had a minimal effect on nutrient intake by pregnant women. Income had a positive relationship to the intake of energy and protein by pregnant women: an additional 1.4 kcal of energy and 0.04 g of protein was consumed for every $100 per year increase in income. These results differ somewhat from those reported for the largely nonpregnant sample of women aged 19 to 50 who participated in CSFII. Their mean intakes of calcium; magnesium; iron; zinc; and vitamins B_6, E, and folate increased slightly with income (Peterkin, 1986). To some extent, the apparent effects of income in the CSFII analysis may be due to other demographic differences, such as household composition and lower proportions of blacks and Hispanics in the higher-income groups.

WIC Participation

The third-trimester mean intake of several nutrients by women who were WIC participants was significantly higher than that of nonparticipants

(Rush et al., 1988). For protein, the intake was 5 g/day higher; for iron, 3.2 mg/day; for calcium, 133 mg/day; and for vitamin C, 32 mg/day. Vitamin A intake was unchanged. Among WIC participants there were also statistically significant higher daily intakes of energy (111 kcal), magnesium (25 mg), thiamin (0.34 mg), riboflavin (0.37 mg), niacin (3.2 mg), vitamin B_6 (0.34 mg), and vitamin B_{12} (1.3 μg). In a smaller study, Suitor et al. (1990) found that WIC participants had significantly higher intakes of protein, calcium, iron, and vitamin B_6 per 1,000 kcal compared with nonparticipants. The strongest explanation for the higher intakes is the greater nutrient density of WIC foods compared with that of women's usual diets; the relative increases for most nutrients were higher than that for energy.

In the National WIC Evaluation (Rush et al., 1988), the effects of WIC on nutrient intake appeared to be generally uniform across sociodemographic groups, except for the greater improvements in calcium intake by blacks. The heaviest cigarette smokers also benefited more; WIC participation increased their intake of most nutrients.

Maternal Age

There are insufficient data from random national surveys to describe the effects of maternal age on nutrient intake during pregnancy, but data from CSFII and NHANES II indicate that intakes of most nutrients and of energy by women decrease with age (Carroll et al., 1983; USDA, 1985). As shown in Table 13-2, there are wide differences among the reported intakes by pregnant teenagers in several small studies (Endres et al., 1985, 1987; Loris et al., 1985). In contrast to the data on nonpregnant women, the National WIC Evaluation (Rush et al., 1988) indicated that younger women consumed less energy (intake increased by 18 kcal/day for each year of age), protein (0.5 g/year), and calcium (8 mg/year).

SUMMARY

Data on the reported dietary nutrient intakes by pregnant women studied in the past decade show that the intakes of eight nutrients consistently average less than the 1989 RDAs, namely, vitamins B_6, D, E, and folate; iron; calcium; zinc; and magnesium. Because of these apparent shortfalls, the subcommittee paid special attention to evidence regarding the need to supplement pregnant women with those nutrients. Somewhat less attention was directed toward protein; thiamin; riboflavin; niacin; and vitamins A, B_{12}, and C, because average dietary intakes generally meet the 1989 RDAs. The most notable relationship between ethnic background and dietary intake is a lower consumption of calcium by blacks, Hispanics, and American Indians. WIC participation is associated with higher intakes of energy and a number of vitamins and minerals.

REFERENCES

Beal, V.A. 1971. Nutritional studies during pregnancy. II. Dietary intake, maternal weight gain, and infant size. J. Am. Diet. Assoc. 58:321-326.

Brandes, J.M. 1967. First-trimester nausea and vomiting as related to outcome of pregnancy. Obstet. Gynecol. 30:427-431.

Brennan, R.E., M.B. Kohrs, J.W. Nordstrom, J.P. Sauvage, and R.E. Shank. 1983a. Composition of diets of low-income pregnant women: comparison of analyzed with calculated values. J. Am. Diet. Assoc. 83:538-545.

Brennan, R.E., M.B. Kohrs, J.W. Nordstrom, J.P. Sauvage, and R.E. Shank. 1983b. Nutrient intake of low-income pregnant women: laboratory analysis of foods consumed. J. Am. Diet. Assoc. 83:546-550.

Butte, N.F., D.H. Calloway, and J.L. Van Duzen. 1981. Nutritional assessment of pregnant and lactating Navajo women. Am. J. Clin. Nutr. 34:2216-2228.

Carroll, M.D., S. Abraham, and C.M. Dresser. 1983. Dietary Intake Source Data: United States, 1976-80. Vital and Health Statistics, Series 11, No. 231. DHHS Publ. No. (PHS) 83-1681. National Center for Health Statistics, Public Health Service, U.S. Department of Health and Human Services, Hyattsville, Md. 483 pp.

Dwyer, J., and C.W. Suitor. 1984. Caveat emptor: assessing needs, evaluating computer options. J. Am. Diet. Assoc. 84:302-312.

Endres, J.M., K. Poell-Odenwald, M. Sawicki, and P. Welch. 1985. Dietary assessment of pregnant adolescents participating in a supplemental-food program. J. Reprod. Med. 30:10-17.

Endres, J., S. Dunning, S. Poon, P. Welch, and H. Duncan. 1987. Older pregnant women and adolescents: nutrition data after enrollment in WIC. J. Am. Diet. Assoc. 87:1011-1019.

Hunt, I.F., N.J. Murphy, A.E. Cleaver, B. Faraji, M.E. Swendseid, A.H. Coulson, V.A.Clark, N. Laine, C.A. Davis, and J.C. Smith, Jr. 1983. Zinc supplementation during pregnancy: zinc concentration of serum and hair from low-income women of Mexican descent. Am. J. Clin. Nutr. 37:572-582.

IOM (Institute of Medicine). 1988. Prenatal Care: Reaching Mothers, Reaching Infants. Report of the Committee to Study Outreach for Prenatal Care, Division of Health Promotion and Disease Prevention. National Academy Press, Washington, D.C. 254 pp.

King, J.C., S.H. Cohenour, C.G. Corruccini, and P. Schneeman. 1978. Evaluation and modification of the basic four food guide. J. Nutr. Educ. 10:27-29.

Klebanoff, M.A., P.A. Koslowe, R. Kaslow, and G.G. Rhoads. 1985. Epidemiology of vomiting in early pregnancy. Obstet. Gynecol. 66:612-616.

Loris, P., K.G. Dewey, and K. Poirier-Brode. 1985. Weight gain and dietary intake of pregnant teenagers. J. Am. Diet. Assoc. 85:1296-1305.

LSRO (Life Sciences Research Office). 1989. Nutrition Monitoring in the United States: An Update Report on Nutrition Monitoring. Prepared for the U.S. Department of Agriculture and the U.S. Department of Health and Human Services. DHHS Publ. No. (PHS) 89-1225. U.S. Government Printing Office, Washington, D.C. (various pagings).

NRC (National Research Council). 1982. Alternative Dietary Practices and Nutritional Abuses in Pregnancy: Proceedings of a Workshop. Report of the Committee on Nutrition of the Mother and Preschool Child, Food and Nutrition Board, Commission on Life Sciences. National Academy Press, Washington, D.C. 211 pp.

NRC (National Research Council). 1989. Recommended Dietary Allowances, 10th ed. Report of the Subcommittee on the Tenth Edition of the RDAs, Food and Nutrition Board, Commission on Life Sciences. National Academy Press, Washington, D.C. 284 pp.

Olson, J.A. 1987. Recommended dietary intakes (RDI) of vitamin A in humans. Am. J. Clin. Nutr. 45:704-716.

Peterkin, B.B. 1986. Women's diets: 1977 and 1985. J. Nutr. Educ. 18:251-257.

Picone, T.A., L.H. Allen, M.M. Schramm, and P.N. Olsen. 1982. Pregnancy outcome in North American women. I. Effects of diet, cigarette smoking, and psychological stress on maternal weight gain. Am. J. Clin. Nutr. 36:1205-1213.

Rush, D., N.L. Sloan, J. Leighton, J.M. Alvir, D.G. Horvitz, W.B. Seaver, G.C. Garbowski, S.S. Johnson, R.A. Kulka, M. Holt, J.W. Devore, J.T. Lynch, M.B. Woodside, and D.S. Shanklin. 1988. The National WIC Evaluation: Evaluation of the Special Supplemental Food Program for Women, Infants, and Children. V. Longitudinal study of pregnant women. Am. J. Clin. Nutr. 48:439-483.

Suitor, C.J.W., J. Gardner, and W.C. Willett. 1989. A comparison of food frequency and diet recall methods in studies of nutrient intake of low-income pregnant women. J. Am. Diet. Assoc. 89:1786-1794.

Suitor, C.W., J.D. Gardner, and M.L. Feldstein. 1990. Characteristics of diet among a culturally diverse group of low-income pregnant women. J. Am. Diet. Assoc. 90:543-549.

Taggart, N. 1961. Food habits in pregnancy. Proc. Nutr. Soc. 20:35-40.

Taper, L.J., J.T. Oliva, and S.J. Ritchey. 1985. Zinc and copper retention during pregnancy: the adequacy of prenatal diets with and without dietary supplementation. Am. J. Clin. Nutr. 41:1184-1192.

Tierson, F.D., C.L. Olsen, and E.B. Hook. 1985. Influence of cravings and aversions on diet in pregnancy. Ecol. Food Nutr. 17:117-129.

Tierson, F.D., C.L. Olsen, and E.B. Hook. 1986. Nausea and vomiting of pregnancy and association with pregnancy outcome. Am. J. Obstet. Gynecol. 155:1017-1022.

USDA (U.S. Department of Agriculture). 1985. Nationwide Food Consumption Survey. Continuing Survey of Food Intakes by Individuals. Women 19-50 Years and Their Children 1-5 Years, 1 Day, 1985. Report No. 85-1. Nutrition Monitoring Division, Human Nutrition Information Service, U.S. Department of Agriculture, Hyattsville, Md. 102 pp.

Villar, J., E. Kestler, P. Castillo, A. Juarez, R. Menendez, and N.W. Solomons. 1988. Improved lactose digestion during pregnancy: a case of physiologic adaptation? Obstet. Gynecol. 71:697-700.

Worthington-Roberts, B., R.E. Little, M.D. Lambert, and R. Wu. 1989. Dietary cravings and aversions in the postpartum period. J. Am. Diet. Assoc. 89:647-651.

14

Iron Nutrition During Pregnancy

IMPORTANCE OF IRON DURING PREGNANCY

Among healthy human beings, pregnant women and rapidly growing infants are most vulnerable to iron deficiency (Bothwell et al., 1979). Both groups have to absorb substantially more iron than is lost from the body, and both are at a considerable risk of developing iron deficiency under ordinary dietary circumstances. During pregnancy, more iron is needed primarily to supply the growing fetus and placenta and to increase the maternal red cell mass (Hallberg, 1988).

Iron deficiency is common among pregnant women in industrialized countries, as shown by numerous studies in which hemoglobin concentrations during the last half of pregnancy were found to be higher in iron-supplemented women than in those given a placebo or no supplement (Table 14-1) (Chanarin and Rothman, 1971; Dawson and McGanity, 1987; Puolakka et al., 1980b; Romslo et al., 1983; Svanberg et al., 1976a; Taylor et al., 1982; Wallenburg and van Eijk, 1984). This higher hemoglobin concentration as a result of an improved iron supply not only increases the oxygen-carrying capacity, but it also provides a buffer against the blood loss that will occur during delivery (Hallberg, 1988).

Iron is essential for the production of hemoglobin, which functions in the delivery of oxygen from the lungs to the tissues of the body, and for the synthesis of iron enzymes, which are required to utilize oxygen for the production of cellular energy (Bothwell et al., 1979).

272

TABLE 14-1 Effects of Iron Supplementation on Mean Hemoglobin Concentration Late in Pregnancy

Dose of Elemental Iron[a]	Number of Subjects		Hemoglobin, g/dl, at 35–40 wk of Gestation			Reference
	Supplemented	Controls	Supplemented	Controls	Difference[b]	
30 mg/day as ferrous fumarate[c]	49	46	12.4	11.4	1.0	Chanarin and Rothman, 1971
100 mg, twice daily, with meals, sustained release	24	26	12.4	11.4	1.0	Svanberg et al., 1976a
100 mg, twice daily, sustained release	16	16	12.7	11.0	1.7	Puolakka et al., 1980b
65 mg (+ 350 µg of folate)	21	24	12.7	11.0	1.6	Taylor et al., 1982
200 mg/day	22	23	12.6	11.3	1.3	Romslo et al., 1983
105 mg, sustained release, at breakfast	21	23	12.6	12.2	0.4	Wallenburg and van Eijk, 1984
65 mg as part of multivitamin-mineral supplement after meals	16	13	12.4	11.4	1.0	Dawson and McGanity, 1987

[a] Ferrous sulfate, unless otherwise stated.

[b] All differences were statistically significant except for Wallenburg and van Eijk (1984).

[c] Doses of 60 mg and 120 mg did not result in higher hemoglobin values.

Definition of Anemia and Iron Deficiency

Anemia is defined as a hemoglobin concentration that is more than 2 standard deviations below the mean for healthy individuals of the same age, sex, and stage of pregnancy. Although iron deficiency is the most common cause of anemia, infection, genetic factors, and many other conditions can also lead to anemia. Iron depletion is generally described in terms of three stages of progressively increasing severity (Bothwell et al., 1979):

1. *depletion of iron stores*
2. *impaired hemoglobin production* (or iron deficiency without anemia)
3. *iron deficiency anemia*

The first stage, depletion of iron, is characterized by a low serum ferritin level. This stage is the most difficult to define because it involves an arbitrary decision about how low iron stores should be before they are considered depleted. This is a particularly thorny issue with respect to pregnancy, because storage iron, estimated from bone marrow aspirates (or less directly by the serum ferritin), is low or absent in most women during the third trimester, whether (Svanberg et al., 1976a) or not (Heinrich et al., 1968; Svanberg et al., 1976a) they have received an iron supplement. For this reason, the subcommittee considered low iron stores in late pregnancy to be physiologic and reserved the term *iron deficiency* for the second and third stages. The second stage, *impaired hemoglobin production*, is recognized by laboratory tests that indicate an insufficient supply of iron to developing red blood cells, such as a low ratio of serum iron to total iron-binding capacity (Fe/TIBC), low mean corpuscular volume (MCV), and/or elevated erythrocyte protoporphyrin (EP), but with a hemoglobin concentration that remains within the normal reference range. *Iron deficiency anemia* (the third stage) refers to an anemia (e.g., hemoglobin values below the 5th percentile in Figure 14-1) that is associated with additional laboratory evidence of iron deficiency, such as a low serum ferritin level, low serum Fe/TIBC, low MCV, or an elevated EP level (also see the section Laboratory Characteristics of Impaired Hemoglobin Production).

Effects of Maternal Anemia on the Newborn

Although some epidemiologic evidence suggests that anemia during pregnancy could be harmful to the fetus, the data are far from conclusive. In a report of more than 54,000 pregnancies in the Cardiff area of South Wales, the risk of low birth weight, preterm birth, and perinatal mortality was found to be higher when the hemoglobin concentration was in the anemic range—<10.4 g/dl before 24 weeks of gestation—compared with a midrange hemoglobin concentration of 10.4 to 13.2 g/dl (Murphy et al., 1986). Elevated hemoglobin values of >13.2 g/dl were also associated

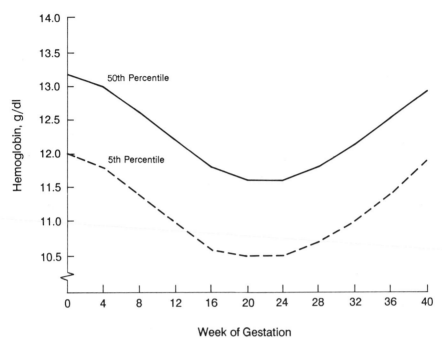

FIGURE 14-1 Normal hemoglobin values during pregnancy. Values from 12 to 40 weeks of gestation are based on data from Svanberg et al. (1976a), Sjöstedt et al. (1977), Puolakka et al. (1980b), and Taylor et al. (1982). The baseline values (zero weeks) are based on LSRO (1984), and the 4- and 8-week values are extrapolated from all these data and from Clapp et al. (1988). Unpublished figure from R. Yip, Centers for Disease Control, 1989, with permission.

with an increased risk of the same poor pregnancy outcomes, perhaps because such values are characteristic of women who develop preeclampsia (hypertension accompanied by generalized pitting edema or proteinuria after week 20 of gestation), who are similarly at risk. Another pertinent study is that of Garn and coworkers (1981), which was based on more than 50,000 pregnancies in the National Collaborative Perinatal Project of the National Institute of Neurologic and Communicative Disorders and Stroke. As in the South Wales study, there was a U-shaped relationship between the maternal hemoglobin or hematocrit level during pregnancy and the pregnancy outcome. When the lowest hemoglobin concentration during any stage of pregnancy was below 10.0 g/dl, the likelihood of low birth weight, preterm birth, and perinatal mortality was increased. A hemoglobin concentration that was high during pregnancy (>13.0 g/dl) was also associated with these poor pregnancy outcomes.

In most populations, iron deficiency is by far the most common cause of anemia before 24 weeks of gestation (Puolakka et al., 1980c). It seems plausible, therefore, that iron deficiency could account for the higher risk to the fetus among the anemic pregnant women in the studies described above. However, a cause-and-effect relationship has not been established. Iron deficiency and anemia are more common in blacks and in those of low socioeconomic status, those with multiple gestations, and those with limited education (LSRO, 1984). Any of these confounding factors could be related to a poor pregnancy outcome independently of iron deficiency.

Additional studies indicate a link between maternal anemia at full term and low birth weight (Klein, 1962; Lieberman et al., 1987; Macgregor, 1963), but interpretation of the results is complicated by the fact that the hemoglobin concentration normally rises in the third trimester of pregnancy (Figure 14-1) if sufficient iron is available (Puolakka et al., 1980b; Sjöstedt et al., 1977; Svanberg et al., 1976a; Taylor et al., 1982). An association between a low maternal hemoglobin concentration at delivery and low birth weight can be expected since lower hemoglobin values are characteristic of an earlier stage of gestation.

The infant of an iron-depleted mother has surprisingly little evidence of anemia or depletion of iron stores. Numerous studies in which serum ferritin was used to estimate the neonatal iron stores of infants from iron-deficient or iron-sufficient or supplemented mothers show relatively little difference (Agrawal et al., 1983; Fenton et al., 1977; Kaneshige, 1981; Kelly et al., 1978; MacPhail et al., 1980; Milman et al., 1987; Puolakka et al., 1980a) or no significant difference (Bratlid and Moe, 1980; Celada et al., 1982; Hussain et al., 1977; Messer et al., 1980; Rios et al., 1975; van Eijk et al., 1978). Hemoglobin concentration in the newborn was unaffected or minimally affected in most studies (Agrawal et al., 1983; Murray et al., 1978; Sisson and Lund, 1958; Sturgeon, 1959). In the study reported by Sturgeon, hemoglobin concentrations of 6-, 12-, and 18-month-old infants of iron-supplemented mothers were similar to those in infants of unsupplemented mothers. Only in two studies, both from developing countries, was it concluded that newborn infants of anemic mothers were also anemic, although to a far lesser degree than their mothers (Nhonoli et al., 1975; Singla et al., 1978). However, comparable studies from similar settings did not confirm this finding (Agrawal et al., 1983; Murray et al., 1978), suggesting that other nutritional deficiencies and such factors as infection (malaria) might explain the disagreement. Overall, there is little or no laboratory evidence that infants of iron-deficient mothers are more likely to be iron deficient, but it is possible that the risk of low birth weight, prematurity, and perinatal mortality may be increased.

PREVALENCE OF IRON DEFICIENCY

Data on the prevalence of iron deficiency among women during the childbearing years in the United States are available mainly from the second (1976-1980) National Health and Nutrition Examination Survey (NHANES II) (LSRO, 1984). Population estimates were based on a combination of laboratory indices—EP, MCV, and Fe/TIBC—in a nationally representative sample of 2,474 women aged 20 to 44 and 697 younger women aged 15 to 19. Serum ferritin assays were done on a subset of approximately 30% of this population; it was a relatively new assay at the time. Too few pregnant women were included in the survey for detailed analysis.

Two sets of laboratory criteria were used to estimate the prevalence of impaired iron status, which was defined as two or three abnormal laboratory test results out of a set of three tests for iron status. This approach had been found to be more reliable in relation to anemia than the use of any single test (Cook et al., 1976). In the so-called MCV model, MCV, Fe/TIBC, and EP were used for the analysis; these laboratory results were available for most subjects. In the ferritin model, the serum ferritin concentration was substituted for the MCV and probably represents an earlier stage of iron deficiency. Impaired iron status in either model can be considered to be equivalent to iron deficiency, taking into consideration that infection and chronic disease can be confounding factors by mimicking the laboratory abnormalities of iron deficiency.

Among nonpregnant women between the ages of 20 and 44, estimated percentages of impaired iron status varied according to model used: 9.6 ± 1.3% (standard error of the mean [SEM]) as determined by the ferritin model, and 5.4 ± 0.5% as determined by the MCV model. Iron deficiency anemia (two or three abnormal values *and* hemoglobin <11.9 g/dl) among nonpregnant white women aged 20 to 44 was less than 2% as determined by both models.

If the prevalence of iron deficiency among pregnant women were no higher than the 5 to 10% reported in NHANES II for nonpregnant women of childbearing age, there would be little basis for considering routine iron supplementation during pregnancy. However, it is generally agreed that both iron needs and prevalence of iron deficiency increase substantially during pregnancy (Hallberg, 1988). In a paper on the worldwide prevalence of anemia written for the World Health Organization, the global prevalence of anemia was estimated at 51% among pregnant women, compared with 35% among women in general, including pregnant women (DeMaeyer and Adiels-Tegman, 1985). Most of the anemia was attributed to iron deficiency. The higher prevalence for pregnant women is consistent with the estimated high iron needs during pregnancy (Bothwell et al., 1979; Hallberg, 1988; see also the section Iron Requirements for Pregnancy).

The most convincing evidence that pregnant women in industrial-ized countries often cannot meet their iron needs from diet alone comes from three careful longitudinal studies from northern European countries. Groups of iron-supplemented and unsupplemented pregnant women were followed with laboratory studies from early pregnancy at 4-week intervals (Puolakka et al., 1980b; Svanberg et al., 1976b; Taylor et al., 1982). In all these studies, the hemoglobin values in the unsupplemented group were significantly lower than those in the supplemented group after 24 to 28 weeks of gestation. The mean difference was 1.0 to 1.7 g/dl between weeks 35 and 40 of gestation. In the latter two studies, the means were more than 2 standard deviations apart during this period, indicating a high preva-lence of impaired hemoglobin production because of a lack of iron in the unsupplemented group. Thus, even though there are no good prevalence data for iron deficiency during pregnancy, it is reasonable to infer that the prevalence is high.

SPECIAL GROUPS AT RISK

Data from 1976-1980 NHANES II and 1982-1984 Hispanic HANES (HHANES) suggest that low socioeconomic status, low level of education, black or Hispanic background, and high parity were associated with iron deficiency (impaired iron status) in the MCV model for nonpregnant women (LSRO, 1984, 1989). It is reasonable to infer that the same factors would play a role, probably to a greater degree, when iron demands are drastically increased during the last half of pregnancy. The following factors are associated with an increased risk of iron deficiency:

- Pregnancy (second two trimesters)
- Menorrhagia (loss of more than 80 ml of blood per month)
- Diets low in both meat and ascorbic acid
- Multiple gestation
- Blood donation more than three times per year
- Chronic use of aspirin

Socioeconomic Indicators

The prevalence of iron deficiency in NHANES II tended to be higher among the poor; the difference was of borderline significance ($p < .1$) for women aged 20 to 44 and significant ($p < .05$) for women aged 15 to 19. The percentages were 5.1 ± 0.5 (SEM) and 3.6 ± 1.0, respectively, for those above the poverty level and 7.8 ± 1.5 and $8.2 \pm 1.8\%$, respectively, for those below the poverty level. Iron deficiency was also more common among women between the ages of 20 and 44 with limited education (13.4

± 2.8%) compared with those with high school (5.4 ± 0.6%) or college (4.2 ± 0.8%) education.

Racial and Ethnic Backgrounds

The prevalence of iron deficiency using the MCV model among 20- to 44-year-old Mexican-American women in HHANES was substantially higher than that among non-Hispanic whites in NHANES II, 11.9 ± 2.0% compared with 5.4 ± 0.5%, respectively. Average parity among the Mexican-American women was considerably higher than that among non-Hispanic whites, and this probably contributed to the higher prevalence of iron deficiency among the Mexican-American women. Impaired iron status with increasing parity was also more prevalent in NHANES II. Iron deficiency was present in 3.1 ± 0.5% of women with no children, in 3.8 ± 0.8% of those with one or two children, in 9.4 ± 1.1% of those with three to four children, and in 11.5 ± 2.1% of those with five or more children. In NHANES II, the same prevalence of iron deficiency (impaired iron status) was found among black women, aged 20 to 44, as among whites in the same age group (5.7 ± 0.9 and 5.0 ± 0.6%, respectively). Among the small sample of teenagers, there was a difference (3.8 ± 0.9 and 12.6 ± 4.7, respectively) of borderline significance—(p <0.1).

Many risk factors, such as poverty, ethnic background, education, and parity, are closely interrelated. Unfortunately, the effects of these interrelationships have not been systematically studied. Most studies have focused on only one factor at a time.

Adolescents

Teenagers may also have an increased risk of iron deficiency because of the high iron requirements imposed by their recent growth spurt (Dawson and McGanity, 1987). In NHANES II, females aged 15 to 19 had a 4.9 ± 1.1% prevalence of iron deficiency as determined by the MCV model and 14.2 ± 3.5% as determined by the ferritin model. The sample was small, and the percentages did not differ significantly from those of the corresponding group of women between the ages of 20 and 44.

IRON METABOLISM IN RELATION TO PREGNANCY

Essential and Storage Iron

The total amount of iron in the average woman's body is about 2.2 g (Bothwell et al., 1979), which is equal to the weight of a dime. Most of this iron can be considered *essential* because it functions in the transport and utilization of oxygen for the production of cellular energy. Two compounds, ferritin and hemosiderin, serve as a reserve. Iron from these compounds can be mobilized for the production of essential compounds when the supply of dietary iron is insufficient. The vulnerability of an individual to iron deficiency depends on the amount of iron stored.

Iron Loss

Catabolized iron is efficiently reutilized, and very little iron is lost from the body except through bleeding. Normal iron losses average approximately 0.9 mg/day in adult men—the population that has been the most thoroughly studied (Green et al., 1968). The corresponding value for women, excluding menstrual losses, is estimated to be about 0.8 mg/day. Menstrual iron losses average about 0.5 mg/day. When this is added to the other losses of 0.8 mg/day, the total is 1.3 mg/day.

Excessive menstrual blood loss (menorrhagia), defined as >80 ml/ month, occurs in about 10% of women (Cole et al., 1971; Hallberg et al., 1966). This is equivalent to 1 mg of iron or more lost per day, more than twice the average menstrual iron loss. Menstrual blood loss of >80 ml/month commonly results in iron deficiency (Hallberg et al., 1966). Consequently, some women face the increased iron demands of pregnancy with an already established iron deficiency. Menstrual blood loss varies markedly among women, but in any given woman, there is relatively little variation in the amount of blood lost from one month to the next (Hallberg et al., 1966). Unfortunately, a careful history can barely distinguish groups of women whose volume of blood loss is expected to differ on the basis of oral contraceptive use (Frassinelli-Gunderson et al., 1985).

Women who take oral contraceptive agents will, on average, halve their menstrual blood loss, whereas those who use intrauterine devices (now rare in the United States) will roughly double it (Hefnawi et al., 1974; Israel et al., 1974). Users of oral contraceptives have substantially higher iron stores than do nonusers, based on serum ferritin values (Frassinelli-Gunderson et al., 1985). In NHANES II, 18% of women aged 20 to 44 took oral contraceptives.

Other common reasons for increased iron losses are blood donation and aspirin ingestion. Women who donate more than three units of blood per year are at high risk of being iron deficient (Finch et al., 1977; Simon et al., 1981), unless they take iron supplements regularly. Aspirin ingestion amounting to 300 mg (one tablet) four times a day increases intestinal blood loss from the normal average of about 0.5 ml/day to 5 ml/day (Pierson et al., 1961). These amounts are equivalent to about 0.2 and 2.0 mg of iron loss per day, respectively.

Regulation of Body Iron

The amount of iron in the body is determined mainly by the percentage of food iron absorbed from the intestine—a percentage that can vary more than 20-fold (Charlton and Bothwell, 1983; Hallberg, 1981). The bioavailability of iron—that is, the proportion absorbed from food—is determined both by the nature of the diet and by a regulatory mechanism in the intestinal mucosa that is responsive to the abundance of storage iron.

Absorption of Nonheme and Heme Iron from Food

Two types of iron are present in food: heme iron, which is found principally in animal products, and nonheme iron, which is found mainly in plant products. Most of the iron in the diet, an average of more than 88% (Raper et al., 1984), is present as nonheme iron and consists primarily of iron salts. The absorption of nonheme iron is strongly influenced by its solubility in the upper part of the small intestine, which in turn depends on the composition of the meal as a whole (Charlton and Bothwell, 1983; Hallberg, 1981).

Iron absorption tends to be poor from meals in which whole-grain cereals and legumes predominate. Phytates in whole-grain cereals, calcium and phosphorus in milk, tannin in tea, and polyphenols in many vegetables all inhibit iron absorption by decreasing the intestinal solubility of nonheme iron from the entire meal. The addition of even relatively small amounts of meat and ascorbic acid-containing foods substantially increases the absorption of iron from the entire meal by keeping nonheme iron more soluble. For example, compared with water, orange juice will roughly double the absorption of nonheme iron from a meal. Tea and coffee, on the other hand, will cut the absorption of nonheme iron by more than half when compared with water (Hallberg, 1981; Rossander et al., 1979). Thus, modifications in the diet offer great scope for improving iron absorption during pregnancy. Consumption of meals containing enhancers of iron absorption, such as meat and ascorbic acid-rich fruits and vegetables, and avoidance of strong inhibitors such as tea should do much to prevent iron deficiency (Monsen et al., 1978). However, there is little information on the effectiveness of dietary counseling in preventing iron deficiency.

Heme iron is derived primarily from the hemoglobin and myoglobin in meat, poultry, and fish. Although heme iron accounts for a smaller proportion of iron in the diet than nonheme iron does, a much greater percentage of heme iron is absorbed, and its absorption is relatively unaffected by other dietary constituents (Hallberg, 1981).

When both forms of iron in the diet are considered, the average total dietary iron absorption by men is about 6% and by women in their child-bearing years, 13% (Charlton and Bothwell, 1983). The higher absorption in women is related to their lower iron stores and helps to compensate for the losses of iron associated with menstruation.

Intestinal Regulation

Entry of soluble nonheme iron into the body is regulated in the mucosal cell of the small intestine (Charlton and Bothwell, 1983), but the mechanism remains uncertain (Davidson and Lönnerdal, 1988; Huebers and Finch, 1987; Peters et al., 1988). If iron stores are low, the intestinal mucosa readily takes up nonheme iron and increases the proportion that is absorbed from the diet. During the course of pregnancy, as iron stores decrease, the absorption of dietary nonheme iron increases (Svanberg et al., 1976b). However, the adequacy of this homeostatic response is limited by the amount of absorbable iron in the diet and the high iron requirements for pregnancy.

IRON REQUIREMENTS FOR PREGNANCY

The body iron requirement for an average pregnancy is approximately 1,000 mg. Hallberg (1988) calculated that 350 mg of iron is lost to the *fetus* and the *placenta* and 250 mg is lost in *blood at delivery*. In addition, about 450 mg of iron is required for the large increase in maternal *red blood cell mass*. Lastly, *basal losses* of iron from the body continue during pregnancy and amount to about 240 mg. Thus, the total iron requirements of a pregnancy (excluding blood loss at delivery) average about 1,040 mg. Permanent iron losses during pregnancy include loss to the fetus and placenta, blood loss at delivery, and basal losses, which together total 840 mg.

The total iron needs of slightly more than 1,000 mg are concentrated in the last two trimesters of pregnancy. This amount is equivalent to about 6 mg of iron absorbed per day in a woman who starts pregnancy with absent or minimal storage iron. This is a large amount of iron to accumulate over a 6-month period, especially when compared with the average total body iron content of 2,200 mg and the 1.3 mg of iron absorbed per day by nonpregnant women.

Although 450 mg of iron for red cell production must be supplied during pregnancy, a large part of this can subsequently augment iron stores after a vaginal delivery, when the red cell mass decreases. The result is analogous to a postpartum injection of iron: serum ferritin levels will spontaneously increase within a few months after delivery in most women who develop mild iron deficiency during late pregnancy because of the iron that is released by the decline in red cell mass (Puolakka et al., 1980b; Svanberg et al., 1976a; Taylor et al., 1982). Postpartum iron status is also improved by the decreased iron loss during this period: less than 0.3 mg/day is lost in human milk, and menstruation is rare in women during their first few months of lactation.

The average blood loss during a cesarean delivery is almost twice that occurring with the average vaginal delivery of a single fetus (Pritchard, 1965; Pritchard et al., 1962; Ueland, 1976); the postpartum improvement in iron status may therefore be less complete after a cesarean delivery.

CHARACTERISTICS OF IRON DEFICIENCY DURING PREGNANCY

To establish reasonable goals for iron nutrition during pregnancy, it is helpful to distinguish between the *potential for iron deficiency as reflected by low iron stores alone* and *iron deficiency that results in impaired hemoglobin production.* In the absence of other laboratory evidence of iron deficiency, low serum ferritin is not associated with any deficits in physiologic function (Bothwell et al., 1979; Dallman, 1986). For this reason, an acceptable goal for iron nutrition during pregnancy is simply to avoid progression beyond low iron stores (first stage of iron depletion) to the stages of impaired hemoglobin production (second stage) or iron deficiency anemia (third stage).

Laboratory Characteristics of Impaired Hemoglobin Production

At this stage of iron depletion, the hemoglobin concentration is typically at the lower end of the normal range but not low enough to meet the definition of anemia. Nevertheless, there is the potential for impairment of physiologic function, because the production of essential iron compounds is decreased. This stage can most reliably be distinguished by a rise in hemoglobin concentration in response to iron treatment, demonstrating that the woman's previous hemoglobin concentration had been below her potential. Iron administration, regardless of dose, will not raise the hemoglobin concentration in the absence of iron deficiency. The hemoglobin response to iron therapy is difficult to use to detect iron deficiency during pregnancy because of the normal changes in blood volume and hemoglobin concentration during this period (Figure 14-1).

Fe/TIBC is typically subnormal in people with impaired hemoglobin production due to iron deficiency. Unfortunately, normal ranges for Fe/TIBC during pregnancy have not been firmly established. Fe/TIBC declines substantially during pregnancy, even in iron-supplemented women (Puolakka et al., 1980b; Svanberg et al., 1976a), and results from the test to determine this ratio indicate large biologic variations (Dallman, 1984;

LSRO, 1984). EP level is elevated with iron deficiency and is a potentially useful test during pregnancy (Schifman et al., 1987), particularly since levels in iron-supplemented women appear to remain stable from early to late gestation (Romslo et al., 1983).

Physiologic Changes in Hemoglobin Concentration and Criteria for Anemia During Pregnancy

For nonpregnant women, the normal mean hemoglobin concentration is 13.5 g/dl, and the 5th percentile value is about 12.0 g/dl (LSRO, 1984). As noted above, however, values change considerably during pregnancy (Figure 14-1). Even women who are adequately supplemented with iron have an almost 2 g/dl decline to a *mean* hemoglobin level of 11.6 g/dl in the second trimester (Puolakka et al., 1980b; Sjöstedt et al., 1977; Svanberg et al., 1976a; Taylor et al., 1982), largely because of the normal expansion of plasma volume (Hytten, 1985; Taylor and Lind, 1979). This increase in plasma volume is detectable as early as 6 to 8 weeks into gestation (Lund and Donovan, 1967). In the last trimester, the hemoglobin concentration gradually rises, reaching a mean value of 12.5 g/dl at 36 weeks of gestation. The World Health Organization criteria for anemia include a uniform value of <11.0 g/dl for all pregnant women instead of <12.0 g/dl, which is used for nonpregnant women (WHO, 1968). The values shown in Figure 14-1 were derived from four carefully performed longitudinal studies of iron-supplemented women (Puolakka et al., 1980b; Sjöstedt et al., 1977; Svanberg et al., 1976a; Taylor et al., 1982). On the basis of these data, cutoff values of 11.0, 10.5, and 11.0 g/dl for the first, second, and third trimesters, respectively, have recently been proposed by the Centers for Disease Control for the screening of pregnant women for anemia (CDC, 1989). If a pregnant woman is judged to be anemic by these criteria (or according to Figure 14-1) and the serum ferritin is <12 μg/liter, she can be presumed to have iron deficiency anemia because other causes of anemia are not characterized by a low serum ferritin level.

The MCV of red blood cells is typically decreased in people with iron deficiency anemia. In the absence of iron deficiency, however, the MCV normally rises by about 5% during pregnancy (Puolakka et al., 1980b; Taylor et al., 1982). Until adjusted MCV reference values for pregnancy are developed, it is doubtful that this determination will have much diagnostic value for pregnant women.

As long as iron deficiency remains prevalent among pregnant women, *the difficulty of predicting the subsequent development of iron deficiency from laboratory tests will argue strongly in favor of routine iron supplementation,* irrespective of the results of a routine screen for anemia. A more definitive screening followed by treatment only of those women with laboratory evidence of iron deficiency is a more difficult, time-consuming, and costly alternative. Tests for hemoglobin and serum ferritin are the most commonly used combination of laboratory tests for the diagnosis of iron deficiency in studies of pregnant women (Charoenlarp et al., 1988; Dawson and McGanity, 1987; Puolakka et al., 1980b; Romslo et al., 1983; Taylor et al., 1982; Wallenburg and van Eijk, 1984). However, even if hemoglobin and serum ferritin values are normal early in pregnancy, this is no assurance that iron deficiency anemia or impaired hemoglobin production (Lewis and Rowe, 1986) will not develop later. The need to repeat the hemoglobin and serum ferritin analyses one or more times later in pregnancy may be a deterrent to applying the screen-and-treat approach to the routine care of pregnant women.

ABSORPTION OF IRON SUPPLEMENTS

The absorption of iron supplements is influenced by the solubility of the iron compound (Brise and Hallberg, 1962a); the dose (Brise and Hallberg, 1962a; Ekenved et al., 1976a; Hahn et al., 1951; Sölvell, 1970); timing of the dose, e.g., with or between meals (Brise, 1962; Ekenved et al., 1976a; Hallberg et al., 1978; Layrisse et al., 1973); delivery of the dose, e.g., alone or as part of a vitamin-mineral supplement (Babior et al., 1985; Seligman et al., 1983); and the abundance of iron stores in the individual (Bezwoda et al., 1979; Brise and Hallberg, 1962a; Nielsen et al., 1976; Norrby, 1974).

When determining the dose of iron supplements, it is important to distinguish between the amount of the iron compound and the equivalent in terms of elemental iron. For example, hydrated ferrous sulfate (USP) contains 20% of iron by weight; therefore, a 300-mg tablet of ferrous sulfate contains 60 mg of iron. The corresponding percentages of iron in other commonly used compounds are 12% in ferrous gluconate and 32% in ferrous fumarate. The *total* absorption of iron from any of these ferrous iron compounds at any specified dose is roughly proportional to its iron content (Brise and Hallberg, 1962a). In the following discussion, doses are specified in terms of elemental iron.

There are two general approaches to evaluating the adequacy of various doses of iron supplements during pregnancy. One involves determining the percentage of iron that is absorbed from a *test dose* of the iron supplement and then extrapolating the results to the conditions of routine supplement use. The second approach, which might be termed a *therapeutic trial*, is to administer a certain dose of the supplement over several months and then to determine the efficacy of the regimen in preventing iron deficiency, based on the hemoglobin concentration and other laboratory tests of iron status.

Absorption from a Test Dose

A large and classic study of iron absorption from iron supplements during pregnancy included 466 women (Hahn et al., 1951), who were studied on their second prenatal visit, before initiation of iron supplements. Eleven different doses of ferrous ^{59}Fe were administered ranging from 1.8 to 120 mg. Figure 14-2 shows the median results for the 18-, 39-, and 120-mg doses. The higher the iron dose, the larger the amount absorbed but the lower the percentage absorbed. Absorption from the 120-mg dose was only about twice that from the 18-mg dose. Similarly, only about 50% more iron was absorbed when the dose was increased by about 200%—from 39 to 120 mg. These data suggest that doses of 120 mg and above may not confer a sufficient benefit to warrant the substantial likelihood of side effects (discussed below). Another noteworthy finding was the increase in iron absorption as pregnancy progressed (Figure 14-2).

Studies of women who donate blood regularly can provide data that are of relevance to pregnant women, because women who donate blood share many of the same characteristics with respect to low iron stores, increased iron requirements, and increased iron absorption. The average blood donation by a woman results in the loss of 200 mg of iron (Finch et al., 1977). Brise and Hallberg (1962a) used a dose of 30 mg of elemental iron as ferrous sulfate to study iron absorption in women after an overnight fast. A reassuringly high absorption of 27% was reported in donors compared with 17% in nondonors.

The relationships among stage of gestation, abundance of iron stores, and iron absorption were evaluated by Heinrich and coworkers (1968) in a large group of unsupplemented pregnant women who were given a very small test dose of ferrous iron (0.56 mg of ^{59}Fe) after an overnight fast between the fourth and ninth months of gestation. Hematologic studies and stainable iron in the bone marrow were also analyzed. Absorption increased gradually from about 40% during the fourth month to 90% during the ninth month of gestation. The results support the study of Hahn and coworkers (1951) in showing a substantial rise in iron absorption during pregnancy in unsupplemented women. The very high percentages that were reported by Heinrich and coworkers (1968) can be anticipated with a small test dose of iron, but should not be extrapolated to ordinary circumstances of diet and supplement use. The results also showed that absorption was greatest in those women with the lowest iron stores.

Iron absorption during the progression of pregnancy was also studied by Svanberg et al. (1976a). Iron absorption in primiparous women was measured from a single test dose of 100 mg of elemental iron, which was given as a solution of ferrous sulfate after an overnight fast at 12, 24, and 35 weeks of gestation. Starting at 12 weeks of gestation, women were

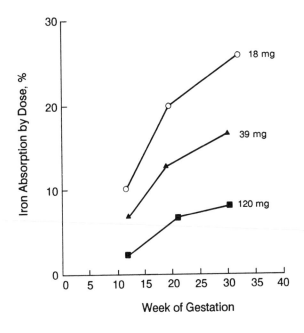

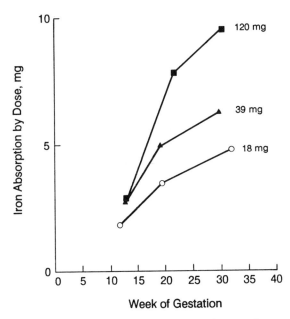

FIGURE 14-2 Absorption of iron in relation to dose and stage of pregnancy. Based on data from Hahn et al. (1951).

randomized to groups receiving either 100 mg of iron as a sustained-release tablet of ferrous sulfate or a placebo twice a day with meals. In accord with the study of Hahn and coworkers (1951), iron absorption in the placebo group increased during the course of pregnancy from about 7% at 12 weeks and 9% at 24 weeks to 14% at 35 weeks of gestation. This rise in absorption was associated with and could be ascribed to a decline in storage iron, as estimated from bone marrow aspirates. There was a smaller rise in mean iron absorption in the iron-treated group, who had values of 6, 7, and 9% at 12, 24, and 35 weeks of gestation, respectively.

Slow-release iron supplements of various types were developed primarily to circumvent the high prevalence of side effects when large doses of iron are used. These preparations are more expensive than ordinary, rapidly soluble iron supplements. In three of the studies summarized in Table 14-1, slow-release forms of ferrous sulfate at doses of 105 to 200 mg of iron per day were effective in preventing iron deficiency during pregnancy (Puolakka et al., 1980b; Svanberg et al., 1976a; Wallenburg and van Eijk, 1984). Ekenved et al. (1976a) found that a slow-release preparation was better absorbed than ordinary ferrous sulfate when given with a meal but less well absorbed under fasting conditions. Several slow-release forms of iron are so poorly absorbed that they are unlikely to confer substantial benefit (Middleton et al., 1966). Consequently, only a *slow-release preparation* of proven effectiveness provides a reasonable alternative should gastrointestinal side effects develop when standard preparations of ferrous iron are used at recommended doses.

Iron tablets (other than slow release preparations) are absorbed more completely when given between rather than with meals (Ekenved et al., 1976a; Hallberg et al., 1978; Layrisse et al., 1973). In the study by Layrisse et al. (1973), 100 mg of iron was given in the form of a ferrous sulfate tablet either after an overnight fast or with a variety of meals characterized by high or low food iron bioavailability. An average of 10 mg (10%) was absorbed after the overnight fast. Irrespective of the type of meal, only an average of 4 to 5 mg was absorbed when the tablet was administered with the meal.

Iron absorption seems to be much greater when a supplement contains only an iron salt than when the iron is part of certain multivitamin-mineral supplements. Calcium carbonate and magnesium oxide appear to be particularly inhibitory to iron absorption (Babior et al., 1985; Seligman et al., 1983). In the 1983 study by Seligman and colleagues, iron absorption improved markedly when calcium as calcium carbonate was decreased from 350 to 250 mg and magnesium as magnesium oxide was decreased from 100 to 25 mg. These findings demonstrate the importance of additional research to test appropriate prenatal multinutrient supplements for in vivo bioavailability. Rough comparisons of iron absorption from various supplements can be most easily derived from the increase in serum iron that occurs after administration of the supplement (Ekenved et al., 1976b).

Since ascorbic acid-rich foods enhance the absorption of dietary iron, one might anticipate that adding ascorbic acid to an iron supplement would also increase iron absorption. However, this was not the case when 50 or 100 mg of ascòrbate was given with 30 mg of iron as ferrous sulfate after an overnight fast (Brise and Hallberg, 1962b). Only with very large doses of 200 mg or more was there an increase in iron absorption. However, such large doses of ascorbate, when given with 60 mg of iron, commonly result in epigastric pain as a side effect (Hallberg et al., 1967a). Even when an iron supplement was given with a meal, the addition of 100 mg of ascorbic acid was not effective in increasing the absorption of ferrous iron (Grebe et al., 1975). Thus, it appears that although ascorbic acid is effective in enhancing absorption of dietary iron, presumably by helping to convert insoluble ferric iron to more soluble ferrous iron, this role is probably less important for supplemental iron given in the ferrous form.

Some commonly consumed foods, such as certain breakfast cereals, are highly fortified to supply the equivalent of the Food and Drug Administration's U.S. Recommended Daily Allowance (U.S. RDA) for iron in a single serving. The extent to which fortification iron is absorbed is likely to vary markedly according to the type of iron and the composition of the product (INACG, 1982). Absorption of added ferrous fumarate is enhanced if the product is also fortified with ascorbic acid (INACG, 1982). This enhancement may be surprising in view of the lack of a similar effect with ascorbic acid added to the much larger amounts of ferrous iron that are contained in supplements. Iron absorption is decreased if the fortified cereal product is rich in phytate (Hallberg et al., 1989). Breakfast cereals in the United States are not typically fortified with ferrous iron, and the reliability of such products in preventing iron deficiency during pregnancy is not established. It is therefore prudent not to rely on fortified products as a substitute for an iron supplement.

Therapeutic Trials

Several longitudinal studies comparing the use of an iron supplement with a placebo or no supplement during pregnancy are summarized in Table 14-1. All of them were performed in northern Europe or North America and most involved middle-income women. The results indicate that 30 mg (Chanarin and Rothman, 1971) or 65 mg (Dawson and McGanity, 1987; Taylor et al., 1982) of elemental iron per day was as effective as any of the higher doses. There are few therapeutic trials in which doses of iron were less than 60 mg/day. Their results are important, however, because the absorption studies of Hahn et al. (1951) indicate that lower doses should be adequate and because the prevalence of intestinal side effects is related to dose (Hallberg et al., 1967b; see also the section Compliance and Side Effects).

Probably the most complete and authoritative of these studies was that of Chanarin and Rothman (1971), who compared groups receiving doses of ferrous fumarate supplying 30, 60, or 120 mg of iron per day with a group given a placebo. An additional group was given one injection of 1 g of iron as intravenous iron dextran, followed by a 60-mg oral dose of iron per day. Women at 20 weeks of gestation were assigned sequentially to the five groups and treated until term; the contents of the prescribed tablets were not known to the investigators. Between 46 and 49 subjects per group completed the study. Figure 14-3 shows the hemoglobin and serum iron values during the course of pregnancy in the 30-mg, 120-mg, and placebo groups. When compared at 37 weeks of gestation, the hemoglobin and serum iron levels of the 30-mg group did not differ significantly from those of the groups receiving higher doses of iron. The investigators concluded that 30 mg of elemental iron per day was effective in maintaining hemoglobin levels throughout pregnancy. More recently, Hiss (1986) also recommended a dose of 30 mg/day in a review on anemia during pregnancy. In support of this dose, he cited the results of Scott and Pritchard (1974), who determined the hemoglobin concentration and stainable iron in bone marrow at the beginning of the second trimester and at delivery in 20 women who were given 30 mg of iron per day as ferrous fumarate throughout that period. The hemoglobin concentration rose from an initial mean of 11.2 g/dl to a final value of 12.6 g/dl, and bone marrow iron at delivery equaled or exceeded the initial values. One study that cast some doubt on the efficacy of low doses is that of de Leeuw and coworkers (1966), who report that 39 mg of ferrous iron per day did not maintain as high a hemoglobin concentration as did a dose of 78 mg/day. Chanarin and Rothman (1971) suggested that compliance may not have been as good as it was in their own well-monitored study.

A relatively modest dose of iron is preferable to a high dose since iron may inhibit the absorption of other nutrients, zinc in particular. Sandström and coworkers (1985) showed that when a multivitamin-mineral supplement is taken on an empty stomach, high iron doses will inhibit the absorption of concurrently administered zinc. It also appears that iron supplementation, even at modest doses (38 to 65 mg/day for 1 to 4 weeks), may result in a slight decline in serum zinc (Hambidge et al., 1987). Possible consequences of the iron-zinc interaction for human nutrition were reviewed by Solomons (1986).

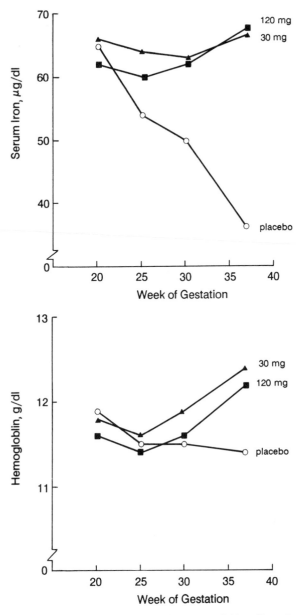

FIGURE 14-3 Serum iron and hemoglobin levels in groups of 46 to 49 randomly assigned women receiving daily either a placebo or various doses of elemental iron as ferrous fumarate given orally. Data from groups receiving 60-mg oral doses of iron or 1 g of parenteral iron followed by 60-mg oral doses of iron per day are not shown but are similar to those of the iron-supplemented groups shown in the figure. Based on data from Chanarin and Rothman (1971).

How Much Extra Iron Must Be Absorbed from a Supplement in Order To Prevent Iron Deficiency?

A reasonable theoretic approach to estimating the requirement for absorbed supplemental iron is to calculate how much iron would be needed to prevent the hemoglobin deficits in unsupplemented women compared with supplemented women. The amount of iron required to prevent such a deficit can be derived most directly from the study of Taylor and Lind (1979), which is summarized in Table 14-1, in which total red cell mass and plasma volume were measured at 12 and 36 weeks of gestation. The final hemoglobin concentration averaged 1.6 g/dl higher in the supplemented than in the unsupplemented group (among the highest differences observed in the studies summarized in Table 14-1). Over this 24-week study period, the red cell mass increased by an average of approximately 450 ml in the supplemented group compared with 180 ml in the unsupplemented women, a difference of 270 ml. Since each milliliter of packed red blood cells contains about 1.2 mg of iron, a 270-ml difference in red cell mass is equivalent to 325 mg of iron. Dividing 325 mg of iron by the 168 days between 12 and 36 weeks of gestation indicates that 1.9 mg of extra iron must be assimilated daily to prevent the deficit in red blood cell mass. After allowing for a higher rate of iron accumulation between 36 and 40 weeks of gestation and adding 25% for greater than average needs, the subcommittee estimated that about 3 mg of supplemental iron in addition to dietary iron should be assimilated daily during the second and third trimesters to prevent iron deficiency in most women. Figure 14-2 suggests that 3 mg of iron can be readily absorbed from a 30-mg daily dose of ferrous iron given between meals.

Duration and Dose

An appropriate time to begin iron supplementation at a dose of 30 mg/day is after about week 12 of gestation (the beginning of the second trimester), when the iron requirements for pregnancy begin to increase. Iron administration at a dose of 60 to 120 mg/day (preferably in divided doses) is indicated if there is laboratory evidence of an already established anemia at any stage of pregnancy. The dose should be decreased to 30 mg/day when the hemoglobin concentration is within the normal range for the stage of gestation (Figure 14-1).

Compliance and Side Effects

One problem with supplement use during pregnancy is uncertainty about compliance (Bonnar et al., 1969), particularly when poverty and certain ethnic beliefs reduce the availability or acceptability of supplements. Early in pregnancy, morning sickness probably contributes to reduced consumption of nutrient supplements. Late in pregnancy, constipation and abdominal discomfort are frequent regardless of whether supplements are used or not. Taking high doses of iron may increase these problems and thus discourage supplement use. Iron appears to be best tolerated when administered at bedtime.

Potential side effects of iron administration include heartburn, nausea, upper abdominal discomfort, constipation, and diarrhea. The most careful studies that focused on side effects involved double-blind administration of large therapeutic doses of iron to large groups of blood donors (Hallberg et al., 1967b; Sölvell, 1970). At a dosage of 200 mg of iron per day as ferrous sulfate divided into three doses per day, approximately 25% of subjects had side effects, compared with 13% of those who received a placebo. When the dose was doubled, side effects increased to 40%. Constipation and diarrhea occurred with the same frequency at the two doses, but nausea and upper abdominal pain were more common at the higher dose. The risk of side effects is proportional to the amount of elemental iron in various soluble ferrous iron compounds and therefore appeared to be primarily a function of the amount of soluble iron in the small intestine. Little information is available about side effects at doses below 200 mg, but it is reasonable to infer that side effects are much less likely at 30 mg/day.

CLINICAL APPLICATIONS

• To prevent iron deficiency, the subcommittee recommends the routine use of 30 mg of ferrous iron per day beginning at about week 12 of gestation, in conjunction with a well-balanced diet that contains enhancers of iron absorption (ascorbic acid, meat).

• To enhance absorption, it is advisable to take supplemental iron between meals with liquids other than milk, tea, and coffee.

• Hemoglobin or hematocrit should routinely be determined at the first prenatal visit in order to detect preexisting anemia. A hemoglobin level below 11.0 g/dl during the first or third trimesters or below 10.5 g/dl during the second trimester is defined as anemia. Anemia accompanied by a serum ferritin concentration of <12 μg/dl can be presumed to be iron deficiency anemia and requires treatment with 60 to 120 mg of ferrous iron daily. When the hemoglobin concentration becomes normal for the stage of gestation, the dose can be decreased to 30 mg/day.

REFERENCES

Agrawal, R.M.D., A.M. Tripathi, and K.N. Agarwal. 1983. Cord blood haemoglobin, iron and ferritin status in maternal anaemia. Acta Paediatr. Scand. 72:545-548.

Babior, B.M., W.A. Peters, P.M. Briden, and C.L. Cetrulo. 1985. Pregnant women's absorption of iron from prenatal supplements. J. Reprod. Med. 30:355-357.

Bezwoda, M.R., T.H. Bothwell, J.D. Torrance, A.P. MacPhail, R.W. Charlton, G. Kay, and J. Levin. 1979. The relationship between marrow iron stores, plasma ferritin concentrations and iron absorption. Scand. J. Haematol. 22:113-120.

Bonnar, J., A. Goldberg, and J.A. Smith. 1969. Do pregnant women take their iron? Lancet 1:457-458.

Bothwell, T.H., R.W. Charlton, J.D. Cook, and C.A. Finch. 1979. Iron Metabolism in Man. Blackwell Scientific Publications, Oxford. 576 pp.

Bratlid, D., and P.J. Moe. 1980. Hemoglobin and serum ferritin levels in mothers and infants at birth. Eur. J. Pediatr. 134:125-127.

Brise, H. 1962. Influence of meals on iron absorption in oral iron therapy. Acta Med. Scand., Suppl. 376:39-45.

Brise, H., and L. Hallberg. 1962a. Absorbability of different iron compounds. Acta Med. Scand., Suppl. 376:23-37.

Brise, H., and L. Hallberg. 1962b. Effect of ascorbic acid on iron absorption. Acta Med. Scand., Suppl. 376:51-58.

CDC (Centers for Disease Control). 1989. CDC criteria for anemia in children and childbearing-aged women. Morbid. Mortal. Week. Rep. 38:400-404.

Celada, A., R. Busset, J. Gutierrez, and V. Herreros. 1982. Maternal and cord blood ferritin. Helv. Paediatr. Acta 37:239-244.

Chanarin, I., and D. Rothman. 1971. Further observations on the relation between iron and folate status in pregnancy. Br. Med. J. 2:81-84.

Charlton, R.W., and T.H. Bothwell. 1983. Iron absorption. Annu. Rev. Med. 34:55-68.

Charoenlarp, P., S. Dhanamitta, R. Kaewvichit, A. Silprasert, C. Suwanaradd, S. Na-Nakorn, P. Prawatmuang, S. Vatanavicharn, U. Nutcharas, P. Pootrakul, V. Tanphaichitr, O. Thanangkul, T. Vaniyapong, T. Toe, A. Valyasevi, S. Baker, J. Cook, E.M. DeMaeyer, L. Garby, and L. Hallberg. 1988. A WHO collaborative study on iron supplementation in Burma and in Thailand. Am. J. Clin. Nutr. 47:280-297.

Clapp, J.F., III, B.L. Seaward, R.H. Sleamaker, and J. Hiser. 1988. Maternal physiologic adaptations to early human pregnancy. Am. J. Obstet. Gynecol. 159:1456-1460.

Cole, S.K., W.Z. Billewicz, and A.M. Thomson. 1971. Sources of variation in menstrual blood loss. J. Obstet. Gynaecol. Br. Commonw. 78:933-939.

Cook, J.D., C.A. Finch, and N.J. Smith. 1976. Evaluation of the iron status of a population. Blood 48:449-455.

Dallman, P.R. 1984. Diagnosis of anemia and iron deficiency: analytic and biological variations of laboratory tests. Am. J. Clin. Nutr. 39:937-941.

Dallman, P.R. 1986. Biochemical basis for the manifestations of iron deficiency. Annu. Rev. Nutr. 6:13-40.

Davidson, L.A., and B. Lönnerdal. 1988. Specific binding of lactoferrin to brush-border membrane: ontogeny and effect of glycan chain. Am. J. Physiol. 254:G580-G585.

Dawson, E.B., and W.J. McGanity. 1987. Protection of maternal iron stores in pregnancy. J. Reprod. Med. 32:478-487.

de Leeuw, N.K.M., L. Lowenstein, and Y.S. Hsieh. 1966. Iron deficiency and hydremia in normal pregnancy. Medicine 45:291-315.

DeMaeyer, D., and M. Adiels-Tegman. 1985. The prevalence of anaemia in the world. World Health Stat. Q. 38:302-316.

Ekenved, G., B. Arvidsson, and L. Sölvell. 1976a. Influence of food on the absorption from different types of iron tablets. Scand. J. Haematol., Suppl. 28:79-88.

Ekenved, G., A. Norrby, and L. Sölvell. 1976b. Serum iron increase as a measure of iron absorption—studies on the correlation with total absorption. Scand. J. Haematol., Suppl. 28:31-49.

Fenton, V., I. Cavill, and J. Fisher. 1977. Iron stores in pregnancy. Br. J. Haematol. 37:145-149.

Finch, C.A., J.D. Cook, R.F. Labbe, and M. Culala. 1977. Effect of blood donation on iron stores as evaluated by serum ferritin. Blood 50:441-447.

Frassinelli-Gunderson, E.P., S. Margen, and J.R. Brown. 1985. Iron stores in users of oral contraceptive agents. Am. J. Clin. Nutr. 41:703-712.

Garn, S.M., S.A. Ridella, A.S. Petzold, and F. Falkner. 1981. Maternal hematologic levels and pregnancy outcomes. Semin. Perinatol. 5:155-162.

Grebe, G., C. Martinez-Torres, and M. Layrisse. 1975. Effect of meals and ascorbic acid on the absorption of a therapeutic dose of iron as ferrous and ferric salts. Curr. Ther. Res. 17:382-397.

Green, R., R. Charlton, H. Seftel, T. Bothwell, F. Mayet, B. Adams, C. Finch, and M. Layrisse. 1968. Body iron excretion in man: a collaborative study. Am. J. Med. 45:336-353.

Hahn, P.F., E.L. Carothers, W.J. Darby, M. Martin, C.W. Sheppard, R.O. Cannon, A.S. Beam, P.M. Densen, J.C. Peterson, and G.S. McClellan. 1951. Iron metabolism in human pregnancy as studied with the radioactive isotope, Fe^{59}. Am. J. Obstet. Gynecol. 61:477-486.

Hallberg, L. 1981. Bioavailability of dietary iron in man. Annu. Rev. Nutr. 1:123-147.

Hallberg, L. 1988. Iron balance in pregnancy. Pp. 115-127 in H. Berger, ed. Vitamins and Minerals in Pregnancy and Lactation. Raven Press, New York.

Hallberg, L., A. Högdahl, L. Nilsson, and G. Rybo. 1966. Menstrual blood loss—a population study. Acta Obstet. Gynecol. Scand. 45:320-351.

Hallberg, L., L. Sölvell, and H. Brise. 1967a. Search for substances promoting the absorption of iron: studies on absorption and side-effects. Acta Med. Scand., Suppl. 459:11-21.

Hallberg, L., L. Ryttinger, and L. Sölvell. 1967b. Side-effects of oral iron therapy: a double-blind study of different iron compounds in tablet form. Acta Med. Scand., Suppl. 459:3-10.

Hallberg, L., E. Björn-Rasmussen, G. Ekenved, L. Garby, L. Rossander, R. Pleehachinda, R. Suwanik, and B. Arvidsson. 1978. Absorption from iron tablets given with different types of meals. Scand. J. Haematol. 21:215-224.

Hallberg, L., M. Brune, and L. Rossander. 1989. Iron absorption in man: ascorbic acid and dose-dependent inhibition by phytate. Am. J. Clin. Nutr. 49:140-144.

Hambidge, K.M., N.F. Krebs, L. Sibley, and J. English. 1987. Acute effects of iron therapy on zinc status during pregnancy. Obstet. Gynecol. 4:593-596.

Hefnawi, F., H. Askalani, and K. Zaki. 1974. Menstrual blood loss with copper intrauterine devices. Contraception 9:133-139.

Heinrich, H.C., H. Bartels, B. Heinisch, K. Hausmann, R. Kuse, W. Humke, and H.J. Mauss. 1968. Intestinale ^{59}Fe-Resorption und prälatenter Eisenmangel während der Gravidität des Menschen. Klin. Wochenschr. 46:199-202.

Hiss, R.G. 1986. Evaluation of the anemic patient. Pp. 1-18 in R.K. Laros, Jr., ed. Blood Disorders in Pregnancy. Lea & Febiger, Philadelphia.

Huebers, H.A., and C.A. Finch. 1987. The physiology of transferrin and transferrin receptors. Physiol. Rev. 67:520-582.

Hussain, M.A.M., T.H. Gaafar, M. Laulicht, and A.V. Hoffbrand. 1977. Relation of maternal and cord blood serum ferritin. Arch. Dis. Child. 52:782-784.

Hytten, F. 1985. Blood volume changes in normal pregnancy. Clin. Haematol. 14:601-612.

INACG (International Nutritional Anemia Consultative Group). 1982. The Effects of Cereals and Legumes on Iron Availability. A Report of the International Nutritional Anemia Consultative Group (INACG). The Nutrition Foundation, Washington, D.C. 44 pp.

Israel, R., S.T. Shaw, Jr., and M.A. Martin. 1974. Comparative quantitation of menstrual blood loss with the Lippes loop, Dalkon shield, and Copper T intrauterine devices. Contraception 10:63-71.

Kaneshige, E. 1981. Serum ferritin as an assessment of iron stores and other hematologic parameters during pregnancy. Obstet. Gynecol. 57:238-242.

Kelly, A.M., D.J. MacDonald, and A.N. McDougall. 1978. Observations on maternal and fetal ferritin concentrations at term. Br. J. Obstet. Gynaecol. 85:338-343.

Klein, L. 1962. Premature birth and maternal prenatal anemia. Am. J. Obstet. Gynecol. 83:588-590.

Layrisse, M., C. Martínez-Torres, J.D. Cook, R. Walker, and C.A. Finch. 1973. Iron fortification of food: its measurement by the extrinsic tag method. Blood 41:333-352.

Lewis, G.J., and D.F. Rowe. 1986. Can a serum ferritin estimation predict which pregnant women need iron? Br. J. Clin. Pract. 40:15-16.

Lieberman, E., K.J. Ryan, R.R. Monson, and S.C. Schoenbaum. 1987. Risk factors accounting for racial differences in the rate of premature birth. N. Engl. J. Med. 317:743-748.

LSRO (Life Sciences Research Office). 1984. Assessment of the Iron Nutritional Status of the U.S. Population Based on Data Collected in the Second National Health and Nutrition Examination Survey, 1976-1980. Federation of American Societies for Experimental Biology, Bethesda, Md. 120 pp.

LSRO (Life Sciences Research Office). 1989. Nutrition Monitoring in the United States: An Update Report on Nutrition Monitoring. Prepared for the U.S. Department of Agriculture and the U.S. Department of Health and Human Services. DHHS Publ. No. (PHS) 89-1225. U.S. Government Printing Office, Washington, D.C. (various pagings).

Lund, C.J., and J.C. Donovan. 1967. Blood volume during pregnancy: significance of plasma and red cell volumes. Am. J. Obstet. Gynecol. 98:393-403.

Macgregor, M.W. 1963. Maternal anaemia as a factor in prematurity and perinatal mortality. Scott. Med. J. 8:134-140.

MacPhail, A.P., R.W. Charlton, T.H. Bothwell, and J.D. Torrance. 1980. The relationship between maternal and infant iron status. Scand. J. Haematol. 25:141-150.

Messer, R.D., A.M. Russo, W.R. McWhirter, D. Sprangemeyer, and J.W. Halliday. 1980. Serum ferritin in term and preterm infants. Aust. Paediatr. J. 16:185-188.

Middleton, E.J., E. Nagy, and A.B. Morrison. 1966. Studies on the absorption of orally administered iron from sustained-release preparations. N. Engl. J. Med. 274:136-139.

Milman, N., K.K. Ibsen, and J.M. Christensen. 1987. Serum ferritin and iron status in mothers and newborn infants. Acta Obstet. Gynecol. Scand. 66:205-211.

Monsen, E.R., L. Hallberg, M. Layrisse, D.M. Hegsted, J.D. Cook, W. Mertz, and C.A. Finch. 1978. Estimation of available dietary iron. Am. J. Clin. Nutr. 31:134-141.

Murphy, J.F., J. O'Riordan, R.G. Newcombe, E.C. Coles, and J.F. Pearson. 1986. Relation of haemoglobin levels in first and second trimesters to outcome of pregnancy. Lancet 1:992-995.

Murray, M.J., A.B. Murray, N.J. Murray, and M.B. Murray. 1978. The effect of iron status of Nigerien mothers on that of their infants at birth and 6 months, and on the concentration of Fe in breast milk. Br. J. Nutr. 39:627-630.

Nhonoli, A.M., F.E. Kihama, and B.D. Ramji. 1975. The relation between maternal and cord serum iron levels and its effect on fetal growth in iron deficient mothers without malarial infection. Br. J. Obstet. Gynaecol. 82:467-470.

Nielsen, J.B., E. Ikkala, L. Sölvell, E. Björn-Rasmussen, and G. Ekenved. 1976. Absorption of iron from slow-release and rapidly-disintegrating tablets—a comparative study in normal subjects, blood donors and subjects with iron deficiency. Scand. J. Haematol., Suppl. 28:89-97.

Norrby, A. 1974. Iron absorption studies in iron deficiency. Scand. J. Haematol., Suppl. 20:1-125.

Peters, T.J., K.B. Raja, R.J. Simpson, and S. Snape. 1988. Mechanisms and regulation of intestinal iron absorption. Ann. N.Y. Acad. Sci. 526:141-147.

Pierson, R.N., Jr., P.R. Holt, R.M. Watson, and R.P. Keating. 1961. Aspirin and gastrointestinal bleeding: chromate[51] blood loss studies. Am. J. Med. 31:259-265.

Pritchard, J.A. 1965. Changes in blood volume during pregnancy and delivery. Anesthesiology 26:393-399.

Pritchard, J.A., R.M. Baldwin, J.C. Dickey, and K.M. Wiggins. 1962. Blood volume changes in pregnancy and the puerperium. II. Red blood cell loss and changes in apparent blood volume during and following vaginal delivery, cesarean section, and cesarean section plus total hysterectomy. Am. J. Obstet. Gynecol. 84:1271-1282.

Puolakka, J., O. Jänne, and R. Vihko. 1980a. Evaluation by serum ferritin assay of the influence of maternal iron stores on the iron status of newborns and infants. Acta Obstet. Gynecol. Scand., Suppl. 95:53-56.

Puolakka, J., O. Jänne, A. Pakarinen, P.A. Järvinen, and R. Vihko. 1980b. Serum ferritin as a measure of iron stores during and after normal pregnancy with and without iron supplements. Acta Obstet. Gynecol. Scand., Suppl. 95:43-51.

Puolakka, J., O. Jänne, A. Pakarinen, and R. Vihko. 1980c. Serum ferritin in the diagnosis of anemia during pregnancy. Acta Obstet. Gynecol. Scand., Suppl. 95:57-63.

Raper, N.R., J.C. Rosenthal, and C.E. Woteki. 1984. Estimates of available iron in diets of individuals 1 year old and older in the Nationwide Food Consumption Survey. J. Am. Diet. Assoc. 84:783-787.

Rios, E., D.A. Lipschitz, J.D. Cook, and N.J. Smith. 1975. Relationship of maternal and infant iron stores as assessed by determination of plasma ferritin. Pediatrics 55:694-699.

Romslo, I., K. Haram, N. Sagen, and K. Augensen. 1983. Iron requirement in normal pregnancy as assessed by serum ferritin, serum transferrin saturation and erythrocyte protoporphyrin determinations. Br. J. Obstet. Gynaecol. 90:101-107.

Rossander, L., L. Hallberg, and E. Björn-Rasmussen. 1979. Absorption of iron from breakfast meals. Am. J. Clin. Nutr. 32:2484-2489.

Sandström, B., L. Davidsson, Å. Cederblad, and B. Lönnerdal. 1985. Oral iron, dietary ligands and zinc absorption. J. Nutr. 115:411-414.

Schifman, R.B., J.E. Thomasson, and J.M. Evers. 1987. Red blood cell zinc protoporphyrin testing for iron-deficiency anemia in pregnancy. Am. J. Obstet. Gynecol. 157:304-307.

Scott, D.E., and J.A. Pritchard. 1974. Anemia in pregnancy. Clin. Perinatol. 1:491-506.

Seligman, P.A., J.H. Caskey, J.L. Frazier, R.M. Zucker, E.R. Podell, and R.H. Allen. 1983. Measurements of iron absorption from prenatal multivitamin-mineral supplements. Obstet. Gynecol. 61:356-362.

Simon, T.L., P.J. Garry, and E.M. Hooper. 1981. Iron stores in blood donors. J. Am. Med. Assoc. 245:2038-2043.

Singla, P.N., S. Chand, S. Khanna, and K.N. Agarwal. 1978. Effect of maternal anaemia on the placenta and the newborn infant. Acta Paediatr. Scand. 67:645-648.

Sisson, T.R.C., and C.J. Lund. 1958. The influence of maternal iron deficiency on the newborn. Am. J. Clin. Nutr. 6:376-385.

Sjöstedt, J.E., P. Manner, S. Nummi, and G. Ekenved. 1977. Oral iron prophylaxis during pregnancy: a comparative study on different dosage regimens. Acta Obstet. Gynecol. Scand., Suppl. 60:3-9.

Solomons, N.W. 1986. Competitive interaction of iron and zinc in the diet: consequences for human nutrition. J. Nutr. 116:927-935.

Sölvell, L. 1970. Oral iron therapy-side effects. Pp. 573-583 in L. Hallberg, H.G. Harwerth, and A. Vannotti, eds. Iron Deficiency: Pathogenesis, Clinical Aspects, Therapy. Academic Press, London.

Sturgeon, P. 1959. Studies of iron requirements in infants. III. Influence of supplemental iron during normal pregnancy on mother and infant. B. The infant. Br. J. Haematol. 5:45-55.

Svanberg, B., B. Arvidsson, A. Norrby, G. Rybo, and L. Sölvell. 1976a. Absorption of supplemental iron during pregnancy—a longitudinal study with repeated bone-marrow studies and absorption measurements. Acta Obstet. Gynecol. Scand., Suppl. 48:87-108.

Svanberg, B., B. Arvidsson, E. Björn-Rasmussen, L. Hallberg, L. Rossander, and B. Swolin. 1976b. Dietary iron absorption in pregnancy—a longitudinal study with repeated measurements of non-haeme iron absorption from whole diet. Acta Obstet. Gynecol. Scand., Suppl. 48:43-68.

Taylor, D.J., and T. Lind. 1979. Red cell mass during and after normal pregnancy. Br. J. Obstet. Gynaecol. 86:364-370.

Taylor, D.J., C. Mallen, N. McDougall, and T. Lind. 1982. Effect of iron supplementation on serum ferritin levels during and after pregnancy. Br. J. Obstet. Gynaecol. 89:1011-1017.

Ueland, K. 1976. Maternal cardiovascular dynamics. VII. Intrapartum blood volume changes. Am. J. Obstet. Gynecol. 126:671-677.

van Eijk, H.G., M.J. Kroos, G.A. Hoogendoorn, and H.C.S. Wallenburg. 1978. Serum ferritin and iron stores during pregnancy. Clin. Chim. Acta 83:81-91.

Wallenburg, H.C.S., and H.G. van Eijk. 1984. Effect of oral iron supplementation during pregnancy on maternal and fetal iron status. J. Perinat. Med. 12:7-11.

WHO (World Health Organization). 1968. Nutritional Anaemias. Report of a WHO Scientific Group. Technical Report Series No. 405. World Health Organization, Geneva. 37 pp.

15

Trace Elements

With the exceptions of iron and iodine, the trace elements are the nutrients most recently identified as essential for humans. The roles of some have not been clearly defined, despite substantial progress over the past 30 years. Periodic reevaluation is needed as the boundaries of knowledge expand. The trace elements included in this chapter are those for which Recommended Dietary Allowances (RDAs) or safe and adequate daily dietary intakes have been established by the Food and Nutrition Board (NRC, 1989), with the exception of iron (see Chapter 14).

Progressive physiologic changes during gestation contribute to the difficulty of interpreting laboratory data. Although mild deficiency of one or more trace elements may be one etiologic factor in a multifactorial problem such as premature delivery or intrauterine growth retardation, a causal role would be difficult to detect. Suboptimal status, or marginal deficiency, of trace elements has been documented in human and animal models, but it is typically difficult to identify. The selection of appropriate subjects, the large number of subjects required, and the difficulties of implementing intervention studies in free-living populations are among the factors that hamper definitive research to determine whether and when increased intakes of specific trace elements may be of any value to the course of pregnancy and to the developing fetus.

With respect to potential toxicity, the trace elements in general have an intermediate position between the fat-soluble vitamins and the water-soluble vitamins (see Chapters 17 and 18). Of greater concern than overt toxicity is the potential for interactions between trace elements. For example, relatively large doses of iron may interfere with the absorption of zinc in pregnant women. Zinc supplementation may compensate for this interaction but may, in turn, affect the metabolism of copper and other micronutrients. The full extent of nutrient-nutrient interactions is not yet completely known.

ZINC

Cell Replication and Differentiation

At the molecular level, zinc is involved extensively in nucleic acid and protein metabolism and, hence, in the fundamental processes of cell differentiation and replication (see the review by Hambidge et al., 1986). Zinc and zinc-dependent enzymes, for example, are involved in the synthesis of deoxyribonucleic acid (DNA), ribonucleic acid (RNA), and ribosomes. Zinc deficiency reduces the activity of these enzymes, but disturbances of cell replication and differentiation appear to be attributable primarily to the adverse effects of zinc deficiency on gene expression (Chesters, 1978; Crossley et al., 1982). For example, zinc fingers (Klug and Rhodes, 1987) play a critical role in the attachment of the transcription proteins to DNA. These fingers are projections, the shape of which is dependent on a zinc atom at the base. This essential step in the initiation of the transcription process is but one example of the numerous ways in which zinc is involved in all stages of the cell cycle.

Reproduction in Animals

In view of the multiple physiologic roles of zinc in cell replication and differentiation, it is not surprising that an adequate supply of this micronutrient is necessary for reproduction. Animal studies have shown that all phases of reproduction in the female, from estrus to parturition and lactation, are affected adversely by zinc deficiency (Hambidge et al., 1986). Severe zinc deficiency in rodents disrupts the estrous cycle and causes infertility (Swenerton and Hurley, 1980). Zinc is necessary for the normal development of the preembryonic conceptus. In the immediate postfertilization period, zinc deficiency can result in abnormal development of preimplantation eggs (Hurley and Schrader, 1975).

In the rat, maternal dietary zinc restriction during embryogenesis has profound teratogenic effects involving many organ systems, especially the skeletal and central nervous systems (Dreosti, 1982; Hurley, 1981). The pattern of malformations depends on the precise period of zinc deprivation and the embryonic events that are occurring at that stage of gestation

(Record et al., 1985). Zinc restriction can result in fetal growth retardation in male fetuses of monkeys and fetuses of both sexes of rats and sheep (Hurley et al., 1985). Zinc deficiency in the postembryonic period has been associated with behavioral abnormalities in the offspring of rats and monkeys (Strobel et al., 1979) and with abnormalities in the ontogeny and postnatal function of the immune system (Haynes et al., 1985). Maternal zinc deficiency also has species-dependent effects on the course of pregnancy and delivery. In rats, zinc deficiency in late pregnancy causes prolonged labor with atonic bleeding (Apgar, 1968). Such effects appear to result from a failure of normal hormonal changes at delivery. Premature delivery may be the most likely complication of maternal zinc deficiency in the ewe and guinea pig (Apgar, 1987).

Reproduction in Humans

There have been a few reported cases of severe human zinc deficiency during pregnancy that resulted from inadequately treated acrodermatitis enteropathica—a hereditary condition in which zinc absorption is impaired. Among these cases, there was a high incidence of major obstetric complications and congenital malformations in the offspring (Hambidge et al., 1975). The prevalence and consequences of milder zinc deficiency during human pregnancy remain poorly defined. In several studies, associations were found between low zinc levels in plasma or tissue and complications of pregnancy and delivery, such as pregnancy-induced hypertension; prolonged labor; intrapartum hemorrhage; and impaired fetal development such as congenital malformations, intrauterine growth retardation (Adeniyi, 1987; Crosby et al., 1977; Fehily et al., 1986), and prematurity (Cherry et al., 1987). Campbell-Brown et al. (1985) reported unusually low dietary zinc levels among Hindu vegetarian women in London, England, whose offspring had low birth weights. However, there was no correlation between the maternal serum zinc level and birth weight. In general, there has been a lack of consistency in the findings of different studies (see reviews by Hambidge, 1989, and Swanson and King, 1987).

In randomized controlled trials of groups believed to be at relatively high risk of zinc deficiency, zinc supplements have had limited and inconsistent effects. For example, in a study of low-income women of Mexican descent, Hunt et al. (1984) found a significantly lower incidence of pregnancy-induced hypertension in the zinc-supplemented group than in the placebo-treated group. They speculated that zinc may reduce the incidence of pregnancy-induced hypertension by affecting prostaglandin metabolism. In a subsequent study of teenage pregnancies in the same population, this effect was not observed (Hunt et al., 1985). Nor was a zinc supplement found to have a beneficial effect on pregnancy-induced hypertension in black adolescent teenagers in New Orleans (Cherry et al., 1987), despite an association between low plasma zinc concentrations and pregnancy-induced hypertension in an earlier study of that population (Cherry et al., 1981). Zinc supplementation was, however, associated with a lower incidence of premature births in that study.

Sample sizes have been inadequate to assess definitively the effect of zinc supplements on intrauterine growth. Nevertheless, the results of one recent study (Mahomed et al., 1989) indicated that an effect on fetal growth is unlikely in an unselected population of pregnant women.

Estimated Zinc Requirements During Pregnancy

Swanson and King (1987) estimate that 100 mg of zinc is retained in maternal and fetal tissues during pregnancy and that 0.7 mg/day is accumulated during the last trimester. At most, 1 mg/day is retained during the third trimester, allowing for intra- and interindividual variation. If fractional absorption is 25% during the third trimester, a maximum of an additional 4 mg of zinc per day is needed. Corresponding increments in dietary requirements during the first and second trimesters would be approximately 0.5 and 1.5 mg of zinc per day, respectively. It is not yet known whether fractional zinc absorption increases during late gestation in humans as it does in rats (Davies and Williams, 1977).

Studies of nonpregnant adults provide information about zinc absorption, utilization, and excretion that is potentially relevant to human pregnancy. Wada et al. (1985) report that nonpregnant adults adapt to a wide range of zinc intakes. Because of this, results of traditional balance studies cannot be used to establish dietary requirements for this micronutrient. The effects of mild zinc deficiency are subtle and nonspecific. Thus, it is extremely difficult to determine the point at which adaptation gives way to accommodation, i.e., when the earliest adverse effects occur. Reliable estimates of dietary zinc requirements for nonpregnant adults therefore remain elusive. Gibson and Scythes (1982), Holden et al. (1979), and Patterson et al. (1984) have reported that zinc intakes by apparently healthy adults in North America average 8 to 10 mg daily. When these data are considered along with those of Swanson and King (1987), it appears likely that 12 to 14 mg of zinc per day is ample in the third trimester of pregnancy. Indeed, the requirement may be substantially lower than this figure, especially if there are adaptive mechanisms specifically related to pregnancy.

Usual Zinc Intakes

Usual daily dietary zinc intakes during pregnancy range from 8.8 ± 3.5 to 14.4 ± 1.5 (standard deviation) mg/day (Campbell, 1988). Among vegetarians, usual zinc intakes may be even lower. For example, Campbell-Brown et al. (1985) reported a mean intake by Hindu vegetarian women of only 7.5 mg/day.

Dosage Range and Toxicity

The level of zinc supplementation that is safe for pregnant women has not been clearly established. Doses used in zinc supplementation studies in pregnant women have ranged from 15 to 45 mg/day, but one unconfirmed report suggests an association between zinc supplements of 45 mg/day during pregnancy and premature delivery (Kumar, 1976). A daily zinc intake of 50 mg is sufficient to impair copper and iron metabolism (Yadrick et al., 1989). One report, based on the metabolic balance technique and a diet low in copper, indicates that copper absorption is slightly impaired at a dietary zinc intake of only 18.5 mg/day (Festa et al., 1985).

Criteria for Status Assessment

There are no pathognomonic clinical features of zinc deficiency in humans, except in cases of very severe zinc deficiency. The potential adverse effects of maternal zinc deficiency on obstetric course (e.g., pregnancy-induced hypertension) and fetal development (e.g., fetal growth retardation) are also nonspecific and are not helpful in diagnosing zinc deficiency. No reliable and sensitive functional indices of zinc status have been found, including the activity of the metalloenzymes. Indicators of T-cell function have been suggested but are nonspecific. In the second trimester, maternal leukocyte zinc concentrations have been associated with fetal growth retardation (Meadows et al., 1981); however, this is a complex technique that is not applicable outside the research laboratory. Moreover, there are valid reasons to doubt that zinc deficiency is reflected in lower leukocyte zinc concentrations (Milne et al., 1985).

The most widely used laboratory assays for assessment of zinc status include measurements of plasma or serum zinc. Plasma measurements are potentially more accurate but technically more difficult to perform. To make valid comparisons among samples, it is necessary to collect them at a predetermined time relative to meals. Prebreakfast samples are least subject to day-to-day variation (Hambidge et al., 1989).

There is a well-established physiologic decline in plasma zinc throughout gestation, starting early in the first trimester (Hambidge et al., 1983). The cause of this decline is probably multifactorial, including hormonal factors and, later in gestation, increased plasma volume. Because of this decline, normal ranges are needed for each stage of gestation; some guidelines for this have been published (Hambidge et al., 1983). Another putative concern about the use of plasma or serum zinc is the lack of adequate sensitivity in identifying women with zinc deficiency. Other tissue zinc assays, such as hair analysis (Hambidge, 1982), have not been demonstrated to be reliable indicators of zinc status in humans.

Because of the limitations of laboratory assays and functional indices, their use in assessing zinc status is not recommended as a routine part of prenatal care. Studies of response to zinc supplementation offer the most definitive approach to confirming zinc deficiency in groups, but not in individuals.

Prevalence of Zinc Deficiency

Without large-scale zinc supplementation studies, the prevalence of maternal zinc deficiency during pregnancy remains speculative.

Effects of Other Supplements and of Nonnutritive Substances

Alcohol consumption increases losses of zinc in the urine and depresses plasma zinc concentrations (Flynn et al., 1981). Infants with fetal alcohol syndrome have been reported to have low plasma zinc levels and increased urine zinc losses (Anonymous, 1986b). It has been hypothesized, but not confirmed, that the lack of zinc plays a role in the abnormal facial appearance that is typical of fetal alcohol syndrome. Placental transport of zinc was disturbed by chronic alcohol ingestion and did not improve with maternal zinc supplementation in an animal model (Ghishan and Greene, 1983).

In pregnant smokers, whose placental cadmium levels are high, the placental zinc-to-cadmium ratio is positively related to infant birth weight (Kuhnert et al., 1988). In an animal model, administration of cadmium was teratogenic only when marginal zinc deficiency was present as well (Sato et al., 1985); low zinc-to-cadmium ratios in the kidney were suggested as a cause of hypertension. Because of these potential interrelationships between zinc and cadmium, it may be especially important to ensure an adequate zinc intake by pregnant smokers.

Interactions between iron and zinc during gastrointestinal absorption have been well documented (Hamilton et al., 1978; Solomons, 1986), but not consistently in pregnant women. However, prenatal iron supplements, especially if administered in doses ≥ 60 mg of elemental iron per day, can lower maternal plasma zinc concentrations (Dawson et al., 1989; Hambidge et al., 1987). Administration of iron and zinc in the same multimineral supplement also impairs zinc absorption (Sandström et al., 1985). Milne et al. (1984) observed that modest folate supplements may impair zinc absorption, whereas Fuller et al. (1988) reported no effect. If folate has any effect on zinc absorption, it is evidently not of sufficient magnitude to be of much practical importance (Krebs et al., 1988).

Recommendations for Supplementation

There is insufficient evidence on which to base a recommendation for routine zinc supplementation during pregnancy. Iron in large doses (>60 mg/day) and possibly in lower doses (Dawson et al., 1989) does appear to depress plasma zinc in pregnant women and should, therefore, be avoided. Zinc supplementation is recommended when >30 mg of supplemental iron is administered per day.

COPPER

Importance in Pregnancy

Copper-containing enzymes such as cytochrome oxidase play key roles in many oxidative processes and, hence, in the production of most of the energy required for metabolism. Certain cuproenzymes are important in the body's defense against free radicals (e.g., superoxide dismutase in cytosol and mitochondria), in the synthesis of connective tissue (e.g., lysyl oxidase), in the transport and utilization of iron (e.g., ferroxidases, including ceruloplasmin), in the synthesis of norepinephrine (dopamine β-hydroxylase), and in other metabolic pathways (Solomons, 1985).

In animal models, maternal copper deficiency can cause infertility, abortion, and stillbirth (Davis and Mertz, 1987). However, low-copper diets have been shown to be teratogenic only when fed in combination with chelators that bind copper and further compromise copper status (Keen et al., 1982). When pregnant ewes graze on severely copper-deficient pastures, enzootic neonatal ataxia (swayback) occurs in their lambs (Davis and Mertz, 1987). This neurologic disorder results from the decreased activity of cytochrome oxidase in the central nervous system. Feeding of a marginally copper-deficient diet to rats beginning 4 months prior to breeding and continuing through gestation and lactation and to the weaned offspring causes no overt problems but does result in ultrastructural abnormalities in arterial elastin that are similar to the early changes of atherosclerosis (Hunsaker et al., 1984).

Copper deficiency has not been documented in humans during pregnancy. It is quite possible that the demonstrated teratogenic effects of the drug penicillamine, which is a copper chelator, may be mediated through copper deficiency, but copper status has not been investigated in the reported cases (Mjølnerød et al., 1971). Serum copper has been reported to be lower in women who deliver prematurely (Kiiholma et al., 1984), and weak correlations have been observed between levels of copper in maternal serum and hair and indices of fetal growth (Vir et al., 1981).

Pregnancy has a major effect on maternal copper metabolism. There are marked increases in serum ceruloplasmin and in plasma copper (Hambidge and Mauer, 1978). Deviations from normal pregnancy-related changes in serum copper are likely to result from an abnormal obstetric course, e.g., placental insufficiency or intrauterine death, rather than from inadequate copper intake.

Estimated Requirements During Pregnancy

During pregnancy, total copper retention is approximately 30 mg, including 17 mg accumulated by the fetus. Most of this copper is accumulated in late gestation, when copper retention has been calculated to average 0.28 mg/day (Campbell, 1988). At 40% fractional absorption (Turnlund et al., 1983), these figures indicate an increased dietary copper requirement of 0.7 mg/day. Most studies of copper requirements in humans have been conducted in males. Requirements for nonpregnant adult females are expected to be slightly lower. Klevay et al. (1980) concluded that a copper intake of 1.3 mg/day is necessary for males to avoid negative balance. However, Turnlund et al. (1989) clearly demonstrated that adults can adapt to a wide range of copper intakes with changes in copper absorption. They showed that a positive copper balance can be achieved by young men on a diet that provides only 0.8 mg of copper per day. Depending on which figures are accepted, estimated copper requirements during pregnancy would be either 1.5 or 2.0 mg/day.

Usual Intakes

Average copper intake by nonpregnant adults is approximately 1 mg/day (Holden et al., 1979; Pennington et al., 1989) and by pregnant women, 1.4 to 1.8 mg/day (see Table 13-2; Campbell, 1988). Additional careful estimates of copper intake during pregnancy are needed.

Dosage Range and Toxicity

No studies of copper supplementation of pregnant women have been reported. Several prenatal multivitamin-mineral preparations currently marketed provide 2 mg of copper per tablet. Spitalny et al. (1984) reported chronic copper toxicity in adults who drank water containing approximately 8 mg of copper per liter.

Criteria for Status Assessment

Copper and ceruloplasmin concentrations are low in copper-deficient, nonpregnant adults. Pregnancy is accompanied by a progressive increase in circulating ceruloplasmin and, hence, in serum copper up to approximately twice the values in nonpregnant individuals (Hambidge and Mauer, 1978). It is not known if and to what extent these pregnancy-related changes are affected by copper deficiency. An unusually low serum ceruloplasmin or copper concentration occurs during pregnancy if there is a failure of normal placental development, regardless of copper intake. Erythrocyte superoxide dismutase activity is a potentially valuable index of copper status (Uauy et al., 1985), but its use in pregnancy has not yet been established.

Prevalence of Deficiency

Nutritional copper deficiency during human pregnancy has not been documented.

Effects of Other Supplements

Even a moderately excessive zinc intake (e.g., 50 mg of elemental zinc per day, which is approximately three times the 1989 RDA) can interfere with copper absorption and metabolism (Yadrick et al., 1989). A negative change in copper balance may occur if an individual takes supplements providing enough zinc to achieve a total intake of 20 to 25 mg/day (Festa et al., 1985). There is a need for further substantiation of this effect, which has been reported only with very low copper intakes.

Recommendations for Supplementation

Although the estimated mean intake of copper is lower than the estimated copper requirements during the last trimester of pregnancy, there is no evidence that any pregnant woman is deficient in copper to the extent that normal fetal growth and development are jeopardized. Therefore, no recommendation is made for prenatal copper supplementation. If a zinc supplement is administered, however, the subcommittee recommends that a 2-mg copper supplement also be given. This relatively high dose should be at least sufficient to compensate for the relatively poor absorption that occurs when copper is administered with zinc.

IODINE

Iodine is an essential component of the thyroid hormones thyroxine and triiodothyronine. Maternal iodine deficiency during pregnancy is the cause of a wide spectrum of iodine deficiency disorders in the fetus and in the offspring (Anonymous, 1983; Hetzel, 1983; Matovinovic, 1983), including stillbirth, abortions, and congenital anomalies; endemic cretinism, characterized by mental deficiency; profound deafness; spastic dysplegia; or less commonly, the myxedematous type of cretinism. Milder disorders include neurologic impairment manifested by suboptimal intellectual performance and motor skill development and hearing loss in children born in geographic areas where there is an endemic deficiency of iodine (Yan-You and Shu-Hua, 1985). To avoid damage to the fetus, iodine deficiency needs to be corrected prior to conception (Hetzel and Hay, 1979).

A 50- to 70-μg intake of iodine per day is sufficient to avoid the risk of hypothyroidism in adult women. The RDA of 150 μg for adult women is sufficient to offset the adverse effects of dietary goitrogens, and an additional 25 μg of iodine per day is recommended during pregnancy (NRC, 1989).

In the Food and Drug Administration's Total Diet Study, the mean iodine intake by women aged 25 to 30 in the United States during 1986 was 170 μg/day—approximately half the typical intake in 1982 but still high relative to requirements (Pennington et al., 1989). There is no evidence of residual iodine deficiency in the United States, and no iodine supplements are recommended. Although excess dietary iodine intake has been associated with both goiters (Mu et al., 1987) and thyrotoxicosis (Connolly, 1973), this is not a contraindication to the moderate use of iodized salt during pregnancy. In certain countries in Africa, Asia, South America, and Europe, iodine deficiency disorders continue to be a major public health problem. Strenuous international efforts are under way to eradicate this disorder by promoting the use of iodized oil or salt (Anonymous, 1986a).

SELENIUM

Selenium is an essential component of the enzyme glutathione peroxidase, which catalyzes the conversion of hydrogen peroxide to water. Thus, selenium is an important component of the body's defenses against free radical damage (Hoekstra, 1975). In animal models, the effects of selenium deficiency are more apparent if there is a concurrent deficiency of other antioxidants, especially vitamin E.

Selenium deficiency has been identified in humans living in a large area of the People's Republic of China where there is a severe geochemical deficiency of this micronutrient. The deficiency is manifested by a frequently fatal cardiomyopathy (Keshan disease) that occurs in young children and women of childbearing age. Although the etiology of this disease is probably multifactorial, a severe dietary deficiency of selenium is the major etiologic factor (Keshan Disease Research Group, 1979a,b). There have been scattered case reports of similar cardiomyopathies (Johnson et al., 1981) and of skeletal myopathies (van Rij et al., 1979) in selenium-deficient patients maintained on prolonged total parenteral nutrition without selenium supplements (Johnson et al., 1981). Milder selenium deficiency in parenterally fed children has been associated with macrocytosis and hair pigment changes (Vinton et al., 1987).

Keshan disease occurs in areas where the average selenium intake by adult males is 8 μg/day (Yang et al., 1987). Where Keshan disease was not evident, the average selenium intake by Chinese men was 19 μg/day. Maximal plasma glutathione peroxidase activity in Chinese men was achieved with 40 μg of selenium per day (Yang et al., 1988). The average weight of a Chinese man is 60 kg, which is similar to that of women in the United States.

Selenium retentions of 10 and 22 μg/day between weeks 10 to 20 and 30 to 40 of gestation, respectively, have been reported (Swanson et al., 1983) in women with a high selenium intake. However, since selenium homeostasis changes over a wide range of selenium intakes, the metabolic balance technique is not helpful in determining human selenium requirements (Levander and Burk, 1986). On a factorial basis, estimates of selenium retention in the fetus have varied from as little as 1 μg/day to an average of 14 μg/day during the last trimester (NRC, 1989). If fractional absorption from the mother's gastrointestinal tract is 80% (Levander, 1983), an additional 18 μg of dietary selenium would be required daily during late gestation. Thus, the estimated selenium requirement during late gestation would be approximately 60 μg/day. The estimated average dietary selenium intake by women aged 25 to 30 during 1985 and 1986 was about 70 μg/day in the United States (Pennington et al., 1989).

Several cases of selenium toxicity in nonpregnant adults resulted from large intakes of selenium supplements that provided about 30 mg per tablet—approximately 200 times more selenium than that advertised on the label (Helzlsouer et al., 1985). Symptoms of selenium toxicity included nausea, vomiting, nail changes, hair loss, fatigue, and irritability.

Whole blood or erythrocyte selenium levels and glutathione peroxidase activity are used to assess selenium status in nonpregnant adults (Levander, 1986). Plasma selenium is also used, although it is subject to short-term changes. However, the value of these indices is limited by the wide range of values found in apparently healthy subjects. In the United States, plasma selenium concentrations in nonpregnant adults usually range from 100 to 200 ng/ml. Adults with evidence of mild and severe selenium deficiency have plasma levels of less than 40 and 10 ng/ml, respectively. Selenium concentrations in plasma, but not in erythrocytes, decline during gestation. There is no indication of a need to conduct laboratory tests to assess selenium status during pregnancy or to advise pregnant women to take supplemental selenium.

MANGANESE

Manganese is a component of two enzymes—mitochondrial superoxide dismutase, an important antioxidant, and pyruvate carboxylase. Manganese-activated enzymes include the glycosyltransferases, which are necessary for the synthesis of polysaccharides and glycoproteins.

When rat dams are raised from the time of weaning on a manganese-deficient diet, the pups experience poor survival and ataxia. These abnormalities can be prevented by correcting the manganese deficiency as late as day 14 of gestation (Hurley, 1981). Offspring of manganese-deficient dams also have low blood glucose concentrations, which are associated with decreased activity of phosphoenolpyruvate carboxykinase—a manganese enzyme involved in gluconeogenesis (Baly et al., 1984). Deficiency impairs mucopolysaccharide synthesis in the developing otoliths of the pig's inner ear, resulting in a lack of coordination (Hurley, 1981).

There are no adequate data on manganese accumulation in the human conceptus. Usual intake by nonpregnant women aged 25 to 30 is approximately 2 mg/day (Pennington et al., 1989). Both positive and negative manganese balances were observed during late pregnancy in women whose daily manganese intake averaged 2 to 7 mg (Armstrong, 1985).

Manganese deficiency has not been observed in human adults, including pregnant women. The intestine (through absorption) and liver (through biliary excretion) provide strong homeostatic controls of body manganese. Thus, manganese supplements are not indicated during pregnancy. Some data indicate that supplemental iron can interfere with manganese absorption (Davidsson et al., 1988). This merits further research. Manganese administered orally to nonpregnant adults appears to be nontoxic in quantities considerably in excess of requirements (NRC, 1989).

CHROMIUM

Chromium is believed to play a physiologic role as a cofactor for insulin, facilitating the initial attachment of the hormone to its peripheral receptors (Mertz, 1969). However, chromium has not been found in the insulin receptor (Kahn, 1985). There have been numerous, but unconfirmed, reports of chromium deficiency in humans, primarily in patients maintained on prolonged parenteral nutrition (Jeejeebhoy et al., 1977). Glucose intolerance has been the most consistently observed effect of very low chromium intake.

Some reports of chromium concentrations in plasma and tissues suggest that pregnancy may be associated with chromium depletion (Davidson and Burt, 1973; Hambidge and Rodgerson, 1969). It is difficult to substantiate these results, however, because accurate analysis of chromium in human tissues is exacting and there is a lack of established laboratory indices of human chromium status. Thus, the extent to which chromium is important in human nutrition remains uncertain, and there are no data suggesting that chromium supplementation is advisable during pregnancy.

MOLYBDENUM

In humans, molybdenum is a component of two enzymes—xanthine oxidase, which is involved in the degradation of adenosine monophosphate, and sulfite oxidase. Molybdenum deficiency has been described only in one patient who was on prolonged total parenteral nutrition. Excess molybdenum intake interferes with copper metabolism (Mills and Davis, 1987). Molybdenum supplementation during pregnancy is contraindicated.

FLUORIDE

Administration of fluoride is the most effective means to prevent dental caries. Public health measures, including fluoridation of the community or school water supplies or oral supplementation, have been directed primarily toward infants and children younger than age 16. Adults may also derive some benefit from a fluoridated water supply or a 1-mg fluoride supplement per day (American Dental Association Council on Dental Therapeutics, 1984).

The precise mechanism by which fluoride exerts its cariostatic (decay-retarding) effects is uncertain. Most fluoride accumulates in the external enamel layer. Both topical and systemic fluoride appear to provide protection against dental caries most effectively in the tooth's first two posteruptive years (Stookey, 1981). During the preeruptive phase, systemic fluoride may have some beneficial effect, but there is no unanimity of opinion on this subject (American Dental Association Council on Dental Therapeutics, 1984).

Maternal fluoride supplementation during pregnancy has been reported to decrease the incidence of caries in the offspring, even when administered in an area with a fluoridated water supply (Glenn and Glenn, 1987). The designs of the studies on which this claim is partially based have been challenged (Driscoll, 1981). Fluoride supplementation during pregnancy has not been endorsed by the American Dental Association and has not been generally accepted as a validated procedure.

Dental fluorosis, or mottled enamel, has been observed in developing teeth in areas where water supplies contain more than twice the optimal fluoride concentration of 1 mg/liter. Excessive fluoride intake should therefore be avoided.

The subcommittee concluded that there is insufficient evidence to warrant recommending fluoride supplementation during pregnancy as a means of benefiting the teeth of the offspring.

SUMMARY

Although dietary intake of zinc and copper may be considerably lower than the RDA, there is no convincing evidence that this has adverse effects on pregnancy outcome. There is also no persuasive evidence that routine antenatal supplements of any trace element other than iron are potentially beneficial for pregnant women in the United States.

CLINICAL IMPLICATIONS

- Laboratory tests to determine trace element status are not sufficiently sensitive or predictive to justify their expense in routine prenatal care.
- The best means of ensuring an optimal intake of trace elements appears to be consumption of a well-balanced and adequate diet rather than use of mineral supplements.
- Although vegetarian diets can provide reasonable quantities of trace elements, flesh foods frequently contribute larger amounts that are more readily absorbed and are thus potentially advantageous during pregnancy.
- There is no persuasive evidence that it is potentially beneficial to routinely supplement pregnant women with any trace element other than iron in the United States.
- Although zinc nutrition during pregnancy has attracted recent professional and public interest, there is insufficient evidence to support a recommendation for routine prenatal zinc supplementation.
- Although the subcommittee concluded that the iodine content of the food supply in the United States is sufficiently high to make iodine supplementation unnecessary, use of iodized salt is not contraindicated.
- The intake of fluoride provided by fluoridated water supplies is encouraged, but fluoride supplements that result in intake above approximately 1 mg/day are not recommended.

REFERENCES

Adeniyi, F.A.A. 1987. The implications of hypozincemia in pregnancy. Acta Obstet. Gynecol. Scand. 66:579-582.

American Dental Association Council on Dental Therapeutics. 1984. Fluoride compounds. Pp. 395-420 in Accepted Dental Therapeutics, 40th ed. American Dental Association, Chicago.

Anonymous. 1983. From endemic goitre to iodine deficiency disorders. Lancet 2:1121-1122.

Anonymous. 1986a. Prevention and control of iodine deficiency disorders. Lancet 2:433-434.

Anonymous. 1986b. Zinc and fetal alcohol syndrome: another dimension. Nutr. Rev. 44:359-360.

Apgar, J. 1968. Comparison of the effect of copper, manganese, and zinc deficiencies on parturition in the rat. Am. J. Physiol. 215:1478-1481.

Apgar, J. 1987. Effect on the guinea pig of low zinc intake during pregnancy. Fed. Proc., Fed. Am. Soc. Exp. Biol. 46:747.

Armstrong, J. 1985. Trace element metabolism in human pregnancy. M. Phil (C.N.A.A.) Thesis. Robert Gordon's Institute of Technology, University of Aberdeen, Scotland.

Baly, D.L., D.L. Curry, C.L. Hurley. 1984. Effect of manganese on insulin secretion and carbohydrate homeostasis in rats. J. Nutr. 114:1438-1446.

Campbell, D.M. 1988. Trace element needs in human pregnancy. Proc. Nutr. Soc. 47:45-53.

Campbell-Brown, M., R.J. Ward, A.P. Haines, W.R.S. North, R. Abraham, and I.R. McFadyen. 1985. Zinc and copper in Asian pregnancies—is there evidence for a nutritional deficiency? Br. J. Obstet. Gynaecol. 92:875-885.

Cherry, F.F., E.A. Bennett, G.S. Bazzano, L.K. Johnson, G.J. Fosmire, and H.K. Batson. 1981. Plasma zinc in hypertension/toxemia and other reproductive variables in adolescent pregnancy. Am. J. Clin. Nutr. 34:2367-2375.

Cherry, F., H. Sandstead, G. Bazzano, L. Johnson, H. Bunce, D. Milne, and J. Mahalko. 1987. Zinc nutriture in adolescent pregnancy: response to zinc supplementation. Fed. Proc., Fed. Am. Soc. Exp. Biol. 46:748.

Chesters, J.K. 1978. Biochemical functions of zinc in animals. World Rev. Nutr. Diet. 32:135-164.

Connolly, R.J. 1973. The changing age incidence of jodbasedow in Tasmania. Med. J. Aust. 2:171-174.

Crosby, W.M., J. Metcoff, J.P. Costiloe, M. Mameesh, H.H. Sandstead, R.A. Jacob, P.E. McClain, G. Jacobson, W. Reid, and G. Burns. 1977. Fetal malnutrition: an appraisal of correlated factors. Am. J. Obstet. Gynecol. 128:22-31.

Crossley, L.G., K.H. Falchuk, and B.L. Vallee. 1982. Messenger ribonucleic acid function and protein synthesis in zinc-deficient *Euglena gracilis*. Biochemistry 21:5359-5363.

Davidson, I.W.F., and R.L. Burt. 1973. Physiologic changes in plasma chromium of normal and pregnant women: effect of a glucose load. Am. J. Obstet. Gynecol. 116:601-608.

Davidsson, L., Å. Cederblad, B. Lönnerdal, and B. Sandström. 1988. Manganese absorption from human milk, cow's milk and infant formulas. Pp. 511-512 in L.S. Hurley, C.L. Keen, B. Lönnerdal, and R.B. Rucker, eds. Trace Elements in Man and Animals 6. Plenum Press, New York.

Davies, N.T., and R.B. Williams. 1977. The effect of pregnancy and lactation on the absorption of zinc and lysine by the rat duodenum *in situ*. Br. J. Nutr. 38:417-423.

Davis, G.K., and W. Mertz. 1987. Copper. Pp. 301-364 in W. Mertz, ed. Trace Elements in Human and Animal Nutrition, 5th ed., Vol. 1. Academic Press, San Diego, Calif.

Dawson, E.B., J. Albers, and W.J. McGanity. 1989. Serum zinc changes due to iron supplementation in teen-age pregnancy. Am. J. Clin. Nutr. 50:848-852.

Dreosti, I.E. 1982. Zinc in prenatal development. Pp. 19-38 in A.S. Prasad, I.E. Dreosti, and B.S. Hetzel, eds. Clinical Applications of Recent Advances in Zinc Metabolism. Current Topics in Nutrition and Disease, Vol. 7. Alan R. Liss, New York.

Driscoll, W.S. 1981. A review of clinical research on the use of prenatal fluoride administration for prevention of dental caries. J. Dent. Child 48:109-117.

Fehily, D., B. Fitzsimmons, D. Jenkins, F.M. Cremin, A. Flynn, and M.H. Soltan. 1986. Association of fetal growth with elevated maternal plasma zinc concentration in human pregnancy. Hum. Nutr.: Clin. Nutr. 40C:221-227.

Festa, M.D., H.L. Anderson, R.P. Dowdy, and M.R. Ellersieck. 1985. Effect of zinc intake on copper excretion and retention in men. Am. J. Clin. Nutr. 41:285-292.

Flynn, A., S.I. Miller, S.S. Martier, N.L. Golden, R.J. Sokol, and B.C. Del Villano. 1981. Zinc status of pregnant alcoholic women: a determinant of fetal outcome. Lancet 1:572-575.

Fuller, N.J., P.H. Evans, M. Howlett, and C.J. Bates. 1988. The effects of dietary folate and zinc on the outcome of pregnancy and early growth in rats. Br. J. Nutr. 59:251-259.

Ghishan, F.K., and H.L. Greene. 1983. Fetal alcohol syndrome: failure of zinc supplementation to reverse the effect of ethanol on placental transport of zinc. Pediatr. Res. 17:529-531.

Gibson, R.S., and C.A. Scythes. 1982. Trace element intakes of women. Br. J. Nutr. 48:241-248.

Glenn, F.B., and W.D. Glenn III. 1987. Optimum dosage for prenatal fluoride supplementation (PNF): part IX. J. Dent. Child. 54:445-450.

Hambidge, K.M. 1982. Hair analyses: worthless for vitamins, limited for minerals. Am. J. Clin. Nutr. 36:943-949.

Hambidge, K.M. 1989. Mild zinc deficiency in human subjects. Pp. 281-296 in C.F. Mills, ed. Zinc in Human Biology. Springer-Verlag, London.

Hambidge, K.M., and A.M. Mauer. 1978. Trace elements. Pp. 157-193 in Laboratory Indices of Nutritional Status in Pregnancy. Report of the Committee on Nutrition of the Mother and Preschool Child, Food and Nutrition Board. National Academy of Sciences, Washington, D.C.

Hambidge, K.M., and D.O. Rodgerson. 1969. Comparison of hair chromium levels of nulliparous and parous women. Am. J. Obstet. Gynecol. 103:320-321.

Hambidge, K.M., K.H. Neldner, and P.A. Walravens. 1975. Zinc, acrodermatitis enteropathica, and congenital malformations. Lancet 1:577-578.

Hambidge, K.M., N.F. Krebs, M.A. Jacobs, A. Favier, L. Guyette, and D.N. Ikle. 1983. Zinc nutritional status during pregnancy: a longitudinal study. Am. J. Clin. Nutr. 37:429-442.

Hambidge, K.M., C.E. Casey, and N.F. Krebs. 1986. Zinc. Pp. 1-137 in W. Mertz, ed. Trace Elements in Human and Animal Nutrition, 5th ed., Vol. 2. Academic Press, Orlando, Fla.

Hambidge, K.M., N.F. Krebs, L. Sibley, and J. English. 1987. Acute effects of iron therapy on zinc status during pregnancy. Obstet. Gynecol. 4:593-596.

Hambidge, K.M., M.J. Goodall, C. Stall, and J. Pritts. 1989. Post-prandial and daily changes in plasma zinc. J. Trace Elem. Electrol. Health Dis. 3:55-57.

Hamilton, D.L., J.E.C. Bellamy, J.D. Valberg, and L.S. Valberg. 1978. Zinc, cadmium, and iron interactions during intestinal absorption in iron-deficient mice. Can. J. Physiol. Pharmacol. 56:384-389.

Haynes, D.C., M.E. Gershwin, M.S. Golub, A.T.W. Cheung, L.S. Hurley, and A.G. Hendrickx. 1985. Studies of marginal zinc deprivation in rhesus monkeys: VI. Influence on the immunohematology of infants in the first year. Am. J. Clin. Nutr. 42:252-262.

Helzlsouer, K., R. Jacobs, and S. Morris. 1985. Acute selenium intoxication in the United States. Fed. Proc., Fed. Am. Soc. Exp. Biol. 44:1670.

Hetzel, B.S. 1983. Iodine deficiency disorders (IDD) and their eradication. Lancet 2:1126-1129.

Hetzel, B.S., and I.D. Hay. 1979. Thyroid function, iodine nutrition and fetal brain development. Clin. Endocrinol. 11:445-460.

Hoekstra, W.G. 1975. Biochemical function of selenium and its relation to vitamin E. Fed. Proc., Fed. Am. Soc. Exp. Biol. 34:2083-2089.

Holden, J.M., W.R. Wolf, and W. Mertz. 1979. Zinc and copper in self-selected diets. J. Am. Diet. Assoc. 75:23-28.

Hunsaker, H.A., M. Morita, and K.G.D. Allen. 1984. Marginal copper deficiency in rats: aortal morphology of elastin and cholesterol values in first-generation adult males. Atherosclerosis 51:1-19.

Hunt, I.F., N.J. Murphy, A.E. Cleaver, B. Faraji, M.E. Swendseid, A.H. Coulson, V.A. Clark, B.L. Browdy, M.T. Cabalum, and J.C. Smith, Jr. 1984. Zinc supplementation during pregnancy: effects on selected blood constituents and on progress and outcome of pregnancy in low-income women of Mexican descent. Am. J. Clin. Nutr. 40:508-521.

Hunt, I.F., N.J. Murphy, A.E. Cleaver, B. Faraji, M.E. Swendseid, B.L. Browdy, A.H. Coulson, V.A. Clark, R.H. Settlage, and J.C. Smith, Jr. 1985. Zinc supplementation during pregnancy in low-income teenagers of Mexican descent: effects on selected blood constituents and on progress and outcome of pregnancy. Am. J. Clin. Nutr. 42:815-828.

Hurley, L.S. 1981. Teratogenic aspects of manganese, zinc, and copper nutrition. Physiol. Rev. 61:249-295.

Hurley, L.S., and R.E. Shrader. 1975. Abnormal development of preimplantation rat eggs after three days of maternal dietary zinc deficiency. Nature 254:427-429.

Hurley, L.S., M.E. Gershwin, and M.S. Golub. 1985. Marginal zinc deprivation in pregnant monkeys and effects on offspring. Pp. 197-200 in C.F. Mills, I. Bremner, and J.K. Chesters, eds. Trace Elements in Man and Animals 5. Commonwealth Agricultural Bureaux, Farnham Royal, U.K.

Jeejeebhoy, K.N., R.C. Chu, E.B. Marliss, G.R. Greenberg, and A. Bruce-Robertson. 1977. Chromium deficiency, glucose intolerance, and neuropathy reversed by chromium supplementation, in a patient receiving long-term total parenteral nutrition. Am. J. Clin. Nutr. 30:531-538.

Johnson, R.A., S.S. Baker, J.T. Fallon, E.P. Maynard III, J.N. Ruskin, Z. Wen, K. Ge., and H.J. Cohen. 1981. An occidental case of cardiomyopathy and selenium deficiency. N. Engl. J. Med. 304:1210-1212.

Kahn, C.R. 1985. The molecular mechanism of insulin action. Annu. Rev. Med. 36:429-451.

Keen, C.L., B. Lönnerdal, and L.S. Hurley. 1982. Teratogenic effects of copper deficiency and excess. Pp. 109-121 in J.R.J. Sorenson, ed. Inflammatory Diseases and Copper. Humana Press, Clifton, N.J.

Keshan Disease Research Group. 1979a. Epidemiologic studies on the etiologic relationship of selenium and Keshan disease. Chin. Med. J. 92:477-482.

Keshan Disease Research Group. 1979b. Observations on effect of sodium selenite in prevention of Keshan Disease. Chin. Med. J. 92:471-476.

Kiilholma, P., M. Grönroos, R. Erkkola, P. Pakarinen, and V. Näntö. 1984. The role of calcium, copper, iron and zinc in preterm delivery and premature rupture of fetal membranes. Gynecol. Obstet. Invest. 17:194-201.

Klevay, L.M., S.J. Reck, R.A. Jacob, G.M. Logan, Jr., J.M. Munoz, and H.H. Sandstead. 1980. The human requirement for copper. I. Healthy men fed conventional, American diets. Am. J. Clin. Nutr. 33:45-50.

Klug, A., and D. Rhodes. 1987. 'Zinc fingers': a novel protein motif for nucleic acid recognition. Trends Biochem. Sci. 12:464-469.

Krebs, N.F., K.M. Hambidge, R.J. Hagerman, P.L. Peirce, K.M. Johnson, J.L. English, L.L. Miller, and P.V. Fennessey. 1988. The effects of pharmacologic doses of folate on zinc absorption and zinc status. Am. J. Clin. Nutr. 47:783.

Kuhnert, B.R., P.M. Kuhnert, and T.J. Zarlingo. 1988. Associations between placental cadmium and zinc and age and parity in pregnant women who smoke. Obstet. Gynecol. 71:67-70.

Kumar, S. 1976. Effect of zinc supplementation on rats during pregnancy. Nutr. Rep. Int. 13:33-36.

Levander, O.A. 1983. Considerations in the design of selenium bioavailability studies. Fed. Proc., Fed. Am. Soc. Exp. Biol. 42:1721-1725.

Levander, O.A. 1986. Selenium. Pp. 209-279 in W. Mertz, ed. Trace Elements in Human and Animal Nutrition, 5th ed., Vol. 2. Academic Press, Orlando, Fla.

Levander, O.A., and R.F. Burk. 1986. Report on the 1986 A.S.P.E.N. Research Workshop on Selenium in Clinical Nutrition. J. Parenter. Enter. Nutr. 10:545-549.

Mahomed, K., D.K. James, J. Golding, R. McCabe. 1989. Zinc supplementation during pregnancy: a double blind randomised controlled trial. Br. Med. J. 299:826-830.

Matovinovic, J. 1983. Endemic goiter and cretinism at the dawn of the third millennium. Annu. Rev. Nutr. 3:341-412.

Meadows, N.J., W. Ruse, M.F. Smith, J. Day, P.W.N. Keeling, J.W. Scopes, R.P.H. Thompson, and D.L. Bloxam. 1981. Zinc and small babies. Lancet 2:1135-1137.

Mertz, W. 1969. Chromium occurence and function in biological systems. Physiol Rev. 49:163-239.

Mills, C.F., and G.K. Davis. 1987. Molybdenum. Pp. 429-463 in W. Mertz, ed. Trace Elements in Human and Animal Nutrition, 5th ed., Vol. 1. Academic Press, San Diego, Calif.

Milne, D.B., W.K. Canfield, J.R. Mahalko, and H.H. Sandstead. 1984. Effect of oral folic acid supplements on zinc, copper, and iron absorption and excretion. Am. J. Clin. Nutr. 39:535-539.

Milne, D.B., N.V.C. Ralston, and J.C. Wallwork. 1985. Zinc content of blood cellular components and lymph node and spleen lymphocytes in severely zinc-deficient rats. J. Nutr. 115:1073-1078.

Mjølnerød, O.K., K. Rasmussen, S.A. Dommerud, and S.T. Gjeruldsen. 1971. Congenital connective-tissue defect probably due to D-penicillamine treatment in pregnancy. Lancet 1:673-675.

Mu, L., L. Derun, Q. Chengyi, Z. Peiying, Q. Qidong, Z. Chunde, J. Qingzhen, W. Huaixing, C.J. Eastman, S.C. Boyages, J.K. Collins, J.J. Jupp, and G.F. Maberly. 1987. Endemic goitre in central China caused by excessive iodine intake. Lancet 1:257-259.

NRC (National Research Council). 1989. Recommended Dietary Allowances, 10th ed. Report of the Subcommittee on the Tenth Edition of the RDAs, Food and Nutrition Board, Commission on Life Sciences. National Academy Press, Washington, D.C. 284 pp.

Patterson, K.Y., J.T. Holbrook, J.E. Bodner, J.L. Kelsay, J.C. Smith, Jr., and C. Veillon. 1984. Zinc, copper, and manganese intake and balance for adults consuming self-selected diets. Am. J. Clin. Nutr. 40:1397-1403.

Pennington, J.A.T., B.E. Young, and D.B. Wilson. 1989. Nutritional elements in U.S. diets: results from the Total Diet Study, 1982 to 1986. J. Am. Diet. Assoc. 89:659-664.

Record, I.R., I.E. Dreosti, S.J. Manuel, R.A. Buckley, and R.S. Tulsi. 1985. Teratological influence of the feeding cycle in zinc-deficient rats. Pp. 210-213 in C.F. Mills, I. Bremner, and J.K. Chesters, eds. Trace Elements in Man and Animals 5. Commonwealth Agricultural Bureaus, Farnham Royal, U.K.

Sandström, B., L. Davidsson, Å. Cederblad, and B. Lönnerdal. 1985. Oral iron, dietary ligands and zinc absorption. J. Nutr. 115:411-414.

Sato, F., T. Watanabe, E. Hoshi, and A. Endo. 1985. Teratogenic effect of maternal zinc deficiency and its co-teratogenic effect with cadmium. Teratology 31:13-18.

Solomons, N.W. 1985. Biochemical, metabolic, and clinical role of copper in human nutrition. J. Am. Coll. Nutr. 4:83-105.

Solomons, N.W. 1986. Competitive interaction of iron and zinc in the diet: consequences for human nutrition. J. Nutr. 116:927-935.

Spitalny, K.C., J. Brondum, R.L. Vogt, H.E. Sargent, and S. Kappel. 1984. Drinking-water-induced copper intoxication in a Vermont family. Pediatrics 74:1103-1106.

Stookey, G.K. 1981. Perspectives on the use of prenatal fluorides: a reactor's comments. J. Dent. Child. 48:126-127.

Strobel, D., H. Sandstead, L. Zimmermann, and A. Reuter. 1979. Prenatal protein and zinc malnutrition in the rhesus monkey, *Macaca mulatta*. Pp. 43-58 in G.C. Ruppenthal and D.J. Reese, eds. Nursery Care of Nonhuman Primates. Plenum Press, New York.

Swanson, C.A., and J.C. King. 1987. Zinc and pregnancy outcome. Am. J. Clin. Nutr. 46:763-771.

Swanson, C.A., D.C. Reamer, C. Veillon, J.C. King, and O.A. Levander. 1983. Quantitative and qualitative aspects of selenium utilization in pregnant and nonpregnant women: an application of stable isotope methodology. Am. J. Clin. Nutr. 38:169-180.

Swenerton, H., and L.S. Hurley. 1980. Zinc deficiency in rhesus and bonnet monkeys, including effects on reproduction. J. Nutr. 110:575-583.

Turnlund, J.R., C.A. Swanson, and J.C. King. 1983. Copper absorption and retention in pregnant women fed diets based on animal and plant proteins. J. Nutr. 113:2346-2352.

Turnlund, J.R., W.R. Keyes, H.L. Anderson, and L.L. Acord. 1989. Copper absorption and retention in young men at three levels of dietary copper by use of the stable isotope ^{65}Cu. Am. J. Clin. Nutr. 49:870-878.

Uauy, R., C. Castillo-Duran, M. Fisberg, N. Fernandez, and A. Valenzuela. 1985. Red cell superoxide dismutase activity as an index of human copper nutrition. J. Nutr. 115:1650-1655.

van Rij, A.M., C.D. Thomson, J.M. McKenzie, and M.F. Robinson. 1979. Selenium deficiency in total parenteral nutrition. Am. J. Clin. Nutr. 32:2076-2085.

Vinton, N.E., K.A.D. Dahlstrom, C.T. Strobel, and M.E. Ament. 1987. Macrocytosis and pseudoalbinism: manifestations of selenium deficiency. J. Pediatr. 111:711-717.

Vir, S.C., A.H.G. Love, and W. Thompson. 1981. Serum and hair concentrations of copper during pregnancy. Am. J. Clin. Nutr. 34:2382-2388.

Wada, L., J.R. Turnlund, and J.C. King. 1985. Zinc utilization in young men fed adequate and low zinc intakes. J. Nutr. 115:1345-1354.

Yadrick, M.K., M.A. Kenney, and E.A. Winterfeldt. 1989. Iron, copper, and zinc status: response to supplementation with zinc or zinc and iron in adult females. Am. J. Clin. Nutr. 49:145-150.

Yang, G.Q., P.C. Qian, L.Z. Zhu, J.H. Huang, S.J. Liu, M.D. Lu, and L.Z. Gu. 1987. Human selenium requirements in China. Pp. 589-607 in G.F. Combs, Jr., O.A. Levander, J.E. Spallholz, and J.E. Oldfield, eds. Selenium in Biology and Medicine. Van Nostrand Reinhold, New York.

Yang, G.Q., K.Y. Ge., J.S. Chen, and X.S. Chen. 1988. Selenium-related endemic diseases and the daily selenium requirements of humans. World Rev. Nutr. Diet. 55:98-152.

Yan-You, W., and Y. Shu-Hua. 1985. Improvement in hearing among otherwise normal schoolchildren in iodine-deficient areas of Guizhou, China, following use of iodised salt. Lancet 2:518-520.

16

Calcium, Vitamin D, and Magnesium

Calcium and magnesium are both present in the diet and the body at levels much higher than those of trace minerals such as iron. Approximately 99% of the calcium and magnesium in the human body is located in the skeleton. For many years, women have been advised to increase their calcium intake substantially during pregnancy, and there has been concern that many pregnant women do not ingest enough calcium to maintain their own skeletons while providing for fetal needs. Vitamin D is discussed in this chapter since calcium metabolism is dependent on this vitamin. Although calcium and phosphorus metabolism are closely linked, phosphorus is not discussed in this report, since usual intakes of the nutrient are well above the Recommended Dietary Allowance (RDA). Neither inadequate nor excessive intake appears to be a problem in pregnant women (NRC, 1989), and phosphorus is not ordinarily contained in multivitamin-mineral supplements.

CALCIUM

Metabolism

Several changes in calcium metabolism associated with pregnancy facilitate the transfer of calcium from mother to fetus while protecting calcium levels in maternal serum and bone. These include changes in calcium-regulating hormones, which affect intestinal absorption, renal reabsorption, and bone turnover of calcium.

Total serum calcium decreases gradually throughout pregnancy. This is associated with and parallels the drop in serum albumin (to which 60% of the serum calcium is attached) that results from expansion of the extracellular fluid volume. When adjustments are made for changes in serum albumin or protein concentration, little or no change in the total serum calcium level is apparent during pregnancy. Serum ionic calcium changes are minimal (Pitkin et al., 1979).

Early studies indicated that the level of parathyroid hormone (PTH) increases progressively; in late pregnancy, it was reported to be approximately 50% higher than prepregnancy levels (Pitkin et al., 1979). However, more recent research indicates that the previously reported hyperparathyroidism of pregnancy may be an artifact of earlier radioimmunoassay methods. A relatively new immunoradiometric assay that is highly specific for the intact, and presumably biologically active, form of PTH indicated that the mean serum PTH level in 81 pregnant women was 14.4 ± 6.3 compared with 24.8 ± 9.0 (standard deviation) ng/ml in 11 nonpregnant women (Davis et al., 1988), indicating a decline during pregnancy.

A calcium-mobilizing peptide that is similar to PTH has been identified in both rat and human mammary tissue and milk (Budayr et al., 1989; Thiede and Rodan, 1988). The partially purified peptide stimulates calcium transport in the sheep placenta (Rodda et al., 1988), but its role in human pregnancy remains to be determined. Changes in maternal calcitonin have been reported to be inconsistent (Pitkin et al., 1979) or increased in early pregnancy and then stable throughout the remainder of pregnancy (Whitehead et al., 1981). A rise in calcitonin may protect the maternal skeleton against resorption. A substantial amount of the calcium needed by the fetus is provided by the increased maternal efficiency of dietary calcium absorption. Elevated 1,25-dihydroxycholecalciferol levels account for some of this increase, but other as yet unidentified factors may be involved (Halloran and DeLuca, 1980).

Placental transfer of calcium is an active process that occurs against a concentration gradient and involves placental calcium-binding protein (Lester, 1986; Umeki et al., 1981). Total and ionized serum calcium levels in the fetus and newborn are substantially higher than those in the mother.

Calcium Balance

Calcium and phosphorus are deposited in the fetus mainly in the last trimester, but the efficiency of maternal intestinal absorption is increased by at least the second trimester (Heaney and Skillman, 1971; Shenolikar, 1970). In a balance study, true absorption of calcium increased from 27% in nonpregnant women to 54% at 5 to 6 months of gestation and 42% at term (Heaney and Skillman, 1971). Urinary calcium increases during pregnancy, probably because of the higher glomerular filtration rate (Pitkin, 1985).

Fetal calcium levels suggest that ionized calcium is transferred from the mother to the fetus at a rate of 50 mg/day at 20 weeks of gestation to a maximum of 330 mg/day at 35 weeks of gestation (Forbes, 1976). The few calcium balance studies that have been conducted in pregnant women fail to show a positive balance this large, suggesting that calcium may be withdrawn from maternal bone or that there are inaccuracies in the studies. Ashe et al. (1979) studied healthy pregnant white women who consumed an average of 1,390 mg of calcium per day from self-selected diets and reported that they had sufficient calcium intake to balance urinary and fecal losses over the course of pregnancy but not to achieve the anticipated positive balance. Young women with a daily intake of approximately 800 mg of calcium retained an estimated 14 g of calcium during pregnancy—only half the amount needed for the fetus (Heaney and Skillman, 1971). In the third trimester, Scottish women had a positive balance of 142 mg/day when intake was 1 g and 305 mg/day when intake was 2 g (Duggin et al., 1974). Interpretation of these balance data is difficult due to the different levels of calcium intake, stage of pregnancy, and duration of the various studies.

Maternal Bone Loss

It is unclear whether the increased efficiency of intestinal calcium absorption during pregnancy prevents a net loss of calcium from the mother. Calcium balance would be expected to be strongly positive in late pregnancy, but as discussed above, the amount of calcium retained has been reported to be insufficient to supply the estimated total fetal needs (Duggin et al., 1974; Heaney and Skillman, 1971), suggesting that some is withdrawn from the mother's bones.

Substantial increases in absorptive efficiency and positive balance begin in the first trimester. This must represent maternal accumulation of calcium, since the fetal calcium content is negligible at this time. It is possible that calcium added to maternal bone during early pregnancy is transferred to the fetus in later gestation. Perhaps because of their inability to detect small changes in skeletal calcium, measurements of maternal bone mineral changes have failed to support this possibility. An increase in the amount of bone alkaline phosphatase activity that is apparent by 10 to 12 weeks of gestation provides indirect evidence that maternal bone formation may be increased (Valenzuela et al., 1987).

Evidence of bone loss during pregnancy is negative in most studies (Christiansen et al., 1976; Frisancho et al., 1971; Goldsmith and Johnston, 1975; Walker et al., 1972). X-ray spectrophotometry of the forearm showed a 4.2% average loss of trabecular bone and a 2% gain in cortical bone over the course of gestation (Lamke et al., 1977). Measurement of bone mineral density by the photon absorption method applied to the distal radius revealed a significant positive association ($R = .77$) between parity and bone density in 1,053 black and white women in California who were uncontrolled for the extent of lactation (Goldsmith and Johnston, 1975). In a retrospective study conducted in New York State, a 1.1% decrease in femoral neck density per live birth was found, but no association was observed between lumbar spine density and parity (Hreshchyshyn et al., 1988). In Bantu and Caucasian South African women, cortical bone thickness in those with seven or more children was similar to that of women with zero to two children, even though the Bantu's daily intake of calcium averaged less than 400 mg (Walker et al., 1972). Bone density of these two groups was not compared. Since the total amount of calcium transferred to the fetus is 30 g, which is equivalent to only 2.5% of maternal skeletal calcium, bone loss would be difficult to detect even with more precise techniques such as dual photon beam absorptiometry.

Severe calcium and phosphorus restriction in rats increases maternal PTH synthesis, plasma 1,25-dihydroxycholecalciferol, and intestinal calcium absorption and reduces urinary calcium excretion. Consequently, the fetal mineralization process remains normal (Verhaeghe et al., 1988). There are few data on the effect of maternal calcium intake on bone mineralization in human fetuses. In malnourished women in India, either 300 or 600 mg of supplemental calcium administered daily from week 20 of gestation significantly increased the density of fetal bones (Raman et al., 1978). The clinical importance of this is not clear, however, because there was no evidence of skeletal abnormalities in infants born to the placebo group. Usual calcium intakes of the women were reported as low but were not quantified.

Supplementation and Hypertension

An inverse relationship between calcium intake and blood pressure has been found in recent studies of nonpregnant adults. Recently, this finding has been extended to pregnant women in small-scale randomized clinical trials conducted in the United States (Maryland) and Argentina (Belizán et al., 1988) as well as in Ecuador (Lopez-Jaramillo et al., 1987). Daily calcium supplementation ranging from 1,500 to 2,000 mg reduced the incidence of pregnancy-induced hypertension in the two South American countries but not in Maryland. A dose-response relationship was suggested by one of the studies (Belizán et al., 1988). In further support of a possible relationship between calcium metabolism and preeclampsia (pregnancy-induced hypertension with proteinuria) are data demonstrating that the presence of hypocalciuria is a diagnostic aid in differentiating preeclampsia from other forms of gestational hypertension (Taufield et al., 1987). The pathophysiologic basis for these associations is unclear, as is the effect of calcium supplementation on pregnancy outcome. More extensive clinical trials are needed to explore this relationship further.

Supplementation and Leg Cramps

Leg cramps in pregnant women are sometimes attributed to calcium deficiency or disturbances in calcium metabolism. The effectiveness of calcium therapy for treating this complaint is doubtful. Treatment with 2 g of calcium per day for 3 weeks produced no improvement in the incidence of leg cramps compared with that in a placebo group given 2 g of ascorbic acid per day (Hammar et al., 1987).

Recommendations

Although pregnant women, on average, drink more milk than those who are neither pregnant nor lactating, the amounts of calcium recommended for pregnancy are often not achieved by dietary sources alone, especially in blacks, Hispanics, and American Indians (see Chapter 13). No adverse consequences of low calcium intake during pregnancy have been documented. However, there is justifiable concern about the possible effects of inadequate calcium intake by pregnant women under age 25 in whom some mineral is most likely still being added to their bones. The subcommittee defined a low calcium intake to be less than 600 mg/day; below this level of intake the average U.S. adult develops a negative calcium balance (Marshall et al., 1976). This is approximately the amount of calcium in a diet that includes only one small serving of a calcium-rich food in addition to nondairy foods.

The subcommittee recommends, therefore, that younger women with low calcium intakes should either increase their intake of food sources of calcium, such as milk or cheese, or, less preferably, add a supplement that provides 600 mg of calcium per day. In the United States, however, there have been no reports on the effect of maternal calcium supplementation on bone mineralization of the mother or the fetus.

Women with lactose intolerance need careful assessment of their calcium intake because they tend to drink little milk and to have relatively low calcium intakes. This condition is most prevalent among women of black, Hispanic, American Indian, and Asian background. These women can usually tolerate sufficient milk to meet their calcium requirements if taken in amounts less than one glass at a time. Alternative strategies are to consume calcium in yogurt, cheese, or low-lactose milk—foods that contain relatively low amounts of lactose. A glass of milk and a slice of hard cheese each contain approximately 300 mg of calcium.

The absorbability of calcium from the most commonly used supplements is similar to that from dairy products. Absorption is improved by consuming calcium supplements with or at the end of a light meal (Heaney et al., 1989), although the possible inhibitory effects of a meal high in phytate or fiber on calcium absorption have not been adequately investigated.

It is unlikely that pregnant women over age 35 would benefit from calcium supplementation to a greater extent than younger women would. Accelerated bone loss does not occur until menopause.

VITAMIN D

Metabolism

Most vitamin D is synthesized from a precursor in the skin after exposure to ultraviolet light from the sun. Relatively few foods are good sources of this vitamin; the major source in the United States is vitamin D-fortified milk. After vitamin D is ingested or synthesized in the skin, the liver converts it to 25-hydroxycholecalciferol, which is the major circulating form and the best indicator of vitamin D nutritional status. In the kidney, it is converted into 1,25-dihydroxycholecalciferol, the biologically active form of the vitamin. Levels of the active metabolite are not highly correlated with 25-hydroxycholecalciferol levels in the physiologic range. The 1,25-dihydroxycholecalciferol circulates both bound to a protein and in a free form; both forms are elevated during pregnancy (Paulson and DeLuca, 1986). Total levels are approximately doubled at term (Markestad et al., 1986). The extent to which the increase is stimulated by PTH, prolactin, or other hormones is unclear. Levels of the precursor 25-hydroxycholecalciferol have been reported as both unchanged (Hillman et al., 1978) and decreased (Reiter et al., 1979) in pregnant women, but in animal studies they have been found to be lower when diet and exposure to ultraviolet light were controlled (Danan et al., 1980). Both of these metabolites, as well as 24,25-dihydroxycholecalciferol, which has no known function, are able to cross the placenta.

Fetal vitamin D status may be influenced by maternal vitamin D status, placental transfer and synthesis, or fetal synthesis of the vitamin. The relative importance of each to fetal vitamin D status has not been determined in humans. Maternal plasma 25-hydroxycholecalciferol levels are higher than levels in the umbilical vein or in the newborn, although levels of the free hormone may be higher in the fetus (Bouillon et al., 1981). Maternal and fetal levels of 25-hydroxycholecalciferol are positively correlated (Delvin et al., 1982), since the fetus obtains this form of the vitamin from its mother. In rats, a placental transport mechanism transfers vitamin D, 25-hydroxycholecalciferol, and 24,25-dihydroxycholecalciferol in similar proportions to the fetus, especially in the third trimester (Clements and Fraser, 1988). In the fetus, the vitamin is stored mainly as 25-hydroxycholecalciferol in muscle. Clements and Fraser (1988) demonstrated that the vitamin D molecules obtained in utero, rather than from maternal milk, are the main source of the vitamin during the first 10 days postpartum in the rat. This implies that, at least in rats, the vitamin D status of the neonate is affected by the maternal vitamin D status during gestation.

Although 1,25-dihydroxycholecalciferol levels are higher in pregnant than in nonpregnant women, this may have little effect on fetal levels, since this metabolite is produced by both the placenta and the fetal kidneys (Delvin et al., 1985). Although most investigators have found no relationship between maternal and fetal levels of 1,25-dihydroxycholecalciferol, a positive correlation has been reported by Gertner et al. (1980). Deficient maternal levels of 1,25-dihydroxycholecalciferol impair placental calcium transport to the fetus in sheep (Lester, 1986) but not in rats (Brommage and DeLuca, 1984). Human placental calcium-binding protein is believed to facilitate placental calcium transport but is not very responsive to 1,25-dihydroxycholecalciferol (Bruns and Bruns, 1983). Thus, the extent to which maternal vitamin D status regulates the placental transport of calcium is not clear, although the vitamin is necessary for the maintenance of maternal calcium status.

Requirements

The dietary requirement for vitamin D is highly dependent on exposure of the skin to ultraviolet light. In winter, the ultraviolet light reaching the earth's surface is insufficient for vitamin D synthesis in the skin at the latitudes of Britain (51°N; Lawson, 1981); Edmonton, Alberta, Canada (52°N; Webb et al., 1988); and Massachusetts (42°N; Webb et al., 1988). Further south (e.g., in Los Angeles; 34°N), some synthesis does occur in winter, but not as much as it does in Puerto Rico (18°N; Webb et al., 1988).

Prevalence of Deficiency

Only a few studies have provided evidence relevant to the prevalence of vitamin D deficiency in the United States. Because of differences in exposure to ultraviolet light, there are seasonal differences in susceptibility to and prevalence of deficiency.

Seasonal Differences

In New York City, a low vitamin D intake (2.5 to 5 μg, or 100 to 200 IU, per day) combined with a lack of sunlight exposure in winter resulted in reduced plasma levels of 25-dihydroxycholecalciferol in both the mother and the umbilical cord (Rosen et al., 1974). In St. Louis, Missouri, maternal serum 25-hydroxycholecalciferol concentrations were three times higher in August than they were in February (42.1 compared with 15.4 ng/ml) in both black and white women (Hillman and Haddad, 1976).

Studies from outside of the United States are more informative. In autumn, both maternal and fetal 25-hydroxycholecalciferol concentrations are substantially higher than they are in spring in Finland (Kuoppala et al., 1986), England (Verity et al., 1981), and even Israel (Nehama et al., 1987). Reported maternal levels in the fall and spring averaged 17.7 and 10.6 ng/ml in Finland, 25.1 and 16.7 ng/ml in England, and approximately 25 and 16.9 ng/ml in Israel, respectively. Respective newborn levels were 11.5 and 7.5 ng/ml, 16.7 and 10.6 ng/ml, and 18.1 and 11.3 ng/ml. These were positively correlated with maternal values (Nehama et al., 1987; Verity et al., 1981). The prevalence of deficiency (<6.8 ng/ml) in the Israeli women was 7% in spring and zero in fall. No British women had levels this low. A much higher prevalence of maternal deficiency (defined as <5 ng/ml) occurred in Finland—47% in spring and 33% in fall. In all countries, the reported prevalence of borderline values, i.e., between 5 and 8 ng/ml, was relatively high after winter.

Racial, Ethnic, and Dietary Differences

In Cleveland, Ohio, vitamin D levels were higher in white mothers and their infants than they were in their black counterparts (Hollis and Pittard, 1984), probably because the rate of vitamin D synthesis is slower in the skin of blacks (Clemens et al., 1982). On the other hand, a study by Hillman and Haddad (1976) in St. Louis, Missouri, showed no differences in the 25-hydroxycholecalciferol levels in black and white pregnant women in either summer or winter. There are numerous examples of low 25-hydroxycholecalciferol levels resulting from clothing that restricts exposure to ultraviolet light, e.g., in Bedouin (Biale et al., 1979) and Saudi Arabian (Serenius et al., 1984) pregnant women.

A disturbingly high prevalence of vitamin D deficiency has been reported among pregnant Asian (mainly Indian and Pakistani) women living in Britain (Maxwell et al., 1981). Vitamin D deficiency was indicated by low plasma 25-hydroxycholecalciferol levels, osteomalacia, elevated alkaline phosphatase levels, and a high incidence of neonatal hypocalcemia. On average, 35% of the women and 32% of the infants had undetectable levels of 25-hydroxycholecalciferol in the first week postpartum (Maxwell et al., 1981). Vegetarian women in this group were at a special disadvantage: 71% of them had undetectable levels of 25-hydroxycholecalciferol in the first week postpartum. This, together with a lack of seasonal fluctuation in the prevalence of deficiency, suggests that diet was a major factor in the etiology of their deficiency.

Effects of Deficiency

Maternal vitamin D deficiency has been associated with neonatal hypocalcemia and tetany in Europe (Paunier et al., 1978), tooth enamel hypoplasia that is more prevalent in British infants born in late winter or spring (Cockburn et al., 1980; Purvis et al., 1973), and maternal osteomalacia (Brooke et al., 1980).

Evidence for Supplementation

Although there are no concomitant seasonal changes in maternal or fetal 1,25-dihydroxycholecalciferol, calcium, or alkaline phosphatase, the evidence of strong seasonal fluctuations in serum 25-hydroxycholecalciferol has provoked suggestions that pregnant women in northern latitudes should receive vitamin D supplementation during pregnancy, at least during winter months (Kuoppala et al., 1986; Nehama et al., 1987; Verity et al., 1981). Supplementation of British women with approximately 10 μg (400 IU) of vitamin D per day increased maternal and newborn 25-hydroxycholecalciferol levels in both spring and fall (Verity et al., 1981). In Finland, supplementation given because of low 25-hydroxycholecalciferol levels quickly improved plasma levels of the vitamin (Kuoppala et al., 1986). Maternal and fetal 25-hydroxycholecalciferol but not 1,25-dihydroxycholecalciferol levels were increased by supplementation of pregnant French women (Mallet et al., 1986).

The ability of supplements to increase maternal and fetal plasma levels of 25-hydroxycholecalciferol is not sufficient justification to recommend their use. However, other beneficial effects of such supplements have been reported. In Britain, for example, daily supplementation of vitamin D-deficient pregnant women of Asian background with 10 μg (400 IU) per day lowered (but did not eliminate) the incidence of neonatal hypocalcemia and convulsions, and it reduced maternal osteomalacia (Brooke et al., 1980). The women supplemented with 25 μg (1,000 IU) per day gained weight faster (63 g/day) than did unsupplemented controls (46 g/day) (Maxwell et al., 1981). Reported effects of supplementation on birth weight range from nonexistent in France (Mallet et al., 1986) to a halving of the incidence of low birth weight among Asian immigrants in London (Maxwell et al., 1981) and an increase in birth weight of 100 to 300 g among infants born in India (Marya et al., 1981). Infants born to Asian women in Britain given 25 μg (1,000 IU) per day during the last trimester weighed significantly more between 3 and 12 months after birth, and they were taller between 9 and 12 months, (Brooke et al., 1981) compared with those born to similar women given placebos.

Dosage

If supplementation with vitamin D is indicated, careful consideration should be given to selecting a dose that is safe and effective. An excessive vitamin D intake can result in hyperabsorption of calcium, hypercalcemia, and calcification of soft tissues. It is not possible to define a minimal toxic dose (Food and Nutrition Board, 1975) because interindividual sensitivity to excess vitamin D intake is quite variable. Toxicity in nonpregnant adults has been reported after repeated 15-mg (600,000-IU) doses (von Beuren et al., 1966).

In human pregnancy, high maternal intakes of vitamin D were implicated as the cause of a syndrome that included mental and physical growth retardation and hypercalcemia in British infants between 1953 and 1957 (Seelig, 1969). In an animal model, Friedman and Mills (1969) gave high amounts of vitamin D to pregnant rabbits and induced fetal hypercalcemia, aortic stenosis, and abnormal skull development. These symptoms are similar to those caused by excessive vitamin D intake in pregnant women (Friedman and Roberts, 1966).

However, high doses of vitamin D given to pregnant women with hypoparathyroidism produced no fetal abnormalities (Goodenday and Gordan, 1971). Very high doses of 1,25-dihydroxycholecalciferol—17 to 36 mg (680,000 to 1,444,000 IU) per day—produced no harmful effects in a pregnant woman with vitamin D-resistant rickets, although her infant had hypercalcemia (Marx et al., 1980). Thus, it is clear that vitamin D is potentially toxic to the fetus if given in large doses during pregnancy, but the level of intake at which this occurs is uncertain.

The relative efficacy of maternal supplementation with vitamin D is greatest during the third trimester (Clements and Fraser, 1988). Supplements of vitamin D_2 (ergocalciferol) and D_3 (cholecalciferol) are processed similarly by the mother and fetus (Markestad et al., 1984).

Daily 10- to 12.5-μg (400- to 500-IU) vitamin D supplements have been reported to be adequate and safe (Cockburn et al., 1980; Markestad et al., 1986; Paunier et al., 1978). In Britain, therapeutic use of 25 μg (1,000 IU) per day administered in the last trimester reduced signs of deficiency without toxicity (Brooke et al., 1980; Heckmatt et al., 1979). In other countries, a few large doses rather than small daily doses have been provided to reduce the need for patient compliance. In northern

France, for example, a single 5-mg (200,000-IU) oral dose of vitamin D_2 in the seventh month of pregnancy increased maternal and umbilical cord levels of 25-hydroxycholecalciferol to the same extent that 25 μg (1,000 IU) of vitamin D_2 daily throughout the last trimester did (Mallet et al., 1986). In India, 30 μg (1,200 IU) per day given to women in their third trimester was less effective than two very large doses of 15 mg (600,000 IU) given in the seventh and eighth months, based on increased serum calcium, reduced alkaline phosphatase, and increased birth weight (Marya et al., 1981). There is a higher risk of overdose when a few large doses are used in place of daily small doses, and there has been insufficient study of when during pregnancy to administer large doses of vitamin D for maximum effectiveness and safety. This approach to the prevention of vitamin D deficiency is not recommended for use in the United States.

Recommendations

The subcommittee does not recommend routine supplementation with vitamin D during pregnancy. The preceding discussion illustrates that vitamin D deficiency is common among pregnant women in Europe and that the consequences are harmful. In most regions of the United States, however, exposure to sunlight is greater than in Europe, and unlike the milk in most European countries, most milk in the United States is fortified with the vitamin. Nevertheless, daily supplementation with 10 μg of vitamin D should be considered for complete vegetarians, whose 25-hydroxycholecalciferol levels are low due to their avoidance of milk, eggs, and fish (Dent and Gupta, 1975; Maxwell et al., 1981). Supplementation with 5 μg of vitamin D per day should be considered for pregnant women whose consumption of vitamin D-fortified milk is low. This concern is compounded during low exposures to ultraviolet light in winter at the most northern latitudes.

MAGNESIUM

Metabolism

The metabolism of magnesium is not regulated by any known hormone. Magnesium is essential for the release of PTH and its action on the intestine, bone, and kidney. A mild magnesium deficiency increases PTH secretion; administration of large doses of PTH stimulates the intestinal absorption and renal retention of magnesium. Magnesium participates in the 25-hydroxylation of cholecalciferol to form 25-hydroxycholecalciferol.

The maternal serum magnesium concentration rises slightly in early pregnancy, returning to nonpregnant levels by late pregnancy (Reitz et al., 1977). Maternal levels are slightly below and correlated with those of the infant at delivery (Cockburn et al., 1980). Seasonal fluctuations (e.g., 5% lower in summer) in maternal blood levels were reported in some studies (Hillman and Haddad 1976), but not in others (Kuoppala et al., 1986; Verity et al., 1981). Vitamin D supplementation has no effect on maternal or umbilical cord blood magnesium concentrations (Cockburn et al., 1980; Verity et al., 1981).

Magnesium is probably actively transported to the fetus (Reitz et al., 1977). The normal fetus contains 1 g of magnesium, which is acquired primarily during the last two trimesters at a rate of about 6 mg/day.

Adequacy of Intake

Magnesium is widely distributed among foods, especially grains, seafood, and green vegetables. The average U.S. diet contains approximately 120 mg/1,000 kcal. When magnesium intake is low, the efficiency of its absorption increases and relatively more of the mineral is retained by the kidneys.

As indicated in Chapter 13, usual magnesium intakes by pregnant women in the United States are substantially lower than the RDA of 300 mg (NRC, 1989). In one study, 10 healthy, white pregnant women living at home consumed 269 mg/day from their usual diet. For only 6% of 47 one-week-long balance periods were they in a positive magnesium balance (Ashe et al., 1979). On average, balance was negative (−40 mg/day). Intake may have been underestimated, however, since magnesium in drinking water was not measured and there were no signs of magnesium deficiency. In fact, magnesium deficiency has never been reported to occur in healthy individuals consuming ordinary diets (Shils, 1988).

On the basis of a medical records study, Conradt et al. (1984) reported that magnesium supplementation during pregnancy was associated with lower frequencies of fetal growth retardation and preeclampsia. This was reevaluated in a double-blind prospective study in Switzerland (Spätling and Spätling, 1988). Before 16 weeks of pregnancy, women were randomly allocated to either an aspartic acid placebo group or to a group receiving a magnesium supplement providing 360 mg/day as magnesium-aspartate-hydrochloride. The investigators reported that the supplemented group had 30% fewer hospitalizations (for any cause), approximately 50% as many premature births and cases of incompetent cervix, and 25% more perinatal hemorrhages than the placebo group. The rate of infant referral to the neonatal intensive care unit was half as high for infants of magnesium-supplemented mothers as for infants of the placebo group. These results were obtained only when the analysis was limited to women who followed the protocol (thus the sample was no longer random), and they require confirmation from other investigators.

Recommendations

Data are insufficient to support a recommendation of magnesium supplementation for pregnant women. Because of the negative balances found in healthy women consuming usual diets and the potential beneficial effects of supplementation observed in one study, however, research on the effects of magnesium supplementation during pregnancy should receive high priority.

Dosage

There are no reported studies on the safety of different doses of magnesium supplements given during pregnancy. Large doses (e.g., 3 to 5 g) of magnesium salts cause catharsis, but there is no evidence of any other adverse effects in nonpregnant adults (Mordes and Wacker, 1978). In studies of iron absorption in nonpregnant women who took vitamin-mineral supplements containing 60 mg of iron as ferrous fumarate, Seligman et al. (1983) report that 100 mg of magnesium as magnesium oxide added to supplements significantly reduced the absorption of the iron.

SUMMARY

There is no evidence that routine calcium, vitamin D, or magnesium supplementation is beneficial to pregnant women in the United States. Inadequate calcium intake by women under age 25 is more likely to affect maternal bone accretion than to cause inadequate calcification of the fetus. Increased intake of calcium-rich foods is preferred to supplementation because such foods are also a source of other valuable nutrients, e.g., riboflavin and vitamin D.

The vitamin D status of pregnant women is influenced not only by dietary vitamin D (especially in winter) but also by geographic location and season because of the low amounts of ultraviolet radiation in winter months in northern latitudes. Consumption of vitamin D-fortified milk is especially important in winter since that is the main dietary source of vitamin D.

CLINICAL IMPLICATIONS

- Ill effects of low maternal calcium intakes on the mother or fetus have not been reported. Nevertheless, there is some concern that low calcium intakes during pregnancy might impair bone mineral deposition, especially in women under age 25.

- A pregnant woman whose calcium intake is less than 600 mg/day—the approximate amount provided by a diet that includes only one small serving of a calcium-rich food—should be advised to increase her consumption of milk, cheese, yogurt, or other food sources of calcium or to take a calcium supplement at mealtimes that provides 600 mg of calcium per day. The strategy of increasing dairy product intake is preferred since such products also supply energy, protein, minerals, and vitamins—all of which are needed in increased amounts by pregnant women. Special attention should be directed toward the adequacy of intake of black, Hispanic, and American Indian women and complete vegetarians.

- For pregnant women who are milk intolerant because of the lack of the enzyme lactase, strategies should be directed to increase calcium intake through the use of low-lactose, calcium-rich foods before supplementation is considered.

- Older pregnant women do not need higher calcium intakes than do those who are younger.

- Evidence does not support the practice of prescribing calcium for leg cramps during pregnancy.

- There is insufficient evidence to support routine supplementation with large amounts of calcium as a possible means of preventing pregnancy-induced hypertension.

- Women who avoid drinking milk have low dietary intakes of vitamin D, since fortified milk is one of the few dietary sources of this nutrient. This is of special concern in winter months, when there is less synthesis of the vitamin in the skin even at southern latitudes and no synthesis at northern latitudes. Based on the known adverse effects of vitamin D deficiency during pregnancy, such women should be counseled to increase their intake of vitamin D-fortified milk or to take supplements providing 10 μg (400 IU) of vitamin D per day.

- There is no justification for routine supplementation with magnesium during pregnancy.

- The subcommittee does not recommend routine supplementation of pregnant women in the United States with calcium, magnesium, or vitamin D.

- The subcommittee does not recommend the routine use of laboratory tests to assess the calcium, magnesium, or vitamin D status in pregnant women. Assessment of vitamin D status using serum 25-hydroxycholecalciferol levels is recommended for research purposes and, specifically, to evaluate the prevalence of maternal vitamin D deficiency in the United States.

REFERENCES

Ashe, J.R., F.A. Schofield, and M.R. Gram. 1979. The retention of calcium, iron, phosphorus, and magnesium during pregnancy: the adequacy of prenatal diets with and without supplementation. Am. J. Clin. Nutr. 32:286-291.

Belizán, J.M., J. Villar, and J. Repke. 1988. The relationship between calcium intake and pregnancy-induced hypertension: up-to-date evidence. Am. J. Obstet. Gynecol. 158:898-902.

Biale, Y., S. Shany, M. Levi, R. Shainkin-Kestenbaum, and G.M. Berlyne. 1979. 25-Hydroxycholecalciferol levels in Beduin women in labor and in cord blood of their infants. Am. J. Clin. Nutr. 32:2380-2382.

Bouillon, R., F.A. Van Assche, H. Van Baelen, W. Heyns, and P. De Moor. 1981. Influence of the vitamin D-binding protein on the serum concentration of 1,25-dihydroxyvitamin D_3. J. Clin. Invest. 67:589-596.

Brommage, R., and H.F. DeLuca. 1984. Placental transport of calcium and phosphorus is not regulated by vitamin D. Am. J. Physiol. 246:F526-F529.

Brooke, O.G., I.R.F. Brown, C.D.M. Bone, N.D. Carter, H.J.W. Cleeve, J.D. Maxwell, V.P. Robinson, and S.M. Winder. 1980. Vitamin D supplements in pregnant Asian women: effects on calcium status and fetal growth. Br. Med. J. 280:751-754.

Brooke, O.G., F. Butters, and C. Wood. 1981. Intrauterine vitamin D nutrition and postnatal growth in Asian infants. Br. Med. J. 283:1024.

Bruns, M.E., and D.E. Bruns. 1983. Vitamin D metabolism and function during pregnancy and the neonatal period. Ann. Clin. Lab. Sci. 13:521-530.

Budayr, A.A., B.P. Halloran, J.C. King, D. Diep, R.A. Nissenson, and G.J. Strewler. 1989. High levels of a parathyroid hormone-like protein in milk. Proc. Natl. Acad. Sci. U.S.A. 86:7183-7185.

Christiansen, C., P. Rødbro, and B. Heinild. 1976. Unchanged total body calcium in normal human pregnancy. Acta Obstet. Gynecol. Scand. 55:141-143.

Clemens, T.L., J.S. Adams, S.L. Henderson, and M.F. Holick. 1982. Increased skin pigment reduces the capacity of skin to synthesise vitamin D_3. Lancet 1:74-76.

Clements, M.R., and D.R. Fraser. 1988. Vitamin D supply to the rat fetus and neonate. J. Clin. Invest. 81:1768-1773.

Cockburn, F., N.R. Belton, R.J. Purvis, M.M. Giles, J.K. Brown, T.L. Turner, E.M. Wilkinson, J.O. Forfar, W.J.M. Barrie, G.S. McKay, and S.J. Pocock. 1980. Maternal vitamin D intake and mineral metabolism in mothers and their newborn infants. Br. Med. J. 281:11-14.

Conradt, A., H. Weidinger, and H. Algayer. 1984. On the role of magnesium in fetal hypotrophy, pregnancy induced hypertension, and pre-eclampsia. Mag. Bull. 6:68-76.

Danan, J.L., A.C. Delorme, C. Benassayag, G. Vallette, and P. Cuisinier-Gleizes. 1980. 25-Hydroxyvitamin D and 24,25-dihydroxyvitamin D in maternal plasma, fetal plasma and amniotic fluid in the rat. Biochem. Biophys. Res. Commun. 95:453-460.

Davis, O.K., D.S. Hawkins, L.P. Rubin, J.T. Posillico, E.M. Brown, and I. Schiff. 1988. Serum parathyroid hormone (PTH) in pregnant women determined by an immunoradiometric assay for intact PTH. J. Clin. Endocrinol. Metab. 67:850-852.

Delvin, E.E., F.H. Glorieux, B.L. Salle, L. David, and J.P. Varenne. 1982. Control of vitamin D metabolism in preterm infants: feto-maternal relationships. Arch. Dis. Child. 57:754-757.

Delvin, E.E., A. Arabian, F.H. Glorieux, and O.A. Mamer. 1985. In vitro metabolism of 25-hydroxycholecalciferol by isolated cells from human decidua. J. Clin. Endocrinol. Metab. 60:880-885.

Dent, C.E., and M.M. Gupta. 1975. Plasma 25-hydroxyvitamin-D levels during pregnancy in Caucasians and in vegetarian and non-vegetarian Asians. Lancet 2:1057-1060.

Duggin, G.G., N.E. Dale, R.C. Lyneham, R.A. Evans, and D.J. Tiller. 1974. Calcium balance in pregnancy. Lancet 2:926-927.

Food and Nutrition Board. 1975. Hazards of overuse of vitamin D. Am. J. Clin. Nutr. 28:512-513.

Forbes, G.B. 1976. Calcium accumulation by the human fetus. Pediatrics 57:976-977.

Friedman, W.F., and L.F. Mills. 1969. The relationship between vitamin D and the craniofacial and dental anomalies of the supravalvular aortic stenosis syndrome. Pediatrics 43:12-18.

Friedman, W.F., and W.C. Roberts. 1966. Vitamin D and the supravalvar aortic stenosis syndrome: the transplacental effects of vitamin D on the aorta of the rabbit. Circulation 34:77-86.

Frisancho, A.R., S.M. Garn, and W. Ascoli. 1971. Unaltered cortical area of pregnant and lactating women: studies of the second metacarpal bone in North and Central American populations. Invest. Radiol. 6:119-121.

Gertner, J.M., M.S. Glassman, D.R. Coustan, and D.B.P. Goodman. 1980. Fetomaternal vitamin D relationships at term. J. Pediatr. 97:637-640.

Goldsmith, N.F., and J.O. Johnston. 1975. Bone mineral: effects of oral contraceptives, pregnancy, and lactation. J. Bone Jt. Surg. 57:657-668.

Goodenday, L.S., and G.S. Gordan. 1971. No risk from vitamin D in pregnancy. Ann. Intern. Med. 75:807-808.

Halloran, B.P., and H.F. DeLuca. 1980. Calcium transport in small intestine during pregnancy and lactation. Am. J. Physiol. 239:E64-E68.

Hammar, M., G. Berg, F. Solheim, and L. Larsson. 1987. Calcium and magnesium status in pregnant women. A comparison between treatment with calcium and vitamin C in pregnant women with leg cramps. Int. J. Vitam. Nutr. Res. 57:179-183.

Heaney, R.P., and T.G. Skillman. 1971. Calcium metabolism in normal human pregnancy. J. Clin. Endocrinol. Metab. 33:661-670.

Heaney, R.P., K.T. Smith, R.R. Recker, and S.M. Hinders. 1989. Meal effects on calcium absorption. Am. J. Clin. Nutr. 49:372-376.

Heckmatt, J.Z., M. Peacock, A.E.J. Davies, J. McMurray, and D.M. Isherwood. 1979. Plasma 25-hydroxyvitamin D in pregnant Asian women and their babies. Lancet 2:546-549.

Hillman, L.S., and J.G. Haddad. 1976. Perinatal vitamin D metabolism. III. Factors influencing late gestational human serum 25-hydroxyvitamin D. Am. J. Obstet. Gynecol. 125:196-200.

Hillman, L.S., E. Slatopolsky, and J.G. Haddad. 1978. Perinatal vitamin D metabolism. IV. Maternal and cord serum 24,25-dihydroxyvitamin D concentrations. J. Clin. Endocrinol. Metab. 47:1073-1077.

Hollis, B.W., and W.B. Pittard III. 1984. Evaluation of the total fetomaternal vitamin D relationships at term: evidence for racial differences. J. Clin. Endocrinol. Metab. 59:652-657.

Hreshchyshyn, M.M., A. Hopkins, S. Zylstra, and M. Anbar. 1988. Associations of parity, breast-feeding, and birth control pills with lumbar spine and femoral neck bone densities. Am. J. Obstet. Gynecol. 159:318-322.

Kuoppala, T., R. Tuimala, M. Parviainen, T. Koskinen, and M. Ala-Houhala. 1986. Serum levels of vitamin D metabolites, calcium, phosphorus, magnesium and alkaline phosphatase in Finnish women throughout pregnancy and in cord serum at delivery. Hum. Nutr.: Clin. Nutr. 40C:287-293.

Lamke, B., J. Brundin, and P. Moberg. 1977. Changes of bone mineral content during pregnancy and lactation. Acta Obstet. Gynecol. Scand. 56:217-219.

Lawson, D.E.M. 1981. Dietary vitamin D: is it necessary? J. Hum. Nutr. 35:61-63.

Lester, G.E. 1986. Cholecalciferol and placental calcium transport. Fed. Proc., Fed. Am. Soc. Exp. Biol. 45:2524-2527.

Lopez-Jaramillo, P., M. Narvaez, and R. Yepez. 1987. Effect of calcium supplementation on the vascular sensitivity to angiotensin II in pregnant women. Am. J. Obstet. Gynecol. 156:261-262.

Mallet, E., B. Gügi, P. Brunelle, A. Hénocq, J.P. Basuyau, and H. Lemeur. 1986. Vitamin D supplementation in pregnancy: a controlled trial of two methods. Obstet. Gynecol. 68:300-304.

Markestad, T., L. Aksnes, M. Ulstein, and D. Aarskog. 1984. 25-Hydroxyvitamin D and 1,25-dihydroxyvitamin D of D_2 and D_3 origin in maternal and umbilical cord serum after vitamin D_2 supplementation in human pregnancy. Am. J. Clin. Nutr. 40:1057-1063.

Markestad, T., M. Ulstein, L. Aksnes, and D. Aarskog. 1986. Serum concentrations of vitamin D metabolites in vitamin D supplemented pregnant women. A longitudinal study. Acta Obstet. Gynecol. Scand. 65:63-67.

Marshall, D.H., B.E.C. Nordin, and R. Speed. 1976. Calcium, phosphorus and magnesium requirement. Proc. Nutr. Soc. 35:163-173.

Marx, S.J., E.G. Swart, Jr., A.J. Hamstra, and H.F. DeLuca. 1980. Normal intrauterine development of the fetus of a woman receiving extraordinarily high doses of 1,25-dihydroxyvitamin D_3. J. Clin. Endocrinol. Metab. 51:1138-1142.

Marya, R.K., S. Rathee, V. Lata, and S. Mudgil. 1981. Effects of vitamin D supplementation in pregnancy. Gynecol. Obstet. Invest. 12:155-161.

Maxwell, J.D., L. Ang, O.G. Brooke, and I.R.F. Brown. 1981. Vitamin D supplements enhance weight gain and nutritional status in pregnant Asians. Br. J. Obstet. Gynaecol. 88:987-991.

Mordes, J.P., and W.E.C. Wacker. 1978. Excess magnesium. Pharmacol. Rev. 29:273-300.

Nehama, H., S. Wientroub, Z. Eisenberg, A. Birger, B. Milbauer, and Y. Weisman. 1987. Seasonal variation in paired maternal-newborn serum 25-hydroxyvitamin D and 24,25-dihydroxyvitamin D concentrations in Israel. Isr. J. Med. Sci. 23:274-277.

NRC (National Research Council). 1989. Recommended Dietary Allowances, 10th ed. Report of the Subcommittee on the Tenth Edition of the RDAs, Food and Nutrition Board, Commission on Life Sciences. National Academy Press, Washington, D.C. 284 pp.

Paulson, S.K., and H.F. DeLuca. 1986. Vitamin D metabolism during pregnancy. Bone 7:331-336.

Paunier, L., G. Lacourt, P. Pilloud, P. Schlaeppi, and P.C. Sizonenko. 1978. 25-Hydroxyvitamin D and calcium levels in maternal, cord and infant serum in relation to maternal vitamin D intake. Helv. Paediatr. Acta 33:95-103.

Pitkin, R.M. 1985. Calcium metabolism in pregnancy and the perinatal period: a review. Am. J. Obstet. Gynecol. 151:99-109.

Pitkin, R.M., W.A. Reynolds, G.A. Williams, and G.K. Hargis. 1979. Calcium metabolism in normal pregnancy: a longitudinal study. Am. J. Obstet. Gynecol. 133:781-790.

Purvis, R.J., W.J. McK. Barrie, G.S. Mackay, E.M. Wilkinson, F. Cockburn, N.R. Belton, and J.O. Forfar. 1973. Enamel hypoplasia of the teeth associated with neonatal tetany: a manifestation of maternal vitamin-D deficiency. Lancet 2:811-814.

Raman, L., K. Rajalakshmi, K.A.V.R. Krishnamachari, and J.G. Sastry. 1978. Effect of calcium supplementation to undernourished mothers during pregnancy on the bone density of the neonates. Am. J. Clin. Nutr. 31:466-469.

Reiter, E.O., G.D. Braunstein, A. Vargas, and A.W. Root. 1979. Changes in 25-hydroxyvitamin D and 24,25-dihydroxyvitamin D during pregnancy. Am. J. Obstet. Gynecol. 135:227-229.

Reitz, R.E., T.A. Daane, J.R. Woods, and R.L. Weinstein. 1977. Calcium, magnesium, phosphorus, and parathyroid hormone interrelationships in pregnancy and newborn infants. Obstet. Gynecol. 50:701-705.

Rodda, C.P., M. Kubota, J.A. Heath, P.R. Ebeling, J.M. Moseley, A.D. Care, I.W. Caple, and T.J. Martin. 1988. Evidence for a novel parathyroid hormone-related protein in fetal lamb parathyroid glands and sheep placenta: comparisons with a similar protein implicated in humoral hypercalcaemia of malignancy. J. Endocrinol. 117:261-271.

Rosen, J.F., M. Roginsky, G. Nathenson, and L. Finberg. 1974. 25-Hydroxyvitamin D. Plasma levels in mothers and their premature infants with neonatal hypocalcemia. Am. J. Dis. Child. 127:220-223.

Seelig, M.S. 1969. Vitamin D and cardiovascular, renal, and brain damage in infancy and childhood. Ann. N.Y. Acad. Sci. 147:539-582.

Seligman, P.A., J.H. Caskey, J.L. Frazier, R.M. Zucker, E.R. Podell, and R.H. Allen. 1983. Measurements of iron absorption from prenatal multivitamin-mineral supplements. Obstet. Gynecol. 61:356-362.

Serenius, F., A.T. Elidrissy, and P. Dandona. 1984. Vitamin D nutrition in pregnant women at term and in newly born babies in Saudi Arabia. J. Clin. Pathol. 37:444-447.

Shenolikar, I.S. 1970. Absorption of dietary calcium in pregnancy. Am. J. Clin. Nutr. 23:63-67.

Shils, M.E. 1988. Magnesium in health and disease. Annu. Rev. Nutr. 8:429-460.

Spätling, L., and G. Spätling. 1988. Magnesium supplementation in pregnancy. A double-blind study. Br. J. Obstet. Gynaecol. 95:120-125.

Taufield, P.A., K.L. Ales, L.M. Resnick, M.L. Druzin, J.M. Gertner, and J.H. Laragh. 1987. Hypocalciuria in preeclampsia. N. Engl. J. Med. 316:715-718.

Thiede, M.A., and G.A. Rodan. 1988. Expression of a calcium-mobilizing parathyroid hormone-like peptide in lactating mammary tissue. Science 242:278-280.

Umeki, S., S. Nagao, and Y. Nozawa. 1981. The purification and identification of calmodulin from human placenta. Biochim. Biophys. Acta 674:319-326.

Valenzuela, G.J., L.A. Munson, N.M. Tarbaux, and J.R. Farley. 1987. Time-dependent changes in bone, placental, intestinal, and hepatic alkaline phosphatase activities in serum during human pregnancy. Clin. Chem. 33:1801-1806.

Verhaeghe, J., M. Thomasset, A. Bréhier, F.A. van Assche, and R. Bouillon. 1988. 1,25(OH)$_2$D$_3$ and Ca-binding protein in fetal rats: relationship to the maternal vitamin D status. Am. J. Physiol. 254:E505-E512.

Verity, C.M., D. Burman, P.C. Beadle, J.B. Holton, and A. Morris. 1981. Seasonal changes in perinatal vitamin D metabolism: maternal and cord blood biochemistry in normal pregnancies. Arch. Dis. Child. 56:943-948.

von Beuren, A.J., J. Apitz, J. Stoermer, H. Schlange, B. Kaiser, W. v. Berg, and G. Jörgensen. 1966. Vitamin-D-hypercalcämische Herz- und Gefäßerkankung. Dtsch. Med. Wochenschr. 19:881-883.

Walker, A.R.P., B. Richardson, and F. Walker. 1972. The influence of numerous pregnancies and lactations on bone dimensions in South African Bantu and Caucasian mothers. Clin. Sci. 42:189-196.

Webb, A.R., L. Kline, and M.F. Holick. 1988. Influence of season and latitude on the cutaneous synthesis of vitamin D$_3$: exposure to winter sunlight in Boston and Edmonton will not promote vitamin D$_3$ synthesis in human skin. J. Clin. Endocrinol. Metab. 67:373-378.

Whitehead, M., G. Lane, O. Young, S. Campbell, G. Abeyasekera, C.J. Hillyard, I. MacIntyre, K.G. Phang, and J.C. Stevenson. 1981. Interrelations of calcium-regulating hormones during normal pregnancy. Br. Med. J. 283:10-12.

17

Vitamins A, E, and K

In this chapter, the subcommittee reviews data relating to supplementation of the fat-soluble vitamins A, E, and K during pregnancy. Vitamin D, another fat-soluble vitamin, is reviewed in conjunction with calcium in Chapter 16, because calcium metabolism is dependent on that vitamin. The fat-soluble vitamins are often considered together since their absorption, transport, and excretion are influenced by their very limited solubility in water.

VITAMIN A

The term *vitamin A* includes a number of closely related compounds with similar biologic activities. This group of compounds is important throughout life because of their participation in a variety of biologic functions, including vision, reproduction, immune function, and cellular growth and differentiation. Two groups of compounds are related to vitamin A: the *retinoids* (called *preformed vitamin A* if they possess vitamin A activity) and the *carotenoids* (called *precursors of vitamin A* or *provitamin A* if they can be metabolized to an active form of the vitamin). The naturally occurring forms of retinoids include retinol, retinaldehyde, and retinoic acid. The primary form of preformed vitamin A is retinyl ester, which is found in foods of animal origin such as liver, fish liver oils, milk, eggs, and butter. Provitamin A carotenoids are mainly of vegetable origin; carrots and dark-green leafy vegetables are especially rich sources. Nutritional needs for vitamin A can be met by ingesting either preformed retinoids with vitamin

A activity or certain carotenoids, such as carotene, that can be metabolized to vitamin A.

After ingestion, between 70 and 90% of preformed vitamin A is absorbed, whereas the absorption of carotenoids is less efficient and more variable, ranging from 20 to 50%. Retinyl esters are hydrolyzed, reesterified, and transported in chylomicrons to the liver. Carotenoids can be converted to retinol and retinyl esters in the intestinal mucosa, and both carotenoids and the retinyl esters derived from them are transported via the chylomicrons to the liver. The major storage site is the liver, which normally contains more than 90% of the total body stores of vitamin A in well-nourished people. Adipose tissue and the kidney are minor storage sites.

The liver releases a complex of retinol and retinol-binding protein (RBP). This complex combines with transthyretin in the blood, is circulated, and may be either extracted by tissues or remetabolized by the liver and excreted in bile.

Importance

From a public health standpoint, vitamin A is of greatest importance in maintaining visual function. Worldwide, vitamin A deficiency results in approximately 250,000 to 500,000 cases of visual impairment per year, primarily in children in developing countries (FAO, 1988; Sommer, 1982). Thus, vitamin A deficiency appears to be a major public health problem in many parts of the world (Araujo et al., 1986, 1987; Sklan, 1987; Stanton et al., 1986; Villard and Bates, 1987) but is not common in the United States.

The most widely recognized effect of vitamin A is in the retina, where it is involved in photochemical reactions with rhodopsin (Wald, 1968). It also functions throughout the body in aiding glycoprotein synthesis and promoting cellular growth and differentiation.

Vitamin A During Pregnancy

There is only limited information regarding the effect of pregnancy on the metabolism and physiology of vitamin A. Some evidence suggests that the retinol-RBP complex may be different in pregnant women than in nonpregnant controls (Sklan et al., 1985). Data from studies of pregnant sheep support the possibility that binding proteins in the fetus may be different from those in the adult (Donoghue et al., 1982).

Quantitation of the rates at which vitamin A is transferred from mother to fetus is difficult and has largely been limited to animals. The rate at which retinoic acid is transferred to the fetal rat may be lower than that of retinyl ester (Shukla et al., 1986). Studies in vitamin A-sufficient pregnant sheep suggest that transport of vitamin A to the fetus increases but that efficiency of transfer decreases when high levels of vitamin A are provided to the ewe (Donoghue et al., 1985), suggesting that there may be some placental regulation of transport.

Several mechanisms proposed for the transfer of retinol to the fetus are based primarily on animal data. One possibility is the direct transfer of the retinol-RBP complex. Alternatively, placental uptake of retinol, transient esterification in the placental tissues, and release of retinol into the fetal circulation may be involved; this was observed in sheep by Donoghue et al. (1982) and in rats by Törmä and Vahlquist (1986). Data on both sheep and rats suggest that a dynamic equilibrium exists between mother and fetus and that there is substantial transfer in both directions (Donoghue et al., 1982, 1985; Ismadi and Olson, 1982).

Once transferred into the fetus, some retinol is stored in the fetal liver. Wallingford and Underwood (1986) reported that maternal vitamin A supplementation did not increase fetal hepatic retinol levels in rats. In human fetuses, such hepatic concentrations are consistently much lower than those in adults (Montreewasuwat and Olson, 1979; Shah et al., 1987; Wallingford and Underwood, 1986) and correlate with maternal serum retinol levels (Shah et al., 1987). An intercountry comparison of fetal liver tissue showed a significant increase in hepatic vitamin A levels in Swedish but not Ethiopian fetuses during the second and third trimesters compared with first-trimester levels (Gebre-Medhin and Vahlquist, 1984).

Units of Measurement

Chemical and pharmacologic diversity among the compounds with vitamin A activity has led to the use of different units to express vitamin A activity—international units (IUs) and retinol equivalents (REs). An IU is defined in terms of the growth-promoting activity of 0.30 μg of all-*trans* retinol or 0.60 μg of all-*trans* β-carotene. The RE was adopted to account for the difference in the intestinal absorption of retinol and carotene. One RE is equal to 1 μg of all-*trans* retinol, and biologically, 1 RE is assumed to be equivalent to 6 μg of all-*trans* β-carotene (NRC, 1989). At present, the RE is preferred, although IUs have been widely used in the past and are still reported. Because of ambiguities in converting from one system to another, the use of IUs is retained in this chapter if that was the unit of measurement used in the report that is referenced.

Criteria for Deficiency

Assessment of vitamin A status is complicated by the chemical and pharmacologic diversity among the compounds with vitamin A activity.

Methods to assess deficiency include biologic measurements such as biochemical measurements of plasma retinol level or liver concentrations of vitamin A and functional tests such as correction of impaired dark adaptation.

Plasma retinol concentrations can be widely used as a basis for clinical determination of vitamin A status. In normal nonpregnant adults, impaired dark adaptation may result at retinol concentrations below 15 μg/dl (Hume and Krebs, 1949), and abnormal electroretinograms may be found at levels below 4 to 11 μg/dl (Sauberlich et al., 1974). Levels below 30 μg/dl have been associated with vitamin A-responsive anemia, and levels of 7 to 37 μg/dl, with follicular keratosis (Sauberlich et al., 1974). In *Recommended Dietary Allowances* (RDAs) it is recommended that nonpregnant adults maintain plasma retinol concentrations higher than 30 μg/dl in order to maintain body stores; levels less than 20 μg/dl are associated with increased risk for development of clinical signs and symptoms of vitamin A deficiency (NRC, 1989).

Pregnancy complicates the interpretation of these values, in part because blood levels of RBP change with pregnancy (NRC, 1978). In research settings, liver stores of vitamin A have been used to assess vitamin A status—100 μg/g is typical of well-nourished, nonpregnant adults.

Measurement of dark adaptation has also been used for screening vitamin A deficiency (Hume and Krebs, 1949). A more recent method of measuring dark adaptation has been reported as a practical and reliable method requiring only limited technology (Villard and Bates, 1986). From a public health standpoint, this type of assessment may be of considerable value.

Vitamin A appears to be important for fetal growth. In a study of mother-infant pairs in an undernourished population, poor maternal vitamin A status was associated with preterm birth, intrauterine growth retardation, and decreased birth weight (Shah and Rajalakshmi, 1984). In a human autopsy series, maternal serum retinol correlated positively with fetal weight (Shah and Rajalakshmi, 1984; Shah et al., 1987). Chytil (1985) provided evidence that vitamin A may be important for lung growth in human fetuses. Similarly, studies in several animal species, including rats and domestic farm animals, suggest positive correlations of vitamin A with fetal growth. In rats, maternal vitamin A deficiency was correlated with decreased fetal body and organ size (Khanna and Reddy, 1983; Reddy and Khanna, 1983; Sharma and Misra, 1986; Takahashi et al., 1975).

Recommended Intakes

Estimates of vitamin A intakes required to maintain desirable retinol levels have been somewhat variable, ranging from 500 to 1,200 RE/day

(FAO 1988; NRC, 1989; Sauberlich et al., 1974). The RDA for vitamin A is 800 RE for nonpregnant women in the childbearing years and is not increased during pregnancy (NRC, 1989).

Vitamin A deficiency is rare in the United States, and evidence suggests that U.S. women have adequate liver stores of the vitamin. Fetal vitamin A requirements are very low until the third trimester, and even then they are estimated to increase maternal vitamin A requirements by only 9% (NRC, 1989). There is no persuasive evidence that the dietary requirement for vitamin A is increased during pregnancy.

Teratogenicity and Toxicity

It is apparent that vitamin A deficiency affects the human fetus; however, an excess of retinoids has also been of considerable concern, particularly regarding the possibility of teratogenicity (see review by Teratology Society, 1987). Isotretinoin, a synthetic relative of vitamin A (Accutane®, 13-*cis*-retinoic acid), has been reported to be teratogenic in animals and humans in the first trimester (Teratology Society, 1987). The typical phenotype includes such central nervous system abnormalities as hydrocephalus or microcephaly, cardiovascular abnormalities, facial anomalies (e.g., of the ear and palate), and altered growth. A high incidence of spontaneous abortion has also been reported.

Large doses of retinol or retinyl esters may result in a similar syndrome (Rosa et al., 1986; Stånge et al., 1978; Teratology Society, 1987; Woollam, 1985). Retinoic acid also appears to be teratogenic (Lammer et al., 1985). The minimum teratogenic dose is not known. A wide range of maternal vitamin A intakes has been reported in these studies. Of particular concern is the association of a first-trimester 2,000-IU vitamin A supplement with phenotypic isotretinoin syndrome (Lungarotti et al., 1987). However, most other observers suggest that an intake of at least 20,000 to 50,000 IU is required for teratogenicity. Whether or not lower doses produce a less evident clinical syndrome is not known.

Ingestion of excessive amounts of preformed vitamin A produces a well-defined syndrome, including headache, vomiting, diplopia, alopecia, liver damage, and skin abnormalities (Bauernfeind, 1980). These toxic reactions appear to require a sustained total dietary intake of preformed vitamin A in excess of 15,000 RE in adults. It is not known whether pregnancy alters the maternal clinical syndrome of vitamin A toxicity.

In contrast, limited data on humans suggest that high intakes of carotenoids are not teratogenic or toxic to either mother or fetus. In nonpregnant adults, very large intakes of carotenoids do not appear to be harmful, primarily because large doses are inefficiently absorbed and converted to vitamin A.

Usual Intake

Usual intakes of vitamin A by pregnant women are discussed in Chapter 13. As mentioned above, the average vitamin A intake in the United States appears to exceed the RDA for both pregnant and nonpregnant women.

Rush et al. (1988) showed that the average vitamin A intake of low-income women in the United States exceeds the RDA, even before the women enter the Supplemental Food Program for Women, Infants, and Children. Finley et al. (1985) reported that the average dietary intake of vitamin A by complete vegetarians appears to be somewhat higher than that of the average U.S. population. However, since there is also a wide range of individual intakes, it may be important to assess vitamin A intakes, particularly in women with unusual diets or who habitually avoid dietary sources of vitamin A.

Recommendations for Supplementation

Since estimated dietary intake in the United States appears to be sufficient to meet the needs of most pregnant women throughout gestation, routine supplementation during pregnancy is not recommended. Carefully supervised supplementation may be desirable for some groups of pregnant women in the United States, for example, for recent emigrants from countries in which vitamin A deficiency is endemic. Information and opinion on the teratogenic risk of various forms of vitamin A are rapidly evolving, and supplementation of vitamin A should be approached with caution until the risk is clarified.

VITAMIN E

Vitamin E is required by most animal species, although the recognition of its importance in humans is relatively recent. This vitamin is biologically important as an antioxidant; i.e., it traps free radicals and prevents oxidation of unsaturated fatty acids. Manifestations of its deficiency include anemia, neuromuscular abnormalities, and reproductive failure. In humans, vitamin E deficiency has been demonstrated in premature infants, manifested primarily by anemia (Oski and Barness, 1967), and in patients with prolonged, marked fat malabsorption, usually accompanied by neurologic abnormalities (Kelleher et al., 1987; Muller, 1986; Sokol et al., 1985). Many other functions have been attributed to vitamin E, both in the medical and lay literature, but these effects remain unproven and controversial.

Two classes of compounds, tocopherols and tocotrienols, include biologically active forms of vitamin E. Both classes are characterized chemically by a similar ring system, but they differ in the saturation of the side chain. The tocopherols (α-, β-, γ-, and δ-), which have a saturated side chain, are widely found in nature. α-Tocopherol is both the most active and the most prevalent biologic form.

Normal bile secretion and pancreatic function are required for intestinal absorption of vitamin E. After absorption, vitamin E is carried in the blood in the lipoproteins, primarily in high-density lipoproteins in women but in low-density lipoproteins in men (Behrens et al., 1982). As a fat-soluble compound, tocopherol is widely distributed in the fatty component of tissues. Its concentration is similar in most tissues if expressed relative to their fat content.

Vitamin E is widely distributed in the polyunsaturated fatty acids (PUFAs) of cell membranes. Deficiency of vitamin E permits oxidation of PUFAs, with consequent damage to membranes and cells. Although vitamin E serves as the primary antioxidant system, ascorbic acid and selenium also serve this purpose.

Importance

Blood tocopherol levels increase during pregnancy, paralleling a rise in total lipid levels (Horwitt et al., 1972; NRC, 1978). Vitamin E deficiency is not known to be of special concern for pregnant women or their fetuses.

Although vitamin E has not been a major issue in obstetrics and is not believed to be related to the risk of preterm birth, it has attracted considerable interest in the care of newborns, particularly those born prematurely. Premature infants occasionally develop a hemolytic anemia, which is generally believed to be due to vitamin E deficiency. Thus, the vitamin is given to premature infants routinely to meet their special needs (AAP/ACOG, 1988). The limited evidence that macrocytic anemia results from vitamin E deficiency is based primarily on hemolysis after an in vitro peroxide stress. This anemia seldom occurs in full-term neonates or infants (Cruz et al., 1983; Hassan et al., 1966; Linderkamp, 1987; Oski and Barness, 1967; Vanderpas and Vertongen, 1985). However, although the clinical syndrome of anemia is well known, more recent studies have questioned whether this anemia results from vitamin E deficiency (Zipursky et al., 1987). Linderkamp (1987) has pointed out, quite correctly, that many features are unique to the red cells of newborn infants—a factor that complicates interpretation of study results.

Vitamin E may be involved in several other serious problems of premature infants, such as bronchopulmonary dysplasia, a common form of lung disease. Early enthusiasm for treating this disorder with therapeutic doses of vitamin E has waned (Ehrenkranz et al., 1979, 1982; McCarthy et al.,

1984; Wender et al., 1981; Zöberlein et al., 1982). Similarly, there is considerable controversy regarding a role for therapeutic doses of vitamin E in reducing retinopathy of prematurity (retrolental fibroplasia), an infrequent but serious condition leading to substantial visual impairment (Bremer et al., 1986; Hittner et al., 1984; Kretzer et al., 1985; Phelps et al., 1987; Rosenbaum et al., 1985). Evidence has also been presented that vitamin E may be protective in reducing intraventricular hemorrhage in newborn infants (Chiswick et al., 1983; Speer et al., 1984) and microcephaly in rats (Tanaka et al., 1986). Studies of the use of vitamin E in the treatment of these clinical problems have produced inconsistent results, and vitamin E supplementation of preterm infants remains highly controversial (see reviews by Karp and Robertson, 1986; Pereira and Barbosa, 1986; and Phelps, 1987). Attempts to treat diseases of preterm infants with intravenous vitamin E have resulted in major morbidity and mortality (Martone et al., 1986). However, this is now attributed to a stabilizer in the preparation, rather than to the vitamin itself (Alade et al., 1986).

There is no evidence that maternal vitamin E supplementation would reduce the incidence of health problems in premature infants. However, if the fetus acquires vitamin E while it is accumulating fat (during the last 8 to 10 weeks of gestation), the premature infant may be especially low in vitamin E. The full-term infant may therefore have larger vitamin E stores than preterm infants, but the stores are still low compared with those of adults (Gross and Melhorn, 1972). Vitamin E status is difficult to interpret in human fetuses and newborns, in part because both serum lipids and serum levels of vitamin E are low (Ali et al., 1986; Desai et al., 1984; Huijbers et al., 1986; Ostrea et al., 1986; Schulz et al., 1986).

Criteria for Deficiency

In clinical assessment, blood concentrations of tocopherol in normal adults range from 0.5 to 1.2 mg/dl. The tocopherol concentration relates directly to the concentration of total plasma lipids and should be expressed in relation to total lipids.

Recommended and Usual Intakes

The RDA for vitamin E is based on estimates of customary intakes of the vitamin from balanced diets in the United States (NRC, 1989). Actual requirements have not been estimated because of methodologic difficulties. There is significant variation in the tocopherol content of foods. Vegetable oils are the richest source of vitamin E in the U.S. diet. Margarine, shortening, wheat germ, whole grains, and nuts contain large amounts of vitamin E. Substantial loss of tocopherol may occur with processing, storage, and food preparation.

Vitamin E appears to be safe over a wide range of intakes, and no chemical or clinical evidence of toxicity has been observed with oral vitamin E in dosages to 800 mg/day in nonpregnant adults (Farrell and Bieri, 1975). Intake varies widely within and among diets, but appears to average 5 to 11 mg/day for adults eating a typical mixed diet. As noted in Chapter 13, the dietary intake of vitamin E may be difficult to assess because of methodologic and reporting problems. The estimated mean intake by pregnant women in the United States ranges from 3 to 9 mg/day, which is below the pregnancy RDA of 10 mg. The vitamin E intake of well-nourished pregnant and lactating women in England has also been reported to be below the RDA, but without evident clinical signs or symptoms (Black et al., 1986).

Recommendations for Supplementation

In pregnant women, there have been no definable deficiency syndromes for vitamin E, and intakes below the RDA have not been accompanied by an obvious clinical morbidity. Thus, supplementation of healthy pregnant women appears to be unnecessary.

Special Considerations

Given the low vitamin E levels and the clinical syndrome of anemia believed to result from vitamin E deficiency, it is routine to give premature infants supplements of vitamin E.

VITAMIN K

Vitamin K is a fat-soluble vitamin that is required for the synthesis of prothrombin and clotting factors VII, IX, and X. Additional vitamin K-dependent proteins are found in bone, kidney, and other tissues. Natural forms include phylloquinone of plant origin and a group of menaquinones of bacterial origin. Menadione is a fat-soluble synthetic compound with vitamin K activity; several water-soluble derivatives of menadione are also available.

Vitamin K can be absorbed from the small intestine. Efficient absorption occurs in the presence of normal biliary and pancreatic function. The vitamin is widely distributed among tissues; the highest concentration is found in the liver. The body pool of vitamin K is small, and its turnover is rapid (Bjornsson et al., 1980).

Vitamin K is contained in a variety of foods, especially leafy vegetables, dairy products, meat, and eggs. Bacterial flora of the small intestine are another source of vitamin K activity. Analyses of liver compounds with vitamin K activity indicate that food and bacteria provide the normal adult with roughly equal amounts of vitamin K (Rietz et al., 1970).

Importance

The specific importance of vitamin K during pregnancy is largely undetermined. It is known that vitamin K levels and the levels of vitamin K-dependent clotting factors are low in the human fetus (Pietersma-de Bruyn and van Haard, 1985). Transport of vitamin K from mother to fetus has received little attention, but it appears to be limited (Hamulyák et al., 1987, Hiraike et al., 1988). The process of fetal and neonatal clotting is very complicated, and specific clinical problems with bleeding in the fetus are rare. The existence of vitamin K deficiency in the fetus is uncertain (Israels et al., 1987).

By contrast, there is considerable evidence that the newborn infant is functionally vitamin K-deficient, as judged both by vitamin K levels and by abnormal clotting (Lane and Hathaway, 1985; Muntean, 1983; Pietersma-de Bruyn and van Haard, 1985; Prentice, 1985). Accordingly, pediatric and obstetric professional groups recommend that all newborns receive parenteral vitamin K immediately after birth (AAP/ACOG, 1988), whether maternal dietary intake is high or low.

Criteria for Deficiency

Data on plasma vitamin K levels are not systematically available. Vitamin K status is traditionally assessed by blood clotting time. Prolongation of clotting resulting from deficiency of vitamin K-dependent factors is considered to be presumptive evidence of vitamin K deficiency.

Recommended and Usual Intake

The requirement for vitamin K is difficult to estimate, partly because of technical problems. Although a 65-μg RDA for vitamin K has been established for adults, a different recommendation has not been made for vitamin K intake during pregnancy (NRC, 1989).

Normal newborns are routinely given 0.5 to 1.0 mg of vitamin K as phytonadione in a single dose immediately following birth. Hemolytic anemia, hyperbilirubinemia, and kernicterus have been reported in newborns who were given menadione (Owen, 1971). These complications are uncommon today, however, since other forms of vitamin K are in current use.

Vitamin K intake has not been investigated in nationwide studies of nutrient intake. Estimates for usual intake from a mixed diet in the United States range from 300 to 500 μg/day (Olson, 1987).

Recommendations for Supplementation

No vitamin K supplement is indicated in the routine care of pregnant women. No general public health problems have been associated with vitamin K deficiency, which is limited to individuals with disorders that cause substantial degrees of malabsorption or alterations of gut flora. There does not appear to be a need to supplement normal pregnant women with vitamin K, but treatment with vitamin K may be advisable as a part of the medical therapy for pregnant women with malabsorption or those who are undergoing treatment with antibiotics. Vitamin K status should be carefully assessed in patients taking prothrombin-depressing anticoagulants, such as coumarin. Vitamin K may also be of special importance in newborns born to women taking anticonvulsant drugs (Yerby, 1987).

CLINICAL IMPLICATIONS

• Routine supplementation with vitamin A, either as retinol (preformed vitamin A) or carotene (its precursor), appears to be unnecessary in the United States, because the usual dietary intake is adequate to meet the needs of most pregnant women.

• Because of uncertainties about the teratogenicity of preformed vitamin A, use of supplemental retinol is discouraged during the first trimester of pregnancy unless there is evidence of deficiency.

• Although it is routine to supplement premature infants with vitamin E, evidence does not support routine supplementation of pregnant women with this vitamin.

• Although it is advisable that all newborns receive vitamin K at birth, evidence does not indicate that pregnant women should be provided with supplemental vitamin K.

REFERENCES

AAP/ACOG (American Academy of Pediatrics/American College of Obstetricians and Gynecologists). 1988. Guidelines for Perinatal Care, 2nd ed. American Academy of Pediatrics, Elk Grove, Ill. 356 pp.

Alade, S.L., R.E. Brown, and A. Paquet, Jr. 1986. Polysorbate 80 and E-Ferol toxicity. Pediatrics 77:593-597.

Ali, J., H.A. Kader, K. Hassan, and H. Arshat. 1986. Changes in human milk vitamin E and total lipids during the first twelve days of lactation. Am. J. Clin. Nutr. 43:925-930.

Araujo, R.L., M.B.D.G. Araujo, R.O. Sieior, R.D.P. Machado, and B.V. Leite. 1986. Diagnostico da situação da hipovitaminose a e da anemia nutricional na população do vale do Jequitinhonha, Minas Gerais, Brasil. Arch. Latinoam. Nutr. 36:642-653.

Araujo, R.L., M.B.D.G. Araujo, R.D.P. Machado, A.A. Braga, B.V. Leite, and J.R. Oliveira. 1987. Evaluation of a program to overcome vitamin A and iron deficiencies in areas of poverty in Minas Gerais, Brazil. Arch. Latinoam. Nutr. 37:9-22.

Bauernfeind, J.C. 1980. The Safe Use of Vitamin A. A Report of the International Vitamin A Consultative Group (IVACG). The Nutrition Foundation, Washington, D.C. 44 pp.

Behrens, W.A., J.N. Thompson, and R. Madère. 1982. Distribution of α-tocopherol in human plasma lipoproteins. Am. J. Clin. Nutr. 35:691-696.

Bjornsson, T.D., P.J. Meffin, S.E. Swezey, and T.F. Blaschke. 1980. Disposition and turnover of vitamin K₁ in man. Pp. 328-332 in J.W. Suttie, ed. Vitamin K Metabolism and Vitamin K-Dependent Proteins. University Park Press, Baltimore.

Black, A.E., S.J. Wiles, and A.A. Paul. 1986. The nutrient intakes of pregnant and lactating mothers of good socio-economic status in Cambridge, UK: some implications for recommended daily allowances of minor nutrients. Br. J. Nutr. 56:59-72.

Bremer, D.L., G.L. Rogers, H. Bell, and R. Lytle. 1986. The efficacy of vitamin E in retinopathy of prematurity. J. Pediatr. Ophthalmol. Strab. 23:132-136.

Chiswick, M.L., M. Johnson, C. Woodhall, M. Gowland, J. Davies, N. Toner, and D. Sims. 1983. Protective effect of vitamin E on intraventricular haemorrhage in the newborn. Ciba Found. Symp. 101:186-200.

Chytil, F. 1985. Vitamin A and lung development. Pediatr. Pulmonol. 1:S115-S117.

Cruz, C.S.D., P.D. Wimberley, K. Johansen, and B. Friis-Hansen. 1983. The effect of vitamin E on erythrocyte hemolysis and lipid peroxidation in newborn premature infants. Acta Paediatr. Scand. 72:823-826.

Desai, I.D., F.E. Martinez, J.E. Dos Santos, and J.E. Dutra de Oliveria. 1984. Transient lipoprotein deficiency at birth: a cause of low levels of vitamin E in the newborn. Acta Vitaminol. Enzymol. 6:71-76.

Donoghue, S., D.W. Richardson, D. Sklan, and D.S. Kronfeld. 1982. Placental transport of retinol in sheep. J. Nutr. 112:2197-2203.

Donoghue, S., D.W. Richardson, D. Sklan, and D.S. Kronfeld. 1985. Placental transport of retinol in ewes fed high intakes of vitamin A. J. Nutr. 115:1562-1571.

Ehrenkranz, R.A., R.C. Ablow, and J.B. Warshaw. 1979. Prevention of bronchopulmonary dysplasia with vitamin E administration during the acute stages of respiratory distress syndrome. J. Pediatr. 95:873-878.

Ehrenkranz, R.A., R.C. Ablow, and J.B. Warshaw. 1982. Effect of vitamin E on the development of oxygen-induced lung injury in neonates. Ann. N.Y. Acad. Sci. 393:452-466.

FAO (Food and Agriculture Organization). 1988. Requirements of Vitamin A, Iron, Folate, and Vitamin B₁₂. Report of a Joint FAO/WHO Expert Consultation. FAO Food and Nutrition Series No. 23. Food and Agriculture Organization, Rome. 107 pp.

Farrell, P.M., and J.G. Bieri. 1975. Megavitamin E supplementation in man. Am. J. Clin. Nutr. 28:1381-1386.

Finley, D.A., K.G. Dewey, B. Lönnerdal, and L.E. Grivetti. 1985. Food choices of vegetarians and nonvegetarians during pregnancy and lactation. J. Am. Diet. Assoc. 85:678-685.

Gebre-Medhin, M., and A. Vahlquist. 1984. Vitamin A nutrition in the human foetus: a comparison of Sweden and Ethiopia. Acta Paediatr. Scand. 73:333-340.

Gross, S., and D.K. Melhorn. 1972. Vitamin E, red cell lipids and red cell stability in prematurity. Ann. N.Y. Acad. Sci. 203:141-162.

Hamulyák, K., M.A. de Boer-van den Berg, H.H. Thijssen, H.C. Hemker, and C. Vermeer. 1987. The placental transport of [3H]vitamin K₁ in rats. Br. J. Haematol. 65:335-338.

Hassan, H., S.A. Hashim, T.B. Van Itallie, and W.H. Sebrell. 1966. Syndrome in premature infants associated with low plasma vitamin E levels and high polyunsaturated fatty acid diet. Am. J. Clin. Nutr. 19:147-157.

Hiraike, H., M. Kimura, and Y. Itokawa. 1988. Distribution of K vitamins (phylloquinone and menaquinones) in human placenta and maternal and umbilical cord plasma. Am. J. Obstet. Gynecol. 158:564-569.

Hittner, H.M., A.J. Rudolph, and F.L. Kretzer. 1984. Suppression of severe retinopathy of prematurity with vitamin E supplementation: ultrastructural mechanism of clinical efficacy. Opthalmology 91:1512-1523.

Horwitt, M.K., C.C. Harvey, C.H. Dahm, Jr., and M.T. Searcy. 1972. Relationship between tocopherol and serum lipid levels for determination of nutritional adequacy. Ann. N.Y. Acad. Sci. 203:223-236.

Huijbers, W.A., J. Schrijver, A.J. Speek, B.A. Deelstra, and A. Okken. 1986. Persistent low plasma vitamin E levels in premature infants surviving respiratory distress syndrome. Eur. J. Pediatr. 145:170-171.

Hume, E.M., and H.A. Krebs. 1949. Vitamin A Requirement of Human Adults. Report of the Vitamin A Subcommittee, Accessory Food Factors Committee, Medical Research Council. Special Report Series No. 264. Her Majesty's Stationery Office, London. 145 pp.

Ismadi, S.D., and J.A. Olson. 1982. Dynamics of the fetal distribution and transfer of Vitamin A between rat fetuses and their mother. Int. J. Vitam. Nutr. Res. 52:112-119.

Israels, L.G., E. Friesen, A.H. Jansen, and E.D. Israels. 1987. Vitamin K1 increases sister chromatid exchange *in vitro* in human leukocytes and *in vivo* in fetal sheep cells: a possible role for "vitamin K deficiency" in the fetus. Pediatr. Res. 22:405-408.

Karp, W.B., and A.F. Robertson. 1986. Vitamin E in neonatology. Adv. Pediatr. 33:127-147.

Kelleher, J., M.G. Miller, J.M. Littlewood, A.M. McDonald, and M.S. Losowsky. 1987. The clinical effect of correction of vitamin E depletion in cystic fibrosis. Int. J. Vitam. Nutr. Res. 57:253-259.

Khanna, A., and T.S. Reddy. 1983. Effect of undernutrition and vitamin A deficiency on the phospholipid composition of rat tissues at 21 days of age.—I. Liver, spleen, and kidney. Int. J. Vitam. Nutr. Res. 53:3-8.

Kretzer, F.L., A.R. McPherson, A.J. Rudolph, and H.M. Hittner. 1985. Pathogenic mechanism of retinopathy of prematurity: a controversial explanation for the efficacy of oral and intramuscular vitamin E supplementation and cryotherapy. Bull. N.Y. Acad. Med. 61:883-900.

Lammer, E.J., D.T. Chen, R.M. Hoar, N.D. Agnish, P.J. Benke, J.T. Braun, C.J. Curry, P.M. Fernhoff, A.W. Grix, Jr., I.T. Lott, J.M. Richard, and S.C. Sun. 1985. Retinoic acid embryopathy. N. Engl. J. Med. 313:837-841.

Lane, P.A., and W.E. Hathaway. 1985. Vitamin K in infancy. J. Pediatr. 106:351-359.

Linderkamp, O. 1987. Blood rheology in the newborn infant. Baill. Clin. Haematol. 1:801-825.

Lungarotti, M.S., D. Marinelli, T. Mariani, and A. Calabro. 1987. Multiple congenital anomalies associated with apparently normal maternal intake of vitamin A: a phenocopy of the isotretinoin syndrome? Am. J. Med. Genet. 27:245-248.

Martone, W.J., W.W. Williams, M.L. Mortensen, R.P. Gaynes, J.W. White, V. Lorch, M.D. Murphy, S.N. Sinha, D.J. Frank, N. Kosmetatos, C.J. Bodenstein, and R.J. Roberts. 1986. Illness with fatalities in premature infants: association with an intravenous vitamin E preparation, E-Ferol. Pediatrics 78:591-600.

McCarthy, K., M. Bhogal, M. Nardi, and D. Hart. 1984. Pathogenic factors in bronchopulmonary dysplasia. Pediatr. Res. 18:483-488.

Montreewasuwat, N., and J.A. Olson. 1979. Serum and liver concentrations of vitamin A in Thai fetuses as a function of gestational age. Am. J. Clin. Nutr. 32:601-606.

Muller, D.P.R. 1986. Vitamin E—its role in neurological function. Postgrad. Med. J. 62:107-112.

Muntean, W. 1983. Vitamin-K-Mangel bei Neugeborenen. Wien. Klin. Wochenschr. 95:1-5.

NRC (National Research Council). 1978. Laboratory Indices of Nutritional Status in Pregnancy. Report of the Committee on Nutrition of the Mother and Preschool Child, Food and Nutrition Board. National Academy of Sciences, Washington, D.C. 195 pp.

NRC (National Research Council). 1989. Recommended Dietary Allowances, 10th ed. Report of the Subcommittee on the Tenth Edition of the RDAs, Food and Nutrition Board, Commission on Life Sciences. National Academy Press, Washington, D.C. 284 pp.

Olson, J.A. 1987. Recommended dietary intakes (RDI) of vitamin K in humans. Am. J. Clin. Nutr. 45:687-692.

Oski, F.A., and L.A. Barness. 1967. Vitamin E deficiency: a previously unrecognized cause of hemolytic anemia in the premature infant. J. Pediatr. 70:211-220.

Ostrea, E.M., Jr., J.E. Balun, R. Winkler, and T. Porter. 1986. Influence of breast-feeding on the restoration of the low serum concentration of vitamin E and β-carotene in the newborn infant. Am. J. Obstet. Gynecol. 154:1014-1017.

Owen, C.A., Jr. 1971. Vitamin K group. XI. Pharmacology and toxicology. Pp. 492-509 in W.H. Sebrell, Jr. and R.S. Harris, eds. The Vitamins: Chemistry, Physiology, Methods, 2nd ed., Vol. III. Academic Press, New York.

Pereira, G.R., and N.M.N. Barbosa. 1986. Controversies in neonatal nutrition. Pediatr. Clin. North Am. 33:65-89.

Phelps, D.L. 1987. Current perspectives on vitamin E in infant nutrition. Am. J. Clin. Nutr. 46:187-191.

Phelps, D.L., A.L. Rosenbaum, S.J. Isenberg, R.D. Leake, and F.J. Dorey. 1987. Tocopherol efficacy and safety for preventing retinopathy of prematurity: a randomized, controlled, double-masked trial. Pediatrics 79:489-500.

Pietersma-de Bruyn, A.L.J.M., and P.M.M. van Haard. 1985. Vitamin K_1 in the newborn. Clin. Chim. Acta 150:95-101.

Prentice, C.R. 1985. Acquired coagulation disorders. Clin. Haematol. 14:413-442.

Reddy, T.S., and A. Khanna. 1983. Effect of undernutrition and vitamin A deficiency on the phospholipid composition of rat tissues at 21 days of age.—II. Lung, heart, and testes. Int. J. Vitam. Nutr. Res. 53:9-12.

Rietz, P., U. Gloor, and O. Wiss. 1970. Menachinone aus menschlicher Leber und Faulschlamm. Int. Z. Vitaminforsch. 40:351-362.

Rosa, F.W., A.L. Wilk, and F.O. Kelsey. 1986. Teratogen update: vitamin A congeners. Teratology 33:355-364.

Rosenbaum, A.L., D.L. Phelps, S.J. Isenberg, R.D. Leake, and F. Dorey. 1985. Retinal hemorrhage in retinopathy of prematurity associated with tocopherol treatment. Opthalmology 92:1012-1014.

Rush, D., N.L. Sloan, J. Leighton, J.M. Alvir, D.G. Horvitz, W.B. Seaver, G.C. Garbowski, S.S. Johnson, R.A. Kulka, M. Holt, J.W. Devore, J.T. Lynch, M.B. Woodside, and D.S. Shanklin. 1988. The National WIC Evaluation: evaluation of the Special Supplemental Food Program for Women, Infants, and Children. V. Longitudinal study of pregnant women. Am. J. Clin. Nutr. 48:439-483.

Sauberlich, H.E., R.E. Hodges, D.L. Wallace, H. Kolder, J.E. Canham, J. Hood, N. Raica, Jr., and L.K. Lowry. 1974. Vitamin A metabolism and requirements in the human studied with the use of labeled retinol. Vitam. Horm. (N.Y.) 32:251-275.

Schulz, H., K. Schroeder, and W. Feldheim. 1986. Studies on the tocopherol status in blood serum of premature babies and infants. Z. Ernaehrungswiss. 25:1-8.

Shah, R.S., and R. Rajalakshmi. 1984. Vitamin A status of the newborn in relation to gestational age, body weight, and maternal nutritional status. Am. J. Clin. Nutr. 40:794-800.

Shah, R.S., R. Rajalakshmi, R.V. Bhatt, M.N. Hazra, B.C. Patel, N.B. Swamy, and T.V. Patel. 1987. Liver stores of vitamin A in human fetuses in relation to gestational age, fetal size and maternal nutritional status. Br. J. Nutr. 58:181-189.

Sharma, H.S., and U.K. Misra. 1986. Postnatal distribution of vitamin A in liver, lung, heart, and brain of the rat in relation to maternal vitamin A status. Biol. Neonate 50:345-350.

Shukla, R.R., V. Kumar, R. Banerjee, and U.K. Misra. 1986. Placental transfer and fetal distribution of 3H-retinoic acid in rats. Int. J. Vitam. Nutr. Res. 56:29-33.

Sklan, D. 1987. Vitamin A in human nutrition. Prog. Food Nutr. Sci. 11:39-55.

Sklan, D., I. Shalit, N. Lasebnik, Z. Spirer, and Y. Weisman. 1985. Retinol transport proteins and concentrations in human amniotic fluid, placenta, and fetal and maternal sera. Br. J. Nutr. 54:577-583.

Sokol, R.J., M.A. Guggenheim, J.E. Heubi, S.T. Iannaccone, N. Butler-Simon, V. Jackson, C. Miller, M. Cheney, W.F. Balistreri, and A. Silverman. 1985. Frequency and clinical progression of the vitamin E deficiency neurologic disorder in children with prolonged neonatal cholestasis. Am. J. Dis. Child. 139:1211-1215.

Sommer, A. 1982. Nutritional Blindness: Xerophthalmia and Keratomalacia. Oxford University Press, New York. 282 pp.

Speer, M.E., C. Blifeld, A.J. Rudolph, P. Chadda, M.E.B. Holbein, and H.M. Hittner. 1984. Intraventricular hemorrhage and vitamin E in the very low-birth-weight infant: evidence for efficacy of early intramuscular vitamin E administration. Pediatrics 74:1107-1112.

Stånge, L., K. Carlström, and M. Eriksson. 1978. Hypervitaminosis A in early human pregnancy and malformations of the central nervous system. Acta Obstet. Gynecol. Scand. 57:289-291.

Stanton, B.F., J.D. Clemens, B. Wojtyniak, and T. Khair. 1986. Risk factors for developing mild nutritional blindness in urban Bangladesh. Am. J. Dis. Child. 140:584-588.

Takahashi, Y.I., J.E. Smith, M. Winick, and D.S. Goodman. 1975. Vitamin A deficiency and fetal growth and development in the rat. J. Nutr. 105:1299-1310.

Tanaka, H., S. Iwasaki, K. Inomata, F. Nasu, and S. Nishimura. 1986. The protective effects of vitamin E on microcephaly in rats X-irradiated in utero: DNA, lipid peroxide and confronting cisternae. Dev. Brain Res. 27:11-17.

Teratology Society. 1987. Teratology Society position paper: recommendations for vitamin A use during pregnancy. Teratology 35:267-275.

Törmä, H., and A. Vahlquist. 1986. Uptake of vitamin A and retinol-binding protein by human placenta in vitro. Placenta 7:295-305.

Vanderpas, J., and F. Vertongen. 1985. Erythrocyte vitamin E is oxidized at a lower peroxide concentration in neonates than in adults. Blood 66:1272-1277.

Villard, L., and C.J. Bates. 1986. Dark adaptation in pregnant and lactating Gambian women: feasibility of measurement and relation to vitamin A status. Hum. Nutr.: Clin. Nutr. 40C:349-357.

Villard, L., and C.J. Bates. 1987. Effect of vitamin A supplementation on plasma and breast milk vitamin A levels in poorly nourished Gambian women. Hum. Nutr.: Clin. Nutr. 41C:47-58.

Wald, G. 1968. The molecular basis of visual excitation. Nature 219:800-807.

Wallingford, J.C., and B.A. Underwood. 1986. Vitamin A deficiency in pregnancy, lactation, and the nursing child. Pp. 101-152 in J.C. Bauernfeind, ed. Vitamin A Deficiency and its Control. Academic Press, Orlando, Fla.

Wender, D.F., G.E. Thulin, G.J.W. Smith, and J.B. Warshaw. 1981. Vitamin E affects lung biochemical and morphologic response to hyperoxia in the newborn rabbit. Pediatr. Res. 15:262-268.

Woollam, D.H.M. 1985. Basic principles of teratology. Pp. 85-116 in R. MacDonald, ed. Scientific Basis of Obstetrics and Gynaecology, 3rd ed. Churchill Livingstone, Edinburgh.

Yerby, M.S. 1987. Problems and management of the pregnant woman with epilepsy. Epilepsia 28, Suppl. 3:S29-S36.

Zipursky, A., E.J. Brown, J. Watts, R. Milner, C. Rand, V.S. Blanchette, E.F. Bell, B. Paes, and E. Ling. 1987. Oral vitamin E supplementation for the prevention of anemia in premature infants: a controlled trial. Pediatrics 79:61-68.

Zöberlein, H.G., V. Freudenberg, and H. Wehinger. 1982. Bronchopulmonale Dysplasie: prospektiv radomisierte Studie zur prophylaktischen Wirkung von Vitamin E. Monatsschr. Kinderheilkd. 130:706-709.

18

Water-Soluble Vitamins

The subcommittee focused primarily on two water-soluble vitamins—vitamin B_6 and folate, which have been associated most frequently with pregnancy complications and adverse outcomes. Furthermore, adequacy of dietary intakes of these vitamins relative to the Recommended Dietary Allowances (RDAs) by women of childbearing age is generally reported to be lower than that of other water-soluble vitamins. Thus, the subcommittee reviewed evidence regarding the importance of vitamin B_6 and folate in pregnant women, the estimated need for these vitamins, and the usual dietary intakes as a basis for its recommendations on supplementation. The other water-soluble vitamins are generally considered to be consumed in adequate amounts from dietary sources and are, therefore, not an important issue with regard to routine supplementation. Thus, the literature pertaining to them is summarized only briefly.

VITAMIN B_6

Vitamin B_6 is a collective term for six metabolically related pyridines, namely, pyridoxal, pyridoxamine, and pyridoxine and their phosphorylated derivatives (e.g., pyridoxal phosphate). These six forms of the vitamin constitute the B_6 vitamers.

Importance

Almost 50 years ago, interest in the relationship of vitamin B_6 to human pregnancy originated with the empirical use of pharmacologic doses of pyridoxine in the treatment of hyperemesis gravidarum—a condition of prolonged, severe nausea and vomiting during pregnancy (Willis et al., 1942). The lack of firm scientific evidence of the efficacy of this treatment is discussed later in this chapter. Evidence has accumulated that vitamin B_6 is required for protein, carbohydrate, and lipid metabolism as well as for erythrocyte, immune, and hormonal functions (see review by Leklem and Reynolds, 1988). Pyridoxal phosphate (PLP), the physiologically active form of the vitamin, is a coenzyme in over 100 known reactions involved primarily in amino acid metabolism. PLP-containing enzymes include aminotransferases, which are essential to the synthesis of nonessential amino acids, and decarboxylases, which are needed in the formation of histamine, serotonin, dopamine, and γ-aminobutyric acid. PLP is also a coenzyme in the formation of aminolevulinic acid, the first step in the synthesis of heme compounds. These vitamin B_6-dependent reactions are of obvious importance to the normal course and outcome of pregnancy.

Estimated Requirements

Even though the vitamin B_6 intake and status of pregnant women have been widely studied, the requirements for this vitamin during pregnancy have not been clearly defined. It is known, however, that increased protein intake during pregnancy necessitates a modest increase in vitamin B_6 intake (Table 18-1), because of the major role of the vitamin in amino acid metabolism (NRC, 1989). Also, fetal uptake of vitamin B_6, especially in late pregnancy, increases the need for the vitamin. All forms of vitamin B_6, especially PLP, cross the placenta into fetal blood where concentrations are two to five times higher than those in maternal blood (Cleary et al., 1975; Contractor and Shane, 1970). Furthermore, the normal elevation of estrogen levels during pregnancy has been reported to increase tryptophan oxygenase activity (Rose, 1978), which in turn increases the need for vitamin B_6.

A total body vitamin B_6 content of approximately 60 mg and a daily turnover rate of approximately 3% have been found in healthy nonpregnant women (Shane and Contractor, 1980). The vitamin B_6 content of blood was estimated to be less than 0.5 mg of pyridoxine equivalents, i.e., the concentration of individual B_6 vitamers calculated as pyridoxine. The amount of vitamin B_6 in maternal and fetal tissues gained has not been determined, but presumably represents only a small part of the estimated increased need for vitamin B_6 during pregnancy. The percentages of

TABLE 18-1 Recommended Dietary Allowances of Water-Soluble Vitamins for Nonpregnant and Pregnant Women and the Rationale for Increased Allowances During Pregnancy[a]

Vitamin	Recommended Dietary Allowance		Rationale for Increased Allowance for Pregnancy
	Nonpregnant Women[b]	Pregnant Women	
Vitamin C	60 mg	70 mg	To provide for fetal needs; at term, fetal plasma levels are 50% higher than maternal levels
Thiamin	1.1 mg	1.5 mg	To accommodate maternal and fetal growth and increased energy allowance during pregnancy
Riboflavin	1.3 mg	1.6 mg	To provide for increased maternal and fetal synthesis
Niacin (NE)[c]	15 mg	17 mg	Based on energy increase of 300 kcal/day for pregnancy
Vitamin B_6	1.6 mg	2.2 mg	Based partially on the additional protein allowance of 10 g/day for pregnancy
Folate	190 μg	400 μg	Based on 50% food folate absorption; to build or maintain maternal folate stores and to provide for increased folate turnover in rapidly growing tissue
Vitamin B_{12}	2.0 μg	2.2 μg	Fetal needs (0.1–0.2 μg/day) based on analyses of stillborn fetuses; metabolic needs of pregnancy estimated at 0.2 μg/day

[a] From NRC (1989).
[b] Based on highest value recommended for females between the ages of 15 and 50 years.
[c] Niacin equivalent (NE) is equal to 1 mg of niacin or 60 mg of tryptophan.

vitamin B_6 absorbed and metabolized to PLP as well as the oxidation and excretion of the vitamin appear to be the same during pregnancy as they are in the nonpregnant state (Contractor and Shane, 1970).

Decreases in both blood levels of vitamin B_6 and vitamin B_6-dependent enzyme activity occur gradually during pregnancy. The most substantial decrease in plasma PLP levels is found between the fourth and eighth months of gestation, paralleling the period of most intensive growth of the fetus (Reinken and Dapunt, 1978). The fetus appears to lack the ability to phosphorylate pyridoxal and is dependent upon a maternal supply of PLP (Shane and Contractor, 1980). Thus, placental transport of PLP from mother to fetus is one mechanism that clearly leads to lower levels of PLP in maternal plasma, sometimes called the biochemical deficiency of vitamin B_6 of late pregnancy.

Criteria for Status Assessment

Overt clinical signs of vitamin B_6 deficiency (Table 18-2) are rare in the United States. In the absence of established markers, assessment procedures rely almost entirely on biochemical tests, including direct measurements of B_6 vitamers in blood or urine and indirect and functional tests to measure changes in PLP-dependent enzymes or activity coefficients (e.g., in vitro stimulation of enzyme activity by addition of PLP). Plasma PLP, which has been studied extensively, has been reported to be an indicator of vitamin B_6 body stores, whereas pyridoxic acid has been said to reflect intake (Leklem and Reynolds, 1988; Shane and Contractor, 1980; van den Berg, 1988). Concentrations of vitamin B_6 and B_6 vitamers in blood decrease with the normal increase in blood volume during mid- and late pregnancy.

An important consideration is the stage of pregnancy during which the tests are administered because of changes in hormonal balance throughout gestation. Such changes can affect enzyme turnover, enzyme-coenzyme binding properties, and redistribution of the B_6 vitamers in tissues. Knowledge about the effects of maternal homeostasis on the above-mentioned tests is limited (Shane and Contractor, 1980).

Studies of pregnant rats suggest that the pregnancy-induced changes in vitamin B_6 status indicators probably reflect a higher retentive capacity and temporary deposition of vitamin B_6 in tissues early in pregnancy as a result of hormone-induced changes (van den Berg and Bogaards, 1987). There is a need to quantify the influence of these secondary effects upon the biochemical indices of vitamin B_6 status in pregnant women and then to set reference standards.

Studies have consistently shown that in comparison with nonpregnant controls, pregnant women have lower plasma levels of vitamin B_6 and PLP (Cleary et al., 1975; Contractor and Shane, 1970; Hamfelt and Tuvemo, 1972; Lumeng et al., 1976; Reinken and Dapunt, 1978; Roepke and Kirksey, 1979a; Schuster et al., 1984), decreased erythrocyte alanine aminotransferase activity, and higher activity coefficients (Lumeng et al., 1976; Schuster et al., 1981), especially during late pregnancy. Other changes include decreased levels of vitamin B_6 in leukocytes, erythrocytes, and urine and increased production of tryptophan or methionine metabolites following a large oral test dose (2 to 5 g) of the amino acid (Sauberlich, 1978). Abnormal results from a combination of two or more laboratory tests, e.g., decreased activity of vitamin B_6-dependent enzymes coupled with high activity coefficients, are considered more indicative of vitamin B_6 inadequacy than is one abnormal measurement.

Usual Intakes

As shown in Chapter 13, Table 13-2, dietary intakes of vitamin B_6 by pregnant women in the United States have often been reported to be lower than the RDA (NRC, 1989). Using 3-day diet records, Roepke and Kirksey (1979a) calculated the mean daily vitamin B_6 intake of 97 middle-class U.S. women at 5 to 7 months of gestation to be 1.24 ± 0.55 (standard deviation [SD]) mg. Reynolds et al. (1984) analyzed the dietary intakes of 36 upper-middle-class U.S. women at 37 weeks of pregnancy and found their mean vitamin B_6 intake was 1.4 ± 0.42 (SD*) mg per day. The ratio of dietary vitamin B_6 to protein in these women was near the then recommended ratio for nonpregnant adults of 0.02 mg of vitamin B_6 to 1 g of protein. The current recommended ratio is 0.016 mg to 1 g (NRC, 1989). Among a group of 60 healthy pregnant Caucasian women, only three consumed 2.6 mg/day or more (Vir et al., 1980). The RDA at that time was 2.6 mg/day, compared with the current RDA of 2.2 mg/day (NRC, 1989). No significant relationship was observed between their vitamin B_6 status and the birth weights or anthropometric measurements of their neonates; however, the small sample size precluded definitive conclusions. In Florida, Schuster et al. (1981) reported that the mean daily vitamin B_6 intake of disadvantaged pregnant women (mostly of black origin) was 1.4 ± 1.0 (SD) mg, a level comparable to that reported for more economically advantaged women (Reynolds et al., 1984). The mean erythrocyte alanine aminotransferase activation coefficient among the Floridian women was 1.35 (compared with a normal value of ≤1.25 for nonpregnant women). Many values were considered by the researchers to be suggestive of vitamin B_6 inadequacy. In a subsequent study (Schuster et al., 1984) of 46 pregnant women from the same population, mean daily vitamin B_6 intake was estimated to be 1.5 mg (0.019 mg/g of protein).

Vitamin B_6 Status and the Course and Outcome of Pregnancy

Over the years, interest in the vitamin B_6 status of pregnant women has been stimulated by such findings as lower PLP concentrations in the

---

*Calculated from reported standard error of the mean.

TABLE 18-2 Biochemical Indices of Water-Soluble Vitamin Nutritional Status and Clinical Manifestations of Deficiency

Vitamin	Biochemical Indices of Nutritional Status		Clinical Manifestations of Deficiency
	Levels of Vitamins or Metabolites in Body Fluids and Tissues	Activity of Vitamin-Dependent Enzymes	
Vitamin C	Vitamin C in plasma, serum, or leukocytes	None	Follicular hyperkeratosis; swollen, bleeding gums; petechial hemorrhages; joint pain; scurvy
Thiamin	Thiamin excretion in urine	Erythrocyte transketolase activity (ETK); ETK activation coefficient	Anorexia, lassitude, muscle weakness, ataxia, dyspnea upon exertion, heart enlargement, tachycardia, beriberi
Riboflavin	Riboflavin excretion in urine	Glutathione reductase activity (GRA); GRA activity coefficient	Lesions of mucocutaneous surfaces of mouth (angular stomatitis, cheilosis, atrophic lingual papillae, glossitis (magenta tongue), seborrheic skin lesions, and surface lesions of genitalia

			diarrhea, neurologic changes (anxiety, depression, fatigue), pellagra
Vitamin B$_6$	Vitamin B$_6$, pyridoxal phosphate, and other B$_6$ vitamers in serum, plasma, or erythrocytes; 4-pyridoxic acid or total vitamin B$_6$ excretion in urine	Erythrocyte alanine aminotransferase activity (E-Ala-AT); E-Ala-AT activation coefficient; erythrocyte aspartate aminotransferase (E-Asp-AT); E-Asp-AT activation coefficient	Weight loss, dermatitis, stomatitis, anemia, peripheral neuritis, depression, confusion, hyperirritability, electroencephalographic anomalies, epileptiform-type convulsions
Folate	Folate in plasma, serum, or erythrocytes	None applicable	Megaloblastic anemia, hypersegmentation of neutrophils, neutropenia, lesions of intestinal tract
Vitamin B$_{12}$	Vitamin B$_{12}$ in plasma, serum, or erythrocytes	None applicable	Megaloblastic anemia, anorexia, weakness, fatigue, dyspnea, leukopenia, neurologic changes, weight loss, gastric mucosal atrophy, pernicious anemia

umbilical cord blood of preeclamptic mothers compared with those in women with normal pregnancies (Brophy and Siiteri, 1975). However, Lu and colleagues (1981) failed to demonstrate any improvement in the course of toxemia following the administration of pyridoxine. Low levels of PLP in maternal plasma have been associated with low birth weight (Reinken and Dapunt, 1978), but this has not been uniformly confirmed (Vir et al., 1980).

Positive associations between vitamin B_6 status and the course and outcomes of pregnancy have been reported, but results of these studies are controversial, because no placebos were used and the subjects were not randomized or blinded. For example, early studies of pregnant women (Dorsey, 1949; Weinstein et al., 1944; Willis et al., 1942) in which pyridoxine doses of 5 to 100 mg/day were claimed to be effective in treating nausea and vomiting were not controlled; therefore, a placebo effect cannot be ruled out. In a study (Hesseltine, 1946) that included a placebo but that was not randomized or blinded, both pyridoxine and placebo were found to control nausea. The American Medical Association Council on Drugs (1979) has stated that there is no scientific evidence that vitamin B_6 is effective in the treatment of nausea. This viewpoint is supported by a recent review of the safety and efficacy of antiemetics in the treatment of nausea during pregnancy (Leathem, 1986). Associations of vitamin B_6 inadequacy with gestational diabetes (Spellacy et al., 1977) and with "pregnancy depression"—described as pessimism, crying, tension without sleep, or appetite disorders (Pulkkinen et al., 1978)—have also been challenged on methodologic grounds.

The active transport of vitamin B_6 from maternal to fetal blood against a concentration gradient in the placenta lessens the effects of maternal vitamin B_6 inadequacy on the newborn, but it also could result in abnormally high levels in the fetus if pregnant women are given enough supplemental pyridoxine to increase their plasma PLP levels to those of nonpregnant women. Shane and Contractor (1975) postulated that this could adversely affect the synthesis of PLP-dependent enzymes by the fetus and might lead to a higher than normal vitamin B_6 requirement by the infant. However, this hypothesis has not been confirmed or refuted experimentally.

Three reports (Roepke and Kirksey, 1979a; Schuster et al., 1981, 1984) have related low vitamin B_6 intakes and low plasma levels as well as low PLP levels at delivery to unsatisfactory Apgar scores of newborns. These scores are based on heart rate, respiratory effort, muscle tone, reflex irritability, and color at 1 and 5 minutes after delivery (Apgar and James, 1962; Apgar et al., 1958), all of which can be influenced by many variables. Maternal pyridoxine supplementation was associated with improved Apgar scores taken at 1 minute; however, statistically significant improvements

TABLE 18-3   Doses of Water-Soluble Vitamins Associated with Acute or Chronic Toxicity in Otherwise Healthy Pregnant and Nonpregnant Humans

	Doses Associated with Toxicity	
Vitamin	Human Pregnancy	Other Human Studies
Vitamin C	250–500 mg/day[a]	>3 g/day for several mo (Hanck, 1982)
Niacin	NR[b]	>3 g/day for 5–6 mo (Robie, 1967)
Vitamin B$_6$	50 mg/day[c]	>500 mg/day for >1 mo (Cohen and Bendich, 1986)
		2 g/day for 4 mo (Schaumburg et al., 1983)
Folate	NR[b]	15 mg/day for 1 mo[d] (Hunter et al., 1970)

[a] Based on three isolated cases; 250 to 500 mg/day taken for 2 weeks in late pregnancy in one case (Mentzer and Collier, 1975) and 400 mg/day during pregnancy in two cases (Cochrane, 1965).

[b] NR = Not reported.

[c] Based on one isolated case; dose given three to four times weekly for nausea in midpregnancy (Hunt et al., 1954).

[d] The findings from this one uncontrolled experiment with 14 adult volunteers by Hunter et al. (1970) were later refuted in research by Hellström (1971).

were not observed in 5-minute scores, which may be more indicative of long-term infant health problems (Schuster et al., 1984).

Since most pregnant women in the United States now consume multivitamin-mineral preparations containing vitamin B$_6$, it is usually not possible to conduct observational studies of relationships between dietary intake of vitamin B$_6$ and the course and outcome of pregnancy.

Toxicity

There are few data on the safety of pyridoxine supplementation during human pregnancy. Oral doses of pyridoxine greater than 500 mg/day for prolonged periods can result in the development of sensory neuropathy in nonpregnant adults (Cohen and Bendich, 1986) (Table 18-3). In the same review of the safety of pyridoxine, no toxic effects were reported for adults given 500 mg/day or less under medical supervision for periods ranging from 6 months to 6 years.

The suggestion that excessive vitamin B$_6$ intake during pregnancy produces a vitamin B$_6$-dependency state in the newborn is based on one isolated case (Hunt et al., 1954). A woman treated with 50 mg of pyridoxine hydrochloride three or four times weekly for nausea during midpregnancy gave birth to an infant who had repeated convulsive seizures that responded to pyridoxine administration. The outcome was normal in an earlier pregnancy, during which the woman had not been given large doses of pyridoxine. Although pyridoxine-responsive convulsive disorders are occasionally observed in newborns, no reports have confirmed an association between them and maternal pyridoxine intake. Vitamin B_6 dependency appears to reflect an inborn error in metabolism rather than an acquired dependency state (Pitkin, 1982).

Recommendations for Supplementation

Most clinical trials of routine pyridoxine supplementation of pregnant women have failed to demonstrate any differences in pregnancy outcome, thereby casting doubt on the benefits of vitamin B_6 supplements. In a double-blind study, Schuster et al. (1984) found that a daily pyridoxine intake of 5.5 to 7.6 mg during pregnancy was required to avoid a decrease in plasma PLP levels at delivery. Without supplemental pyridoxine, mean levels decreased approximately 30% by 30 weeks of gestation and 25% at delivery over initial values. Lumeng et al. (1976) reported that pyridoxine intakes between 4 and 10 mg/day were needed to maintain plasma PLP at levels similar to those in the first trimester of pregnancy. Since physiologic changes during pregnancy may have accounted for the lower PLP levels, it is questionable whether pyridoxine supplementation should be used to produce levels similar to those in the nonpregnant state. Furthermore, the 4- to 10-mg/day doses of pyridoxine reported to maintain prepregnancy vitamin B_6 status during pregnancy exceed the amount obtainable from food.

For women at high risk for inadequate nutrient intake, e.g., substance abusers, pregnant adolescents, and women bearing multiple fetuses, the subcommittee recommends a daily multivitamin supplement containing 2 mg of vitamin B_6. This level is slightly less than the current RDA of 2.2 mg during pregnancy (NRC, 1989).

Long-term use (>30 months) of oral contraceptives containing high levels of estrogen (e.g., 100 g of mestranol or ethinyl estradiol) was associated with significantly lower maternal and umbilical cord serum vitamin B_6 levels than those in women who took no oral contraceptives, and evidence indicates that their vitamin B_6 reserves may be decreased in early pregnancy (Roepke and Kirksey, 1979b). Donald and Bossé (1979), Leklem (1986), and Leklem et al. (1975) concluded that oral contraceptive use, for short periods, does not significantly increase the need for vitamin B_6. Concern has been expressed about women who routinely take oral contraceptives for several years to postpone their pregnancies (Miller, 1986). However, no data are available regarding the vitamin B_6 status of women taking the currently available oral contraceptives with low doses of estrogens (20 to 35 mg/day).

FOLATE

Folate is a generic descriptor of a group of compounds with chemical structures and nutritional properties similar to those of folic acid (pteroyl-glutamic acid).

Importance

In India, more than 50 years ago, Wills (1931) successfully treated macrocytic anemia in pregnant women with yeast extract; the active substance was later identified as folate. The etiologic role of folate deficiency in megaloblastic anemia of pregnancy and the efficacy of folate therapy in the treatment of this disease are now well established. The fundamental roles of folate in cell replication and metabolism continue to be active areas of investigation.

Folates function in intermediary metabolism as coenzymes in the transfer of single carbon units (formyl, methyl, and formimino) from one compound to another. This step is vital to many metabolic processes, including the metabolism of several amino acids and the synthesis of purine and thymidylate—compounds essential to nucleic acid synthesis. In light of these fundamental roles of folate, a deficiency of this vitamin in the early weeks of pregnancy might be expected to impair cell growth and replication and to result in anomalies in the fetus and placenta, leading to subsequent spontaneous abortion, fetal malformation, or small-for-gestational-age infants (Hibbard, 1975). However, scientific evidence for these associations is inconclusive.

Folate Status and the Course and Outcomes of Pregnancy

Inconsistent results have been obtained in clinical studies to determine the association of mild to moderate folate deficiencies with spontaneous abortion, preterm delivery, fetal malformations, and low birth weight. This is due in part to imprecise definitions of folate status as well as methodologic weaknesses in some of the studies in which no placebos were used and subjects were not randomized or blinded. Some investigators (Hibbard, 1975; Iyengar and Rajalakshmi, 1975) have reported a high incidence of obstetric complications such as spontaneous abortions, toxemia, preterm and small-for-gestational-age infants, and antepartum hemorrhage in folate-deficient populations, whereas others (Giles, 1966; Scott and Usher, 1966) have failed to observe such relationships.

Adverse pregnancy outcomes have been linked with impaired folate status in disadvantaged populations in which folate deficiency and adverse birth outcomes are relatively common. In Johannesburg, South Africa, for example, an oral 500-μg/day supplement of folic acid was associated with a 50% reduction in small-for-gestational-age newborns among Bantu women consuming a low-folate diet; a similar effect was not observed among white women, who consumed more fruits and vegetables (Baumslag et al., 1970). In low-income, malnourished women in Hyderabad, India, oral supplementation with 500 μg of folic acid and 60 mg of elemental iron daily was associated with a 50% reduction in the number of low-birth-weight infants (Iyengar and Rajalakshmi, 1975). A daily folate supplement of 500 μg was needed to maintain erythrocyte folate levels during pregnancy in Gambian women to ensure folate adequacy in the early stages of a subsequent pregnancy (Bates et al., 1986).

Unfortunately, several variables that might influence pregnancy outcomes were not always controlled in these studies. For example, subjects in the experimental groups were not uniformly controlled for age, weight, height, parity, previous pregnancy complications, socioeconomic status, prenatal care, or nutrient intake other than folate. There is no firm scientific evidence that the prophylactic use of folate lessens the complications or adverse outcomes of human pregnancy, with the exception of megaloblastic anemia.

Administration of folate antagonists such as aminopterin (4-amino folic acid) or methotrexate (methyl derivative of aminopterin) has consistently produced teratogenic effects in developing fetuses in both animals and humans. For example, when aminopterin was used as an abortifacient in humans, spontaneous abortions occurred in approximately 75% of the cases and the remaining fetuses were born grossly malformed (Goetsch, 1962; Thiersch, 1952, 1960), e.g., with fusion defects such as cleft lip and palate, hydrocephalus, and other major central nervous system deformities. The association of neural tube defects with folate and other nutrient deficiencies is discussed in Chapter 21.

Estimated Requirements for Pregnancy

Despite the crucial roles of folate in the synthesis of deoxyribonucleic acid (DNA) and in cell replication, the magnitude of the increased needs for folate during pregnancy has not been clearly defined. Dietary requirements rise with increased demands for the vitamin related to increased maternal erythropoiesis, uterine and mammary tissue growth, and placental and fetal growth. Requirements are further increased by greater urinary losses of the vitamin during pregnancy compared with those during nonpregnancy (Fleming, 1972; Landon and Hytten, 1971), but the percentage of folate absorption during pregnancy is unchanged (Iyengar and Babu, 1975).

The size of the folate body pool and equilibrium of the vitamin in relation to folate intake have not been assessed. Liver folate is a major portion of the body folate pool and the level of liver folate parallels the total body pool size (see review by Chanarin, 1979). Liver folate stores >3 μg/g (Hoppner and Lampi, 1980) and <1 μg/g (Gailani et al., 1970) have been suggested to reflect folate adequacy and deficiency, respectively. A dietary folate intake of 3 μg/kg of body weight has been reported to support adequate liver folate stores and to provide for a margin of safety in nonpregnant women (NRC, 1989; Reisenauer and Halsted, 1987).

To determine more precisely the magnitude of the increased folate need during pregnancy, a more complete understanding of cellular folate homeostasis and tissue folate requirements is required (Reisenauer and Halsted, 1987).

Criteria for Status Assessment

In advanced stages, folate deficiency is manifested as megaloblastic anemia, neutropenia, an increased number of hypersegmented polymorphs, and megaloblastic changes in bone marrow (Table 18-2). In earlier stages, these clinical signs may not be present, but the deficiency may be detected by biochemical indicators. The sequence of signs in the development of folate deficiency was observed in a healthy adult male placed on a folate-free diet (Herbert, 1962). In the first stage, serum folate dropped below normal levels. This was followed by an increased number of lobes on the nuclei of the polymorphonuclear leukocytes (hypersegmentation of neutrophils). After 4 months of folate deprivation, erythrocyte folate levels fell below normal and, subsequently, bone marrow became megaloblastic and anemia was evident.

Measurements of folate levels in serum and erythrocytes are the most widely used biochemical indices of folate status. Low serum levels have been used to indicate depleted folate stores (LSRO, 1984) but serve as a basis for treatment only when other signs have been observed. The decrease in serum folate levels during pregnancy has been partially attributed to blood volume expansion, increased urinary excretion of folate, and hormonal influences on folate metabolism. In some women, the continued depression of folate levels in serum and erythrocytes at 6 months postpartum suggested a chronic inadequacy of folate that failed to meet pregnancy needs and then was intensified postpartum (Bruinse et al., 1985). A study in Spain (Zamorano et al., 1985) showed that well-nourished, unsupplemented pregnant women did not have significant decreases in serum folate levels during their pregnancies.

Folate requirements increase rapidly during late pregnancy. This is reflected in decreased plasma folate levels, but not by the more slowly changing folate erythrocyte index (Chanarin, 1979). Nevertheless, researchers usually regard erythrocyte folate levels as the preferred indicator of folate status (Sauberlich, 1978). Erythrocyte folate levels are less sensitive than plasma indices to short-term changes in folate balance (Chanarin and Perry, 1977); a decrease in erythrocyte folate appears to reflect depletion of body folate stores. Neutrophil hypersegmentation (five or more nuclear lobes), ordinarily an early indicator of folate deficiency, is a poor indicator of folate status in pregnant women, since the number of lobes tends to decrease normally during pregnancy (Herbert et al., 1975).

Less commonly used assessment methods include folate functional tests, urinary excretion of formiminoglutamate, and the suppression of thymidine incorporation into DNA by deoxyuridine. Vitamin B_{12} deficiency may, however, complicate these tests, since it interferes with normal folate metabolism. Measurement of the increase in reticulocytes in response to folate administration may be a useful indicator of folate status. Giles and Shuttleworth (1958) showed that folic acid supplements produced a peak increase in reticulocytes—from 0 up to 5 to 10% of circulating red blood cells—in most folate-deficient patients within 5 to 10 days after treatment.

Usual Intake

Folates are present in a variety of foods and occur in especially high levels in liver, fortified or whole grain breads and cereals, dried peas and beans, leafy vegetables, fruit (Subar et al, 1989), and yeast. In usual U.S. diets, most folate (approximately 75%) is found as polyglutamates (Butterworth et al., 1963). Human requirements can be met by a variety of chemical folate forms as long as the essential subunit structure of pteridine, p-aminobenzoic acid, and glutamic acid remains intact. If this structure is broken, biologic activity is lost. Heat, oxidation, and ultraviolet light can cleave the folate molecule, destroying its nutritional value. Thus, certain conditions of storage or cooking can reduce the folate content of foods.

Studies of the intestinal absorption of folate in humans show that monoglutamyl and polyglutamyl folate, the predominant forms in food, have similar bioavailabilities of about 50 to 70%; intestinal hydrolysis of polyglutamyl folate does not appear to limit its absorption (Chandler et al., 1986; Halsted, 1979; Halsted et al., 1986). Absorption of folate monoglutamate and folate polyglutamate was approximately 90% and 50 to 90%, respectively, in the absence of food intake but was lower when taken with various foods (Colman et al., 1975; Tamura and Stokstad, 1973). Food composition and intestinal absorption data suggest that the bioavailability of folate in typical U.S. diets is approximately one-half to two-thirds that of supplemental folic acid ingested separately from food (Sauberlich et al., 1987).

Estimates of dietary folate for population subgroups in the United States are limited. Furthermore, food composition data for folates are incomplete and uncertain. In the United States, the first large-scale dietary survey to include folate was the Continuing Survey of Food Intake by Individuals (CSFII), which began in 1985 (USDA, 1987). CSFII data obtained that year indicated that the mean folate intake by women between the ages of 19 and 34 (all income levels) was 217 μg daily. A special analysis of NHANES II data (Subar et al., 1989) found a mean folate intake of 206 μg daily by women in the same age group. These results are similar to the 227 μg/capita per day estimate of Anderson and Talbot (1981), which was based on the average per-capita use of principal U.S. foods. Ordinarily, per-capita estimates are high, since they have not accounted for food wastage and losses during cooking and storage.

In Boston, Huber et al. (1988) studied 566 pregnant women who were primarily white, middle class, and age 20 or older. Only 48 women in this group derived folate entirely from diet; mean folate intake of this small subgroup was 257 μg/day. In contrast, women who consumed folate supplements (91.5%) had a mean intake of 1,087 μg/day. Intake ranged as high as 6,759 μg/day, which is 16 times the 1989 RDA (NRC, 1989). In comparison to supplemented women, mean serum and erythrocyte folate levels in unsupplemented women were significantly lower, but no other evidence of folate inadequacy was reported.

Prevalence of Inadequacy

In the United States, folate deficiency has not been clearly identified as a general medical problem (Anderson and Talbot, 1981), nor has its prevalence among pregnant women been determined by biochemical or other indices. Colman et al. (1975) have nevertheless suggested that the added burden of pregnancy increases the potential risk and prevalence of folate deficiency. The estimated prevalence of compromised folate status depends, in part, upon the population subgroup studied and the criteria used in making the diagnosis, as discussed below.

A high prevalence of folate inadequacy was reported among pregnant, low-income, predominantly black or Puerto Rican women living in New York City (Herbert et al., 1975) and in Florida (Bailey et al., 1980). In Florida, 48% of the study population was classified as folate deficient based on serum folate and 29% based on erythrocyte folate concentrations. In the New York sample, approximately 20% of the subjects were considered to be folate deficient based on serum folate and 16% on the basis of erythrocyte folate levels. No adjustments were made in these studies for the physiologic decline in these indices after midpregnancy. Furthermore, subjects with serum folate levels defined as deficient (i.e., <3 ng/ml) had no clinical manifestations of the deficiency.

Laboratory data on folate from the second National Health and Nutrition Examination Survey (NHANES II) (LSRO, 1984) show that within the U.S. population, the highest prevalence of low folate levels (serum level <3.0 ng/ml) and erythrocyte levels (<140 ng/ml) and, thus, the greatest risk of folate deficiency occurs among females (including a small number of pregnant women) aged 20 to 44. Of this population group, 15% had low serum folate, 13%, low erythrocyte folate, and 6%, both low serum and erythrocyte folate. The prevalence of low serum and erythrocyte folate was significantly greater among smokers than among nonsmokers and among nonusers of vitamin-mineral supplements than among users. Pregnancy, oral contraceptive use, and parity were also associated with low folate values among 22- to 44-year-old women.

Dosage Range and Toxicity

The safety of large doses of folic acid during pregnancy has not been systematically evaluated (Table 18-3). Low acute and chronic toxicity has been observed in nonpregnant adults. Folic acid is readily excreted in urine.

Large doses of folic acid may inhibit the absorption of other nutrients by competitive interaction (Ghishan et al., 1986; Simmer et al., 1987). They can also obscure the diagnosis of onset or relapse of pernicious anemia, which is extremely rare in women of childbearing age.

Ek (1980) has shown that plasma and erythrocyte folate levels in the fetus were two to four times higher than those in the mother. Since the effects of large maternal doses of folate on the developing fetus are not known, the subcommittee recommends that if folate supplements are used, they not exceed 300 μg/day as folic acid. This dose is higher than the total daily amount of folic acid needed by pregnant women (i.e., 200 μg/day), including those with poor folate stores, essentially no dietary folate, and multiple fetuses (Chanarin, 1985; Colman et al., 1975; NRC, 1989; Pritchard et al., 1969).

Recommendations for Supplementation

Pregnant women in the United States tend to consume less than the current RDA (NRC, 1989) of 400 μg of folate per day from food, have increased urinary losses of folate, and, especially if they are not supplemented, have a steady decrease in serum and erythrocyte folate levels. However, adequate folate for pregnancy can be obtained by regular consumption of fruits and vegetables in a well-selected diet (NRC, 1989). Thus, the subcommittee does not recommend routine folate supplementation during pregnancy but encourages daily use of fruits, vegetables, and whole grains and continued research to improve both the measurement of dietary folate and the assessment of requirements.

The subcommittee recommends modest supplementation for some segments of the U.S. population at risk of folate inadequacy, including some pregnant women who lack the knowledge or financial resources to purchase adequate food or who are abusers of alcohol, cigarettes, or drugs; or those who have malabsorption syndromes (LSRO, 1984). Pregnant adolescents and women bearing more than one fetus may also be at risk of folate deficiency. For these subpopulations, the subcommittee recommends folate supplements of 300 μg daily during pregnancy. This level has been recommended by several investigators (e.g., Chanarin, 1985; Colman et al., 1975; Hansen and Rybo, 1967; and Letsky, 1985).

OTHER WATER-SOLUBLE VITAMINS

The need for other water-soluble vitamins (vitamin C, thiamin, riboflavin, niacin, vitamin B_{12}, pantothenic acid, and biotin) is, in most cases, easily met by diet in the United States. Substantial amounts of thiamin, riboflavin, and niacin are provided by enriched and fortified grain and bakery products. Microfloral synthesis of pantothenic acid and biotin augment the dietary intake of those vitamins.

Blood levels of water-soluble vitamins typically decline progressively during pregnancy, and fetal blood levels become several times greater than those in maternal blood, reflecting active placental transport of the vitamins. These changes appear to be largely physiologic, and as shown in the few controlled clinical trials described in this section, they have not been associated with adverse effects on the course and outcomes of pregnancy.

Vitamin C

Importance and Estimated Requirements

Vitamin C is a collective term for two compounds—ascorbic acid (the predominant form) and dehydroascorbic acid. This vitamin functions as a chemical reducing agent; it reacts with free-radical derivatives of oxygen; and it is essential to several key hydroxylation reactions in the synthesis of procollagen, norepinephrine, and 5-hydroxytryptophan. Vitamin C is an electron donor in the metabolism of tyrosine, folate, histamine, and some drugs and is involved in the synthesis of carnitine and bile acids, release of corticosteroids, and incorporation of iron into ferritin (see reviews by Jaffe, 1984, and Olson and Hodges, 1987). It also plays a role in leukocyte function, immune responses, wound healing, and allergic reactions. Small amounts of vitamin C enhanced by two- to fourfold the intestinal absorption of nonheme iron from plant sources (Cook and Monsen, 1977). Vitamin C deficiency impairs the synthesis of collagen (a protein that gives structure to bones, cartilage, muscle, and blood vessels) (Barnes, 1975), which ultimately leads to the development of scurvy.

During pregnancy, plasma levels of vitamin C normally fall approximately 10 to 15% (Rivers and Devine, 1975), but they have not generally been associated with poor pregnancy outcomes. The decrease has been attributed largely to hormonal adjustments and blood volume expansion during pregnancy rather than to the increased vitamin C demands by maternal and fetal tissues. Increased intake of vitamin C may prevent or mitigate the fall in plasma levels (Vobecky et al., 1974). As a result of the placental concentration gradient, vitamin C levels in fetal blood at term may be 50% higher than those in maternal blood (Khattab et al., 1970). The amount of vitamin C estimated to meet the increased maternal and fetal needs during pregnancy is 10 mg/day more than that required to meet needs in the nonpregnant state (NRC, 1989) (Table 18-1).

Assessment Methodology

Some laboratory indicators of vitamin C nutritional status and clinical manifestations of deficiency are presented in Table 18-2. Among the status indicators, measurement of plasma vitamin C levels is the most practical procedure (Jacob et al., 1987; Sauberlich, 1978) and the most widely used, e.g., in NHANES II (McDowell et al., 1981). There is only limited information on leukocyte ascorbate levels during pregnancy. In contrast to levels in plasma, leukocyte levels have the possible advantage of reflecting slowly changing tissue levels (Jacob et al., 1987) and are therefore affected less by hemodilution or by changes in intake such as those that would accompany vomiting in early pregnancy. However, the methods of estimating leukocyte ascorbate levels are limited primarily to research settings, because they are complex and require relatively large samples of blood. Useful functional indicators of vitamin C status associated with marginally low and very high vitamin C intakes are needed, because such intakes are likely to be more common than deficiency during pregnancy.

Dosage Range and Toxicity

Vitamin C may have pharmacologic actions unrelated to its nutritional functions, but this has not been substantiated in well-controlled clinical studies (see reviews by Briggs, 1984, and Schrauzer, 1979). In nonpregnant adults, megadoses of vitamin C (>3 g/day) have occasionally resulted in stomach cramps, nausea, and diarrhea, particularly when ingested under fasting conditions, and in allergic skin rash and a few isolated cases of intestinal and urinary lithiasis (Smith, 1978). Large doses of vitamin C may also contribute to false results in some clinical tests (e.g., false-positive results for urinary glucose) and may alter the potencies of certain drugs (Briggs, 1978; Flodin, 1988; Houston and Levy, 1975; Ovesen, 1979).

The frequency of reported toxic manifestations of megadoses of vitamin C (Table 18-3) is low relative to the number of persons who routinely ingest large amounts of the vitamin (Rivers, 1987). Because the vitamin is actively transported from placental to fetal blood, megadoses taken during pregnancy could lead to markedly elevated ascorbate levels in the fetus and a potential for adverse effects.

Vitamin C dependency is purported to result from megadoses of vitamin C consumed over time, but has not been confirmed experimentally (Hornig and Moser, 1981). This condition has been described (Alhadeff et al., 1984; Rhead and Schrauzer, 1971) as occurring in individuals who become adapted over time to megadoses of vitamin C by an increased rate of metabolism and excretion; then, following an abrupt lowering of vitamin C intake, they develop signs of deficiency. Concern that fetal vitamin C dependency can be induced in utero by excessive intakes of the vitamin during pregnancy is based on only one anecdotal report (Cochrane, 1965). Two infants, whose mothers were reported to be supplemented with 400 mg of ascorbic acid daily during pregnancy, developed scurvy during the first few weeks postnatally. However, this was observed in a region of Canada where infantile scurvy was relatively frequent. There is no clear evidence that the scorbutic findings were related to excessive maternal intake of vitamin C.

Other Considerations

Some subpopulations follow practices that increase their need for, or result in low dietary intake of, vitamin C. These include users of street drugs and cigarettes (see Chapter 20), heavy users of alcohol, long-term users of oral contraceptives (Irwin and Hutchins, 1976), and regular users of aspirin and salicylates (Flodin, 1988). Women bearing more than one fetus (e.g., twins or triplets) may also require somewhat higher amounts of vitamin C. For women at risk of deficiency, an ascorbic acid supplement of 50 mg/day is recommended if increased consumption of fruits and vegetables is unlikely.

Heavy smokers ($\geq$20 cigarettes/day) need perhaps twice as much vitamin C as nonsmokers to maintain a similar body pool of vitamin C (Kallner et al., 1981). Smokers have decreased plasma ascorbate levels, which are associated with an increased rate of vitamin C metabolism rather than with changes in absorption or urinary excretion.

Thiamin, Riboflavin, and Niacin

Importance and Estimated Requirements

Among the B-complex vitamins, thiamin, riboflavin, and niacin function primarily in the release of energy in cells. Thiamin as thiamin pyrophosphate is essential to key reactions in energy metabolism, especially carbohydrate metabolism. Riboflavin functions primarily as a component of flavin mononucleotide and flavin adenine dinucleotide, both of which catalyze oxidation-reduction reactions. Niacin is a collective term for nicotinic acid, nicotinamide, and niacinamide. Nicotinamide functions as a component of two important coenzymes, nicotinamide adenine dinucleotide and nicotinamide adenine dinucleotide phosphate. Niacin is present in all cells and participates in several metabolic processes, including glycolysis, fatty acid metabolism, and tissue respiration. Because of this involvement of thiamin, riboflavin, and niacin in energy metabolism, these vitamins are needed during pregnancy in amounts proportional to the increased energy requirements (Table 18-1). Niacin intake is usually reported in niacin equivalents, since some of the amino acid tryptophan is converted to niacin in vivo. A niacin equivalent is equal to 1 mg of niacin or 60 mg of tryptophan. Pregnant women have been reported to have an enhanced capacity to convert tryptophan to niacin (Wertz et al., 1958), which could lessen the need for increased dietary niacin during pregnancy. In animal experiments, severe deficiencies of thiamin, riboflavin, or niacin result in fetal death, low birth weight, and congenital defects. However, no analogous findings in humans have been demonstrated.

Assessment Methodology

Laboratory indicators of thiamin, riboflavin, and niacin status are given in Table 18-2 (see the review by Sauberlich, 1978). The most widely used procedures for assessing thiamin nutritional status are measurements of urinary thiamin levels, of erythrocyte transketolase activity and its stimulation by thiamin pyrophosphate added in vitro, and of erythrocyte glutathione reductase activity. The latter measurement is simple and reproducible and requires only a small sample of blood. Measurement of two major metabolites of niacin in urine, N^1-methylnicotinamide and N^1-methyl-2-pyridone-5-carboxylamide (2-pyridone), has been the usual means of assessing niacin status. Although the ratio of 2-pyridone to N^1-methylnicotinamide appears to be the most practical index of niacin status, its reliability and usefulness in pregnant women is not fully established (Sauberlich, 1978).

There is a steady decrease in urinary riboflavin excretion during pregnancy and a progressive increase to 20% in the activation of erythrocyte glutathione reductase following in vitro incubation with the vitamin (Heller et al., 1974). When compared with nonpregnant norms, these findings indicate riboflavin inadequacy. However, the findings were not associated with adverse effects on the course or outcomes of pregnancy.

Usual Intake

CSFII (USDA, 1987) showed that adult women consumed 116% of the 1.2-mg RDA for riboflavin (NRC, 1989). In the same survey, preformed niacin in diets consumed by women aged 19 to 50 averaged 16 mg/day and calculated niacin equivalents (NE) were 27 mg/day, both of which exceeded the 1980 RDA of 13 NE (NRC, 1980). The 1989 RDA is 15 NE (NRC, 1989). Enriched and fortified grains, cereals, and bakery products contribute substantial amounts of thiamin, riboflavin, and niacin to the U.S. diet (Cook and Welsh, 1987). The data in Chapter 13, Table 13-2, also suggest that the usual intake of these nutrients is adequate.

Dosage Range and Toxicity

In nonpregnant humans, no toxic effects have been reported for thiamin, riboflavin, and niacin following long-term high-dose (100 to 200 mg/day) oral supplements of the vitamins, except for some gastric upset. No cases of riboflavin toxicity in humans have been reported, perhaps because the gastrointestinal tract has a limited capacity to absorb riboflavin (McCormick, 1988). Nicotinic acid is not toxic at physiologic levels, but pharmacologic doses of 3 to 9 g/day result in vasodilation (flushing), various metabolic effects, and gastrointestinal problems (Hankes, 1984). Nicotinamide is generally well tolerated (Flodin, 1988).

Vitamin B_{12}

Vitamin B_{12} is a group of cobalamins, i.e., cobalt-containing corrinoids with a tetrapyrrole structure resembling that of iron porphyrins. The predominant forms of the vitamin in plasma and tissues are methylcobalamin, adenosylcobalamin, and hydroxycobalamin. Cyanocobalamin is present in very small amounts in the body. Since it is the most stable form, it is used in vitamin supplements. Both cobalamin and folate function in the transport of single carbon atoms in reactions that are necessary for the synthesis of nucleic acids and the metabolism of certain amino acids. Thus, normal cell division and protein synthesis during pregnancy are dependent upon an adequacy of both vitamins.

Vitamin B_{12} is supplied by animal protein foods, including meat, fish, eggs, and milk. The needs of pregnancy can be easily met by body stores or by diets that provide modest amounts of animal protein foods. Vegetarian diets that include eggs, milk, and cheese provide adequate vitamin B_{12} for pregnancy needs (Immerman, 1981). Since a healthy fetus is estimated to contain about 50 μg of vitamin B_{12}, compared with maternal stores of approximately 3,000 μg, the drain on maternal stores for vitamin B_{12} is usually slight (Immerman, 1981). The 1989 RDA of 2.2 μg/day during pregnancy (Table 18-1) is based on estimates of fetal needs of 0.1 to 0.2 μg/day and increased metabolism during pregnancy (NRC, 1989). An effective enterohepatic circulation recycles vitamin B_{12} from bile and other intestinal secretions, accounting for its long biologic half-life.

Clinical deficiency of vitamin B_{12} is usually secondary to abnormalities of gastrointestinal function. Deficiency caused by diet is very rare but is occasionally observed in adult vegans—complete vegetarians—who have followed an egg- and milk-free vegetarian diet for many years. If these individuals had previously consumed animal foods, their accumulated liver stores could protect them for several years (Immerman, 1981). In a few isolated cases, infants born to mothers who were complete vegetarians have manifested signs of vitamin B_{12} deficiency during the first few months of life (Higginbottom et al., 1978; Sklar, 1986). In view of these findings, the subcommittee recommends a daily vitamin B_{12} supplement of 2.0 μg for complete vegetarians.

Neither oral nor injectable cyanocobalamin has been found to be toxic to nonpregnant adults when administered in quantities several thousand times the daily requirement (LSRO, 1978), but the effects of excessive vitamin B_{12} intake on the fetus have not been investigated.

Pantothenic Acid

Pantothenic acid is present in all living cells, mostly in the form of coenzyme A—an essential cofactor in the transfer of acetyl groups. A second active form of the vitamin is acyl carrier protein—a component of fatty acid synthetase complex. The vitamin is widely distributed in foods, especially in meats, whole-grain cereals, nuts, and legumes. Synthesis of pantothenic acid by intestinal bacteria possibly supplements the dietary intake of this vitamin. Spontaneous deficiency of pantothenic acid has not been observed in humans, except in cases of extreme malnutrition. Experimentally induced deficiency symptoms are intermittent diarrhea, insomnia, leg cramps, and paresthesias. Song et al. (1985) suggest that pregnant women need greater amounts of pantothenate than do nonpregnant women to maintain plasma levels and that such amounts are obtainable from food. Pantothenic acid toxicity in humans has not been reported. Occasional diarrhea is the only side effect reported to result from daily calcium pantothenate doses of 10 to 20 mg (Fox, 1984).

Biotin

Biotin is a sulfur-containing vitamin and a coenzyme for several important carboxylation reactions. Because it is synthesized by intestinal bacteria, spontaneous deficiency has not been observed in humans. A deficiency was produced experimentally in nonpregnant humans by feeding them large amounts of raw egg whites, which contain avidin—a biotin-binding protein. Symptoms of deficiency include seborrheic dermatitis, anorexia, muscle pain, and alopecia. Since biotin is widely distributed in food, needs are easily met by diet. Microflora synthesis also contributes to the biotin requirement. Blood levels of biotin fall progressively during pregnancy, but this has not been associated with adverse outcomes (Bonjour, 1984). No toxic effects of biotin were observed in nonpregnant humans following oral doses as high as 10 to 40 mg/day in the treatment of carboxylase deficiencies (Packman et al., 1981, 1985), but studies of toxicity during pregnancy have not been reported.

CLINICAL IMPLICATIONS

• Data do not provide a firm basis for recommending routine supplementation of the general U.S. population of pregnant women with water-soluble vitamins.

• Laboratory tests for assessment of water-soluble vitamin status are not sufficiently precise or practical to be recommended for routine prenatal care.

• When dietary sources are inadequate, daily supplementation with 300 μg of folate, 2 mg of vitamin B_6, and 50 mg of vitamin C is recommended.

• For complete vegetarians, a daily vitamin B_{12} supplement of 2.0 μg is recommended.

• Special attention should be given to improving the diet of and administering supplements to pregnant adolescents, women bearing more than one fetus, users of cigarettes or street drugs, heavy users of alcohol, and pregnant women at nutritional risk because of poor nutritional knowledge or insufficient financial resources to purchase adequate food.

• Supplemental water-soluble vitamins exceeding the RDA should be avoided during pregnancy, since evidence of their therapeutic efficacy is inconclusive and there is a potential risk for detrimental nutrient-nutrient interactions and for toxicity, especially to the fetus.

REFERENCES

Alhadeff, L., C.T. Gualtieri, and M. Lipton. 1984. Toxic effects of water-soluble vitamins. Nutr. Rev. 42:33-40.

American Medical Association Council on Drugs. 1979. American Medical Association Drug Evaluations, 4th ed. Publishing Sciences, Littleton, Mass. 417 pp.

Anderson, S.A., and J.M. Talbot. 1981. IV. Folate status in the North American population. Pp. 11-25 in A Review of Folate Intake, Methodology, and Status. Life Sciences Research Office, Federation of American Societies for Experimental Biology, Rockville, Md.

Apgar, V., and L.S. James. 1962. Further observations on the newborn scoring system. Am. J. Dis. Child. 104:419-428.

Apgar, V., D.A. Holaday, L.S. James, I.M. Weisbrot, and C. Berrien. 1958. Evaluation of the newborn infant—second report. J. Am. Med. Assoc. 168:1985-1988.

Bailey, L.B., C.S. Mahan, and D. Dimperio. 1980. Folacin and iron status in low-income pregnant adolescents and mature women. Am. J. Clin. Nutr. 33:1997-2001.

Barnes, M.J. 1975. Function of ascorbic acid in collagen metabolism. Ann. N.Y. Acad. Sci. 258:264-277.

Bates, C.J., N.J. Fuller, and A.M. Prentice. 1986. Folate status during pregnancy and lactation in a West African rural community. Hum. Nutr.: Clin. Nutr. 40C:3-13.

Baumslag, N., T. Edelstein, and J. Metz. 1970. Reduction of incidence of prematurity by folic acid supplementation in pregnancy. Br. Med. J. 1:16-17.

Bonjour, J.P. 1984. Biotin. Pp. 403-435 in L.J. Machlin, ed. Handbook of Vitamins: Nutritional, Biochemical and Clinical Aspects. Marcel Dekker, New York.

Briggs, M.H. 1978. Effect of specific nutrient toxicities in animals and man: vitamin C. Pp. 65-70 in M. Rechcigl, Jr., ed. CRC Handbook Series in Nutrition and Food. Section E: Nutritional Disorders, Vol. I. Effect of Nutrient Excesses and Toxicities in Animals and Man. CRC Press, West Palm Beach, Fla.

Briggs, M. 1984. Vitamin C and infectious disease: a review of the literature and the results of a randomized, double-blind, prospective study over 8 years. Pp. 39-81 in M.H. Briggs, ed. Recent Vitamin Research. CRC Press, Boca Raton, Fla.

Brophy, M.H., and P.K. Siiteri. 1975. Pyridoxal phosphate and hypertensive disorders of pregnancy. Am. J. Obstet. Gynecol. 121:1075-1079.

Bruinse, H.W., H. van den Berg, and A.A. Haspels. 1985. Maternal serum folacin levels during and after normal pregnancy. Eur. J. Obstet., Gynecol. Reprod. Biol. 20:153-158.

Butterworth, C.E., Jr., R. Santini, Jr., and W.B. Frommeyer, Jr. 1963. The pteroylglutamate components of American diets as determined by chromatographic fractionation. J. Clin. Invest. 42:1929-1939.

Chanarin, I. 1979. Distribution of folate deficiency. Pp. 7-10 in M.I. Botez and E.H. Reynolds, eds. Folic Acid in Neurology, Psychiatry, and Internal Medicine. Raven Press, New York.

Chanarin, I. 1985. Folate and cobalamin. Clin. Haematol. 14:629-641.

Chanarin, I., and J. Perry. 1977. Mechanisms in the production of megaloblastic anemia. Pp. 156-168 in Folic Acid: Biochemistry and Physiology in Relation to the Human Nutrition Requirement. Proceedings of a Workshop on Human Folate Requirements. Report of the Food and Nutrition Board. National Academy of Sciences, Washington, D.C.

Chandler, C.J., T.T.Y. Wang, and C.H. Halsted. 1986. Pteroylpolyglutamate hydrolase from human jejunal brush borders. J. Biol. Chem. 261:928-933.

Cleary, R.E., L. Lumeng, and T.K. Li. 1975. Maternal and fetal plasma levels of pyridoxal phosphate at term: adequacy of vitamin B_6 supplementation during pregnancy. Am. J. Obstet. Gynecol. 121:25-28.

Cochrane, W.A. 1965. Overnutrition in prenatal and neonatal life: a problem? Can. Med. Assoc. J. 93:893-899.

Cohen, M. and A. Bendich. 1986. Safety of pyridoxine—a review of human and animal studies. Toxicol. Lett. 34:129-139.

Colman, N., J.V. Larsen, M. Barker, E.A. Barker, R. Green, and J. Metz. 1975. Prevention of folate deficiency by food fortification. III. Effect in pregnant subjects of varying amounts of added folic acid. Am. J. Clin. Nutr. 28:465-470.

Contractor, S.F., and B. Shane. 1970. Blood and urine levels of vitamin B_6 in the mother and fetus before and after loading of mother with vitamin B_6. Am. J. Obstet. Gynecol. 107:635-640.

Cook, J.D., and E.R. Monsen. 1977. Vitamin C, the common cold, and iron absorption. Am. J. Clin. Nutr. 30:235-241.

Cook, D.A., and S.O. Welsh. 1987. The effect of enriched and fortified grain products on nutrient intake. Cereal Foods World 32:191-196.

Donald, E.A., and T.R. Bossé. 1979. The vitamin B_6 requirement in oral contraceptive users. II. Assessment by tryptophan metabolites, vitamin B_6, and pyridoxic acid levels in urine. Am. J. Clin. Nutr. 32:1024-1032.

Dorsey, C.W. 1949. The use of pyridoxine and suprarenal cortex combined in the treatment of the nausea and vomiting of pregnancy. Am. J. Obstet. Gynecol. 58:1073-1078.

Ek, J. 1980. Plasma and red cell folate values in newborn infants and their mothers in relation to gestational age. J. Pediatr. 97:288-292.

Fleming, A.F. 1972. Urinary excretion of folate in pregnancy. J. Obstet. Gynaecol. Br. Commonw. 79:916-920.

Flodin, N.W. 1988. Pharmacology of Micronutrients. Current Topics in Nutrition and Disease, Vol. 20. Alan R. Liss, New York. 340 pp.

Fox, H.M. 1984. Pantothenic acid. Pp. 437-457 in L.J. Machlin, ed. Handbook of Vitamins: Nutritional, Biochemical, and Clinical Aspects. Marcel Dekker, New York.

Gailani, S.D., R.W. Carey, J.F. Holland, and J.A. O'Malley. 1970. Studies of folate deficiency in patients with neoplastic diseases. Cancer Res. 30:327-333.

Ghishan, F.K., H.M. Said, P.C. Wilson, J.E. Murrell, and H.L. Greene. 1986. Intestinal transport of zinc and folic acid: a mutual inhibitory effect. Am. J. Clin. Nutr. 43:258-262.

Giles, C. 1966. An account of 335 cases of megaloblastic anaemia of pregnancy and the puerperium. J. Clin. Pathol. 19:1-11.

Giles, C., and E.M. Shuttleworth. 1958. Megaloblastic anaemia of pregnancy and the puerperium. Lancet 2:1341-1347.

Goetsch, C. 1962. An evaluation of aminopterin as an abortifacient. Am. J. Obstet. Gynecol. 83:1474-1477.

Halsted, C.H. 1979. The intestinal absorption of folates. Am. J. Clin. Nutr. 32:846-855.

Halsted, C.H., W.H. Beer, C.J. Chandler, K. Ross, B.M. Wolfe, L. Bailey, and J.J. Cerda. 1986. Clinical studies of intestinal folate conjugates. J. Lab. Clin. Med. 107:228-232.

Hamfelt, A., and T. Tuvemo. 1972. Pyridoxal phosphate and folic acid concentration in blood and erythrocyte aspartate aminotransferase activity during pregnancy. Clin. Chim. Acta 41:287-298.

Hanck, A. 1982. Tolerance and effects of high doses of ascorbic acid. Dosis facit venenum. Int. J. Vit. Nutr. Res., Suppl. 23:221-238.

Hankes, L.V. 1984. Nicotinic acid and nicotinamide. Pp. 329-377 in L.J. Machlin, ed. Handbook of Vitamins: Nutritional, Biochemical, and Clinical Aspects. Marcel Dekker, New York.

Hansen, H., and G. Rybo. 1967. Folic acid dosage in profylactic treatment during pregnancy. Acta Obstet. Gynecol. Scand., Suppl. 7:107-112.

Heller, S., R.M. Salkeld, and W.F. Körner. 1974. Riboflavin status in pregnancy. Am. J. Clin. Nutr. 27:1225-1230.

Hellström, L. 1971. Lack of toxicity of folic acid given in pharmacological doses to healthy volunteers. Lancet 1:59-61.

Herbert, V. 1962. Experimental nutritional folate deficiency in man. Trans. Assoc. Am. Physicians 75:307-320.

Herbert, V., N. Colman, M. Spivack, E. Ocasio, V. Ghanta, K. Kimmel, L. Brenner, J. Freundlich, and J. Scott. 1975. Folic acid deficiency in the United States: folate assays in a prenatal clinic. Am. J. Obstet. Gynecol. 123:175-179.

Hesseltine, H.C. 1946. Pyridoxine failure in nausea and vomiting of pregnancy. Am. J. Obstet. Gynecol. 51:82-86.

Hibbard, B.M. 1975. Folates and the fetus. S. Afr. Med. J. 49:1223-1226.

Higginbottom, M.C., L. Sweetman, and W.L. Nyhan. 1978. A syndrome of methylmalonic aciduria, homocystinuria, megaloblastic anemia and neurologic abnormalities in a vitamin B_{12}-deficient breast-fed infant of a strict vegetarian. N. Engl. J. Med. 299:317-323.

Hoppner, K., and B. Lampi. 1980. Folate levels in human liver from autopsies in Canada. Am. J. Clin. Nutr. 33:862-864.

Hornig, D.H., and U. Moser. 1981. The safety of high vitamin C intakes in man. Pp. 225-248 in J.N. Counsell and D.H. Hornig, eds. Vitamin C (Ascorbic Acid). Applied Science Publishers, London.

Houston, J.B., and G. Levy. 1975. Modification of drug biotransformation by vitamin C in man. Nature 255:78-79.

Huber, A.M., L.L. Wallins, and P. DeRusso. 1988. Folate nutriture in pregnancy. J. Am. Diet. Assoc. 88:791-795.

Hunt, A.D., Jr., J. Stokes, Jr., W.W. McCrory, and H.H. Stroud. 1954. Pyridoxine dependency: report of a case of intractable convulsions in an infant controlled by pyridoxine. Pediatrics 13:140-145.

Hunter, R., J. Barnes, H.F. Oakeley, and D.M. Matthews. 1970. Toxicity of folic acid given in pharmacological doses to healthy volunteers. Lancet 1:61-63.

Immerman, A.M. 1981. Vitamin B_{12} status on a vegetarian diet. World Rev. Nutr. Diet. 37:38-54.

Irwin, M.I., and B.K. Hutchins. 1976. A conspectus of research on vitamin C requirements of man. J. Nutr. 106:821-880.

Iyengar, L., and S. Babu. 1975. Folic acid absorption in pregnancy. Br. J. Obstet. Gynaecol. 82:20-23.

Iyengar, L., and K. Rajalakshmi. 1975. Effect of folic acid supplement on birth weights of infants. Am. J. Obstet. Gynecol. 122:332-336.

Jacob, R.A., J.H. Skala, and S.T. Omaye. 1987. Biochemical indices of human vitamin C status. Am. J. Clin. Nutr. 46:818-826.

Jaffe, G.M. 1984. Vitamin C. Pp. 199-244 in L.J. Machlin, ed. Handbook of Vitamins: Nutritional, Biochemical, and Clinical Aspects. Marcel Dekker, New York.

Kallner, A.B., D. Hartmann, and D.H. Hornig. 1981. On the requirements of ascorbic acid in man: steady-state turnover and body pool in smokers. Am. J. Clin. Nutr. 34:1347-1355.

Khattab, A.K., S.A. Al Nagdy, K.A.H. Mourad, and H.I. El Azghal. 1970. Foetal maternal ascorbic acid gradient in normal Egyptian subjects. J. Trop. Pediatr. 16:112-115.

Landon, M.J., and F.E. Hytten. 1971. The excretion of folate in pregnancy. Br. J. Obstet. Gynaecol. Br. Commonw. 78:769-775.

Leathem, A.M. 1986. Safety and efficacy of antiemetics used to treat nausea and vomiting in pregnancy. Clin. Pharmacol. 5:660-668.

Leklem, J.E. 1986. Vitamin B_6 requirement and oral contraceptive use—a concern? J. Nutr. 116:475-477.

Leklem, J.E., and R.D. Reynolds. 1988. Challenges and directions in the search for clinical applications of vitamin B_6. Pp. 437-454 in J.E. Leklem and R.D. Reynolds, eds. Current Topics in Nutrition and Disease, Vol. 19. Clinical and Physiological Applications of Vitamin B_6. Alan R. Liss, New York.

Leklem, J.E., R.R. Brown, D.P. Rose, H. Linkswiler, and R.A. Arend. 1975. Metabolism of tryptophan and niacin in oral contraceptive users receiving controlled intakes of vitamin B_6. Am. J. Clin. Nutr. 28:146-156.

Letsky, E.A. 1985. Folic acid in pregnancy. Farm. Terap. 2:147-152.

LSRO (Life Sciences Research Office). 1978. Evaluation of the Health Aspects of Vitamin B_{12} as a Food Ingredient. Federation of American Societies for Experimental Biology, Bethesda, Md. 26 pp.

LSRO (Life Sciences Research Office). 1984. Assessment of the Folate Nutritional Status of the U.S. Population Based on Data Collected in the Second National Health and Nutrition Examination Survey, 1976-1980. Federation of American Societies for Experimental Biology, Bethesda, Md. 96 pp.

Lu, J.Y., D.L. Cook, J.B. Javia, Z.A. Kirmani, C.C. Liu, D.N. Makadia, T.A. Makadam, O.B. Omasayie, D.P. Patel, V.J. Reddy, B.W. Walker, C.S. Williams, and R.A. Chung. 1981. Intakes of vitamins and minerals by pregnant women with selected clinical symptoms. J. Am. Diet. Assoc. 78:477-482.

Lumeng, L., R.E. Cleary, R. Wagner, P.L. Yu, and T.K. Li. 1976. Adequacy of vitamin B_6 supplementation during pregnancy: a prospective study. Am. J. Clin. Nutr. 29:1376-1383.

McCormick, D.B. 1988. Riboflavin. Pp. 362-369 in M.E. Shils and V.R. Young, eds. Modern Nutrition in Health and Disease, 7th ed. Lea & Febiger, Philadelphia.

McDowell, A., A. Engel, J.T. Massey, and K. Maurer. 1981. Plan and Operation of the Second National Health and Nutrition Examination Survey, 1976-80. Vital and Health Statistics, Series 1, No. 15. DHHS Publ. No. (PHS) 81-1317. National Center for Health Statistics, Public Health Service, U.S. Department of Health and Human Services, Hyattsville, Md. 144 pp.

Mentzer, W.C., Jr., and E. Collier. 1975. Hydrops fetalis associated with erythrocyte G-6-PD deficiency and maternal ingestion of fava beans and ascorbic acid. J. Pediatr. 86:565-567.

Miller, L.T. 1986. Do oral contraceptive agents affect nutrient requirements-vitamin B_6? J. Nutr. 116:1344-1345.

NRC (National Research Council). 1980. Recommended Dietary Allowances, 9th ed. Report of the Committee on Dietary Allowances, Food and Nutrition Board, Division of Biological Sciences, Assembly of Life Sciences. National Academy Press, Washington, D.C. 185 pp.

NRC (National Research Council). 1989. Recommended Dietary Allowances, 10th ed. Report of the Subcommittee on the Tenth Edition of the RDAs, Food and Nutrition Board, Commission on Life Sciences. National Academy Press, Washington, D.C. 284 pp.

Olson, J.A., and R.E. Hodges. 1987. Recommended dietary intakes (RDI) of vitamin C in humans. Am. J. Clin. Nutr. 45:693-703.

Ovesen, L. 1979. Drugs and vitamin deficiency. Drugs 18:278-298.

Packman, S., L. Sweetman, H. Baker, and S. Wall. 1981. The neonatal form of biotin-responsive multiple carboxylase deficiency. J. Pediatr. 99:418-420.

Packman, S., M.S. Golbus, M.J. Cowan, L. Sweetman, W. Nyhan, B.J. Burri, and H. Baker. 1985. Prenatal treatment of biotin-responsive multiple carboxylase deficiency. Ann. N.Y. Acad. Sci. 447:414-416.

Pitkin, R.M. 1982. Megadose nutrients during pregnancy. Pp. 203-211 in Alternative Dietary Practices and Nutritional Abuses in Pregnancy: Proceedings of a Workshop. Report of the Committee on Nutrition of the Mother and Preschool Child, Food and Nutrition Board, Commission on Life Sciences. National Academy Press, Washington, D.C.

Pritchard, J.A., D.E. Scott, and P.J. Whalley. 1969. Folic acid requirements in pregnancy-induced megaloblastic anemia. J. Am. Med. Assoc. 208:1163-1167.

Pulkkinen, M.O., J. Salminen, and S. Virtanen. 1978. Serum vitamin B_6 in pure pregnancy depression. Acta Obstet. Gynecol. Scand. 57:471-472.

Reinken, L., and O. Dapunt. 1978. Vitamin B_6 nutriture during pregnancy. Int. J. Vitam. Nutr. Res. 48:341-347.

Reisenauer, A.M., and C.H. Halsted. 1987. Human folate requirements. J. Nutr. 117:600-602.

Reynolds, R.D., M. Polansky, and P.B. Moser. 1984. Analyzed vitamin B_6 intakes of pregnant and postpartum lactating and nonlactating women. J. Am. Diet. Assoc. 84:1339-1344.

Rhead, W.J., and G.N. Schrauzer. 1971. Risks of long term ascorbic acid overdose. Nutr. Rev. 29:262-263.

Rivers, J.M. 1987. Safety of high-level vitamin C ingestion. Ann. N.Y. Acad. Sci. 498:445-454.

Rivers, J.M., and M.M. Devine. 1975. Relationships of ascorbic acid to pregnancy and oral contraceptive steroids. Ann. N.Y. Acad. Sci. 258:465-482.

Robie, T.R. 1967. Cyroheptadine: an excellent antidote for niacin-induced hyperthermia. J. Schizophr. 1:133-139.

Roepke, J.L.B., and A. Kirksey. 1979a. Vitamin B_6 nutriture during pregnancy and lactation. I. Vitamin B_6 intake, levels of the vitamin in biological fluids, and condition of the infant at birth. Am. J. Clin. Nutr. 32:2249-2256.

Roepke, J.L.B., and A. Kirksey. 1979b. Vitamin B_6 nutriture during pregnancy and lactation. II. The effect of long-term use of oral contraceptives. Am. J. Clin. Nutr. 32:2257-2264.

Rose, D.P. 1978. The interactions between vitamin B_6 and hormones. Pp. 53-99 in P.L. Munson, E. Diczfalusy, J. Glover, and R.E. Olson, eds. Vitamins and Hormones: Advances in Research and Applications, Vol. 36. Academic Press, New York.

Sauberlich, H.E. 1978. Vitamin indices. Pp. 109-156 in Laboratory Indices of Nutritional Status in Pregnancy. Report of the Committee on Nutrition of the Mother and Preschool Child, Food and Nutrition Board. National Academy of Sciences, Washington, D.C.

Sauberlich, H.E., M.J. Kretsch, J.H. Skala, H.L. Johnson, and P.C. Taylor. 1987. Folate requirement and metabolism in nonpregnant women. Am. J. Clin. Nutr. 46:1016-1028.

Schaumburg, H., J. Kaplan, A. Windebank, N. Vick, S. Rasmus, D. Pleasure, and M.J. Brown. Sensory neuropathy from pyridoxine abuse: a new megavitamin syndrome. N. Engl. J. Med. 309:445-448.

Schrauzer, G.N. 1979. Vitamin C: conservative human requirements and aspects of overdosage. Int. Rev. Biochem. 27:167-188.

Schuster, K., L.B. Bailey, and C.S. Mahan. 1981. Vitamin B_6 status of low-income adolescent and adult pregnant women and the condition of their infants at birth. Am. J. Clin. Nutr. 34:1731-1735.

Schuster, K., L.B. Bailey, and C.S. Mahan. 1984. Effect of maternal pyridoxine-HCl supplementation on the vitamin B_6 status of mother and infant and on pregnancy outcome. J. Nutr. 114:977-988.

Scott, K.E., and R. Usher. 1966. Fetal malnutrition: its incidence, causes, and effects. Am. J. Obstet. Gynecol. 94:951-963.

Shane, B., and S.F. Contractor. 1975. Assessment of vitamin B_6 status. Studies on pregnant women and oral contraceptive users. Am. J. Clin. Nutr. 28:739-747.

Shane, B., and S.F. Contractor. 1980. Vitamin B_6 status and metabolism in pregnancy. Pp. 137-171 in G.P. Tryfiates, ed. Vitamin B_6 Metabolism and Role in Growth. Foods & Nutrition Press, Westport, Conn.

Simmer, K., C. James, and R.P.H. Thompson. 1987. Are iron-folate supplements harmful? Am. J. Clin. Nutr. 45:122-125.

Sklar, R. 1986. Nutritional vitamin B_{12} deficiency in a breast-fed infant of a vegan-diet mother. Clin. Pediatr. 25:219-221.

Smith, L.H. 1978. Risk of oxalate stones from large doses of vitmain C. N. Engl. J. Med. 298:856.

Song, W.O., B.W. Wyse, and R.G. Hansen. 1985. Pantothenic acid status of pregnant and lactating women. J. Am. Diet. Assoc. 85:192-198.

Spellacy, W.N., W.C. Buhi, and S.A. Birk. 1977. Vitamin B_6 treatment of gestational diabetes mellitus: studies of blood glucose and plasma insulin. Am. J. Obstet. Gynecol. 127:599-602.

Subar, A.F., G. Block, and L.D. James. 1989. Folate intake and food sources in the US population. Am. J. Clin. Nutr. 50:508-516.

Tamura, T., and E.L.R. Stokstad. 1973. The availability of food folate in man. Br. J. Haematol. 25:513-532.

Thiersch, J.B. 1952. Therapeutic abortions with a folic acid antagonist, 4-aminopteroylglutamic acid (4-amino P.G.A.) administered by the oral route. Am. J. Obstet. Gynecol. 63:1298-1304.

Thiersch, J.B. 1960. Teratogenic effects of pteroylglutamic acid deficiency in the rat: discussion. Pp. 152-154 in G.E.W. Wolstenholme and C.M. O'Connor, eds. Ciba Foundation Symposium on Congenital Malformations. Little, Brown, Boston.

USDA (U.S. Department of Agriculture). 1987. Nationwide Food Consumption Survey. Continuing Survey of Food Intakes by Individuals. Women 19-50 Years and Their Children 1-5 Years, 1 Day, 1986. Report No. 86-1. Nutrition Monitoring Division, Human Nutrition Information Service, U.S. Department of Agriculture, Hyattsville, Md. 98 pp.

van den Berg, H. 1988. Vitamin and mineral status in healthy pregnant women. Pp. 93-108 in H. Berger, ed. Vitamins and Minerals in Pregnancy and Lactation. Vevey/Raven Press, New York.

van den Berg, H., and J.J. Bogaards. 1987. Vitamin B_6 metabolism in the pregnant rat: effect of progesterone on the (re)distribution in maternal vitamin B_6 stores. J. Nutr. 117:1866-1874.

Vir, S.C., A.H. Love, and W. Thompson. 1980. Vitamin B_6 status during pregnancy. Int. J. Vitam. Nutr. Res 50:403-411.

Vobecky, J.S., J. Vobecky, D. Shapcott, and L. Munan. 1974. Vitamin C and outcome of pregnancy. Lancet 1:630.

Weinstein, B.B., Z. Wohl, G.J. Mitchell, and G.F. Sustendal. 1944. Oral administration of pyridoxine hydrochloride in the treatment of nausea and vomiting of pregnancy. Am. J. Obstet. Gynecol. 47:389-394.

Wertz, A.W., M.E. Lojkin, B.S. Bouchard, and M.B. Derby. 1958. Tryptophan-niacin relationships in pregnancy. J. Nutr. 64:339-353.

Willis, R.S., W.W. Winn, A.T. Morris, A.A. Newsom, and W.E. Massey. 1942. Clinical observations in treatment of nausea and vomiting in pregnancy with vitamins B_1 and B_6. Am. J. Obstet. Gynecol. 44:265-271.

Wills, L. 1931. Treatment of "pernicious anaemia of pregnancy" and "tropical anaemia," with special reference to yeast extract as a curative agent. Br. Med. J. 1:1059-1064.

Zamorano, A.F., F. Arnalich, E.S. Casas, A. Sicilia, C. Solis, J.J. Vazquez, and R. Gasalla. 1985. Levels of iron, vitamin B_{12}, folic acid, and their binding proteins during pregnancy. Acta Haematol. 74:92-96.

19

Protein and Amino Acids

Protein is a macronutrient of major importance in human nutrition. Plant and animal proteins are composed of more than 20 individual amino acids. Within the body, amino acids are used for a wide variety of structural proteins and enzymes; and they serve as a source of energy, carbon, and nitrogen.

Protein has an energy value of approximately 5.5 kcal/g. Of this, approximately 4 kcal/g is used during metabolism; the unmetabolized portion is excreted as urea and other compounds. For meeting metabolic needs and promoting satisfactory rates of protein synthesis, the diet must provide amino acids of adequate quality and quantity.

Amino acids and nitrogen are available to mammals through degradation of proteins and other nitrogenous compounds. Mammals can synthesize nonessential amino acids de novo, if energy and suitable forms of carbon and nitrogen are available. Thus, net requirements for nonessential amino acids can be met both by dietary protein and by endogenous synthesis of amino acids. Ordinarily, the following amino acids are considered to be *essential* amino acids, because they cannot be synthesized by mammals: histidine, isoleucine, leucine, lysine, methionine + cystine, phenylalanine + tyrosine, threonine, tryptophan, and valine (NRC, 1989). Thus, these must be provided in adequate amounts by the diet. Other amino acids, such as arginine and taurine, may functionally appear to be essential during fetal and infant development in some species (Gaull, 1983; Sturman, 1986; Visek, 1986), because the metabolic pathways have not yet fully developed to adult levels and because the amount needed to cover growth and net new

TABLE 19-1 Factorial Estimate of Protein Components of Weight Gain in a Normal Full-Term Pregnancy[a]

Component	Weight, g	Protein, g
Fetus	3,400	440
Placenta	650	100
Amniotic fluid	800	3
Uterus	970	166
Blood	1,250	81
Extracellular fluid	1,680	135
Total	8,750	925

[a] Modified from Calloway (1974), after Hytten and Leitch (1971), with permission.

protein accretion is high. Developmental immaturity of biochemical pathways may also limit conversion of pairs of metabolically related essential amino acids, such as conversion of phenylalanine to tyrosine.

In postnatal life, ingested protein is hydrolyzed to amino acids, which are absorbed and carried via the portal system to the liver. The amino acids then enter the systemic circulation and are distributed throughout the body. The liver is an especially active site for synthesis of protein from amino acids. Since considerable reutilization of amino acids occurs, there is synthesis and degradation of more protein daily than has been ingested.

IMPORTANCE

Pregnancy complicates the already complex metabolism of amino acids. Expansion of blood volume and growth of the maternal tissues require substantial amounts of protein (Table 19-1). Growth of the fetus and placenta also places protein demands on the pregnant woman. Thus, additional protein is essential for the maintenance of a successful pregnancy. However, a review of the processes controlling these changes in maternal protein metabolism is beyond the scope of this chapter.

Maternal protein restriction, alone and in combination with energy restriction, results in consistently decreased fetal growth in many species (Fattet et al., 1984; Hill, 1984; Lederman and Rosso, 1980; Pond et al, 1988; Rosso, 1977a,b, 1980; Rosso and Streeter, 1979). These models demonstrate not only decreased body weight and growth but also decreased numbers of cells and a variety of biochemical changes. A particular concern is that the developing fetus may or may not adequately compensate for some of the effects of maternal protein deprivation, and effects may even span generations.

AMINO ACID UTILIZATION

The fetus receives a continuous stream of amino acids from the mother via the placenta (Battaglia, 1986); the amino acids cross the placenta by a complex series of transport systems, probably including both active and facilitated transport systems. Transport systems may differ on the maternal and fetal sides of the placenta, and different classes of amino acids are transported by different placental systems (Battaglia, 1986; Eaton and Yudilevitch, 1981; Lemons and Schreiner, 1983; Schneider et al., 1979; Smith, 1986; Yudilevitch and Sweiry, 1985). Amino acid concentrations are typically somewhat higher in the fetus than in the mother (Cetin et al., 1988; Soltesz et al., 1985; Yudilevitch and Sweiry, 1985). Moreover, the placenta is very active metabolically, and in laboratory animals, it plays an important role in nitrogen metabolism (Meschia et al., 1980). Because of the complexity of the transport processes and placental metabolism, it is difficult to predict the effect of altered maternal protein intake on fetal amino acid metabolism, both in terms of the total quantitative amino acid flux and in terms of relative changes in the fluxes of individual amino acids.

The fetus must handle rapid entry of both exogenous and endogenous amino acids, and it must provide for the rapid accretion of new protein (Battaglia, 1986). Studies in the unstressed fetal lamb have shown rapid turnovers of leucine and lysine in amounts severalfold higher than umbilical uptakes of the amino acids from the placenta (Battaglia, 1986). More recently, turnover measurements of the nonessential amino acid glycine have suggested the interconversion of glycine and serine in the fetal liver (Marconi et al., 1989). The sheep fetus also appears to catabolize amino acids to urea at a rapid rate (Lemons et al., 1976).

Several investigators have studied the effect of direct amino acid infusion in experimentally induced growth retardation in fetal animals (Charlton and Johengen, 1985; Fattet et al., 1984; Mulvihill et al., 1985). These studies have demonstrated at least partial restitution of birth weight with direct nutritional supplementation. However, there is no evidence that amino acid supplementation of normally grown fetuses significantly increases birth weights above those achieved by controls.

ESTIMATED REQUIREMENTS

Information regarding total protein requirements during pregnancy has been provided through the factorial approach, balance studies, turnover studies, and epidemiologic surveys (see Chapter 12). As noted above, there are theoretical and experimental differences of opinion regarding requirements for protein and amino acids.

The results of body composition studies in human and nonhuman species have formed the basis for estimation of protein accretion in the *fetus*. Hytten and Leitch (1971) reviewed classic studies of human body composition (Kelly et al., 1951; Widdowson and Dickerson, 1964) and estimated fetal protein requirements to be approximately 440 g over the course of pregnancy and the placental protein requirement to be an additional 100 g (Table 19-1). Other reviewers, using much of the same published data on humans, estimated a nitrogen accumulation of 50 to 60 g for a full-term 3,300-g fetus (Sparks, 1984; Ziegler et al., 1976). The data on which such factorial estimates are based are limited, however, and lacking in important details such as accurate gestational age. The results differ because of differences in mathematical modeling and data bases (Hytten and Leitch, 1971; Sparks, 1984; Ziegler et al., 1976). At the standard estimate of 6.25 g of protein per gram of nitrogen, this would amount to 310 to 375 g of protein per human fetus at full term—somewhat lower than previous estimates. Both approaches estimating fetal amino acid and nitrogen requirements demonstrate that the fetus and placenta present a substantial demand for amino acids from the mother.

Nitrogen is found in many compounds other than protein. Nucleic acids and polyamines are two such compounds that may be of particular relevance to the growing fetus. In detailed studies of the chemical composition of the guinea pig fetus, approximately 20% of the nitrogen content was found in compounds other than protein (Sparks et al., 1985). If this is also true of the human fetus, its protein content and requirements may be lower than current estimates.

Using the factorial approach and assuming a 40-week gestation and a 3,300-g newborn, Hytten and Leitch (1971) estimated that 925 g is the *total* increment in body protein during pregnancy (Table 19-1). More recent nitrogen balance studies (Appel and King, 1979; Johnstone et al., 1981) suggest that nitrogen retention approaches the factorial estimate, if adjustment is made for unmeasured losses.

Turnover studies have indicated that protein turnover increases early and remains elevated throughout pregnancy (de Benoist et al., 1985; Fitch and King, 1987; Jackson, 1987). Some investigators have expressed technical concerns about using turnover measurements to estimate protein requirements during pregnancy (Fitch and King, 1987). All human studies to date have used nonessential amino acids to measure the turnover of protein in pregnant women, further complicating the interpretation of these data.

The deposition of protein is not necessarily linear throughout pregnancy. Early during pregnancy, the fetal component is minimal, whereas the requirement for maternal volume expansion and tissue growth may be substantial. Late in pregnancy, the fetus may account for the major increase in protein needs. The additional requirement averaged over gestation appears to be roughly 3 to 4 g of protein per day. If it is assumed that there is a 15% variation in birth weight and that dietary protein is converted at 70% efficiency, the requirement for protein would be an additional 6.0 g/day averaged over pregnancy, but the demand is highest (10.7 g/day) in the last trimester (NRC, 1989). On the basis of these and other considerations, a maternal protein intake of 10 g/day over the Recommended Dietary Allowance (RDA) for protein (i.e., a total of 60 g/day) is recommended throughout pregnancy. This subcommittee notes that most foods that are good sources of protein (e.g., grains, flesh foods, milk, cheese, and dried peas and beans) are also good sources of many other nutrients and thus their use should be encouraged as part of a balanced diet during pregnancy.

USUAL INTAKES

As discussed in Chapter 13, usual protein intakes by pregnant women in the United States range from 75 to 110 g/day. The estimated average intakes of protein by low-income women enrolled in the Supplemental Food Program for Women, Infants, and Children (WIC) were higher than the 1980 RDA of 74 g/day, even before participation in the program (Rush et al., 1988). However, inadequate energy intake may contribute to protein deficiency if there is compensatory catabolism of protein and amino acids to meet energy needs. Thus, the adequacy of dietary protein must be considered in the context of total nutrient intake.

CRITERIA FOR DEFICIENCY

Deficiency of protein is difficult to assess, both because of protein's dynamic and complex metabolism and because protein deficiency is generally associated with deficiencies of other nutrients and energy. Classic signs of protein deficiency include poor growth, muscular weakness, poor hair growth, and low serum albumin, which may result in edema. Classic protein deficiency is rare in the general U.S. population, occurring primarily in people with serious illness or injury rather than as a result of poor dietary intake. However, protein-energy malnutrition is relatively common in other areas of the world, especially among children, and it is associated with decreased birth weight. It is difficult, however, to isolate the effect of protein malnutrition from that of energy intake.

The results of most common laboratory tests used to assess protein deficiency show changes during pregnancy. With the increase in plasma volume, there is a decreased concentration of albumin and certain other blood constituents. However, some blood proteins, especially those whose levels are influenced by estrogen, increase during pregnancy. Urea nitrogen and alpha amino nitrogen levels decrease.

SUPPLEMENTATION STUDIES

A large body of literature documents the results of protein supplementation programs during pregnancy in regions where malnutrition is found. Many of these studies are examined in Chapter 7. In Guatemala, studies were conducted to determine the effects of a protein-energy supplement and a low energy supplement on maternal and newborn outcomes among chronically malnourished rural women (Delgado et al., 1982; Lechtig et al., 1975, 1978) (see Chapter 7, Table 7-2B). In these widely cited studies, investigators found minimal change in birth weight and no effect on gestational duration among women receiving either supplement. Post hoc analysis demonstrated a significant positive effect of spontaneous energy intake on birth weight and maternal weight gain regardless of the protein content of the supplement.

In Colombia, investigators examined the effect of a supplement containing 20 g of protein and 150 kcal of energy given to poor urban women in Bogota. They found an approximately 50-g increase in birth weight in the supplemented group and no effect on gestational duration (Mora et al., 1979). In Taiwan, supplementation with both protein and calories failed to statistically increase the birth weights of infants born to poor rural women (Adair and Pollitt, 1985; Adair et al., 1983; McDonald et al., 1981; Wohlleb et al., 1983).

Studies in the developed world have also demonstrated minimal changes in birth weight as a result of protein supplementation. In the United Kingdom, protein-energy supplementation of pregnant Asian women in Birmingham led to significantly higher maternal weight gains than did energy supplements alone; however, only the supplement that contained vitamins in addition to protein and energy was associated with a significant increase in birth weight (Viegas et al, 1982a,b). Rush et al. (1980) found significant decreases in both gestational length and birth weight and marginally significant increases in mortality and preterm birth rate with high-density protein supplementation of poor women in Harlem, New York. Adams and colleagues (1978) reported that a high-protein supplement given to women in San Francisco resulted in a 45-g decrease in birth weight, compared with controls, and a 140-g decrease in birth weight, compared with infants of mothers who were provided with energy supplements. Reviews of WIC have demonstrated minimal effects of program participation on birth weight, gestational duration, or the incidence of low birth weight (Kennedy and Kotelchuck, 1984; Metcoff et al., 1985; Rush et al., 1988).[*]

In a comprehensive review of the literature on supplementation, Rush and colleagues (1984) reported an inverse relationship between birth weight

---

[*] An average WIC package for pregnant women provides 90 to 1,000 kcal of energy and 40 to 50 g of protein daily.

and protein density in supplements. An increase in prematurity has not been generally associated with supplements that provide protein-to-energy ratios comparable to those found in usual diets.

To summarize, in many studies, protein-energy supplements have been given to pregnant women in an effort to determine the effect on maternal and fetal outcomes. In many of them, no significant changes were found in either birth weight or gestational duration; in others, small changes—from a 30- to 100-g increase in birth weight—were observed. The biologic importance of changes of this magnitude (1 to 3% of the full-term birth weight) is not certain. It is difficult to interpret these studies because of variations in baseline nutritional status, composition of the supplements, and other characteristics; it is particularly problematic to separate the effect of the protein from that of the energy in the supplements.

RECOMMENDATIONS REGARDING SUPPLEMENTATION

On the basis of the estimated additional needs for protein and energy during pregnancy and the usual intake of these nutrients from the U.S. diet, the subcommittee concludes that the additional requirement for protein during pregnancy can be met from dietary sources. Because evidence suggests possible harm from specially formulated high-protein supplements, the use of special protein powders or specially formulated high-protein beverages should be discouraged.

CLINICAL IMPLICATIONS

- A moderate increase in the use of food sources of protein, such as whole grains, milk, and legumes, as part of a balanced diet, is encouraged during pregnancy since these foods are valuable sources of other nutrients.
- Assessment of adequacy of protein status is most important in women whose energy intake is low.
- Use of specially formulated protein supplements (e.g., protein powders) is not recommended during pregnancy.

REFERENCES

Adair, L.S., and E. Pollitt. 1985. Outcome of maternal nutritional supplementation: a comprehensive review of the Bacon Chow study. Am. J. Clin. Nutr. 41:948-978.
Adair, L.S., E. Pollitt, and W.H. Mueller. 1983. Maternal anthropometric changes during pregnancy and lactation in a rural Taiwanese population. Hum. Biol. 55:771-787.
Adams, S.O., G.D. Barr, and R.L. Huenemann. 1978. Effect of nutritional supplementation in pregnancy. I. Outcome of pregnancy. J. Am. Diet. Assoc. 72:144-147.

Appel, J., and J.C. King. 1979. Protein utilization in pregnant and non-pregnant women. Fed. Proc., Fed. Am. Soc. Exp. Biol. 38:388.

Battaglia, F.C. 1986. Placental transport and utilization of amino acids and carbohydrates. Fed. Proc., Fed. Am. Soc. Exp. Biol. 45:2508-2512.

Calloway, D.H. 1974. Nitrogen balance during pregnancy. Pp. 79-94 in M. Winick, ed. Nutrition and Fetal Development. John Wiley & Sons, New York.

Cetin, I., A.M. Marconi, P. Bozzetti, L.P. Sereni, C. Corbetta, G. Pardi, and F.C. Battaglia. 1988. Umbilical amino acid concentrations in appropriate and small for gestational age infants: a biochemical difference present in utero. Am. J. Obstet. Gynecol. 158:120-126.

Charlton, V., and M. Johengen. 1985. Effects of intrauterine nutritional supplementation on fetal growth retardation. Biol. Neonate 48:125-142.

de Benoist, B., A.A. Jackson, J. St. E. Hall, and C. Persaud. 1985. Whole-body protein turnover in Jamaican women during normal pregnancy. Hum. Nutr.: Clin. Nutr. 39C:167-179.

Delgado, H.L., V.E. Valverde, R. Martorell, and R.E. Klein. 1982. Relationship of maternal and infant nutrition to infant growth. Early Hum. Dev. 6:273-286.

Eaton, B.M., and D.L. Yudilevich. 1981. Uptake and asymmetric efflux of amino acids at maternal and fetal sides of placenta. Am. J. Physiol. 241:C106-C112.

Fattet, I., F.D. Hovell, E.R. Ørskov, D.J. Kyle, K. Pennie, and R.I. Smart. 1984. Undernutrition in sheep. The effect of supplementation with protein on protein accretion. Br. J. Nutr. 52:561-574.

Fitch, W.L., and J.C. King. 1987. Protein turnover and 3-methylhistidine excretion in non-pregnant, pregnant and gestational diabetic women. Hum. Nutr.: Clin. Nutr. 41C:327-339.

Gaull, G.E. 1983. Taurine in human milk: growth modulator of conditionally essential amino acid? J. Pediatr. Gastroenterol. Nutr. 2:S266-S271.

Hill, D.E. 1984. Experimental alteration of fetal growth in animals. Mead Johnson Symp. Perinat. Dev. Med. 23:29-36.

Hytten, F.E., and I. Leitch. 1971. The Physiology of Human Pregnancy, 2nd ed. Blackwell Scientific Publications, Oxford. 599 pp.

Jackson, A.A. 1987. Measurement of protein turnover during pregnancy. Hum. Nutr.: Clin. Nutr. 41C:497-498.

Johnstone, F.D., D.M. Campbell, and I. MacGillivray. 1981. Nitrogen balance studies in human pregnancy. J. Nutr. 111:1884-1893.

Kelly, H.J., R.E. Sloan, W. Hoffman, and C. Saunders. 1951. Accumulation of nitrogen and six minerals in the human fetus during gestation. Hum. Biol. 23:61-74.

Kennedy, E.T., and M. Kotelchuck. 1984. The effect of WIC supplemental feeding on birth weight: a case-control analysis. Am. J. Clin. Nutr. 40:579-585.

Lechtig, A., J.P. Habicht, H. Delgado, R.E. Klein, C. Yarbrough, and R. Martorell. 1975. Effect of food supplementation during pregnancy on birthweight. Pediatrics 56:508-520.

Lechtig, A., R. Martorell, H. Delgado, C. Yarbrough, and R.E. Klein. 1978. Food supplementation during pregnancy, maternal anthropometry and birth weight in a Guatemalan rural population. J. Trop. Pediatrics. 24:217-222.

Lederman, S.A., and P. Rosso. 1980. Effects of protein and carbohydrate supplements on fetal and maternal weight and on body composition in food-restricted rats. Am. J. Clin. Nutr. 33:1912-1916.

Lemons, J.A., and R.L. Schreiner. 1983. Amino acid metabolism in the ovine fetus. Am. J. Physiol. 244:E459-E466.

Lemons, J.A., E.W. Adcock III, M.D. Jones, Jr., M.A. Naughton, G. Meschia, and F.C. Battaglia. 1976. Umbilical uptake of amino acids in the unstressed fetal lamb. J. Clin. Invest. 58:1428-1434.

Marconi, A.M., F.C. Battaglia, G. Meschia, and J.W. Sparks. 1989. A comparison of amino acid arteriovenous differences across the liver and placenta of the fetal lamb. Am. J. Physiol. 257:E909-E915.

McDonald, E.C., E. Pollitt, W. Mueller, A.M. Hsueh, and R. Sherwin. 1981. The Bacon Chow study: maternal nutritional supplementation and birth weight of offspring. Am. J. Clin. Nutr. 34:2133-2144.

Meschia, G., F.C. Battaglia, W.W. Hay, and J.W. Sparks. 1980. Utilization of substrates by the ovine placenta in vivo. Fed. Proc., Fed. Am. Soc. Exp. Biol. 39:245-249.

Metcoff, J., P. Costiloe, W.M. Crosby, S. Dutta, H.H. Sandstead, D. Milne, C.E. Bodwell, and S.H. Majors. 1985. Effect of food supplementation (WIC) during pregnancy on birth weight. Am. J. Clin. Nutr. 41:933-947.

Mora, J.O., B. de Paredes, M. Wagner, L. de Navarro, J. Suescum, N. Christiansen, and M.G. Herrera. 1979. Nutritional supplementation and the outcome of pregnancy. I. Birth weight. Am. J. Clin. Nutr. 32:455-462.

Mulvihill, S.J., A. Albert, A. Synn, and E.W. Fonkalsrud. 1985. In utero supplemental fetal feeding in an animal model: effects on fetal growth and development. Surgery 98:500-505.

NRC (National Research Council). 1989. Recommended Dietary Allowances, 10th ed. Report of the Subcommittee on the Tenth Edition of the RDAs, Food and Nutrition Board, Commission on Life Sciences. National Academy Press, Washington, D.C. 284 pp.

Pond, W.G., J.T. Yen, and L.H. Yen. 1988. Body weight deficit in the absence of reduction in cerebrum weight and nucleic acid content in progeny of swine restricted in protein intake during pregnancy. Proc. Soc. Exp. Biol. Med. 188:117-121.

Rosso, P. 1977a. Maternal-fetal exchange during protein malnutrition in the rat. Placental transfer of α-amino isobutyric acid. J. Nutr. 107:2002-2005.

Rosso, P. 1977b. Maternal-fetal exchange during protein malnutrition in the rat. Placental transfer of glucose and a nonmetabolizable glucose analog. J. Nutr. 107:2006-2010.

Rosso, P. 1980. Placental growth, development, and function in relation to maternal nutrition. Fed. Proc., Fed. Am. Soc. Exp. Biol. 39:250-254.

Rosso, P., and M.R. Streeter. 1979. Effects of food or protein restriction on plasma volume expansion in pregnant rats. J. Nutr. 109:1887-1892.

Rush, D., Z. Stein, and M. Susser. 1980. A randomized controlled trial of prenatal nutritional supplementation in New York City. Pediatrics 65:683-697.

Rush, D., A. Kristal, C. Navarro, P. Chauhan, W. Blanc, R. Naeye, and M.W. Susser. 1984. The effects of dietary supplementation during pregnancy on placental morphology, pathology, and histomorphometry. Am. J. Clin. Nutr. 39:863-871.

Rush, D., N.L. Sloan, J. Leighton, J.M. Alvir, D.G. Horvitz, W.B. Seaver, G.C. Garbowski, S.S. Johnson, R.A. Kulka, M. Holt, J.W. Devore, J.T. Lynch, M.B. Woodside, and D.S. Shanklin. 1988. The National WIC Evaluation: evaluation of the Special Supplemental Food Program for Women, Infants, and Children. V. Longitudinal study of pregnant women. Am. J. Clin. Nutr. 48:439-483.

Schneider, H., K.H. Möhlen, and J. Dancis. 1979. Transfer of amino acids across the in vitro perfused human placenta. Pediatr. Res. 13:236-240.

Smith, C.H. 1986. Mechanisms and regulation of placental amino acid transport. Fed. Proc., Fed. Am. Soc. Exp. Biol. 45:2443-2445.

Soltesz, G., D. Harris, I.Z. Mackenzie, and A. Aynsley-Green. 1985. The metabolic and endocrine milieu of the human fetus and mother at 18-21 weeks of gestation. I. Plasma amino acid concentrations. Pediatr. Res. 19:91-93.

Sparks, J.W. 1984. Human intrauterine growth and nutrient accretion. Semin. Perinatol. 8:74-93.

Sparks, J.W., J.R. Girard, S. Callikan, and F.C. Battaglia. 1985. Growth of fetal guinea pig: physical and chemical characteristics. Am. J. Physiol. 248:E132-E139.

Sturman, J.A., A.D. Gargano, J.M. Messing, and H. Imaki. 1986. Feline maternal taurine deficiency: effect on mother and offspring. J. Nutr. 116:655-667.

Viegas, O.A.C., P.H. Scott, T.J. Cole, P. Eaton, P.G. Needham, and B.A. Wharton. 1982a. Dietary protein energy supplementation of pregnant Asian mothers at Sorrento, Birmingham. I. Unselective during second and third trimesters. Br. Med. J. 285:589-592.

Viegas, O.A.C., P.H. Scott, T.J. Cole, P. Eaton, P.G. Needham, and B.A. Wharton. 1982b. Dietary protein energy supplementation of pregnant Asian mothers at Sorrento, Birmingham. II. Selective during third trimester only. Br. Med. J. 285:592-595.

Visek, W.J. 1986. Arginine needs, physiological state and usual diets. A reevaluation. J. Nutr. 116:36-46.

Widdowson, E.M., and J.W.T. Dickerson. 1964. Chemical composition of the body. Pp. 1-247 in C.L. Comar and F. Bronner, eds. Mineral Metabolism: An Advanced Treatise. Vol. II, The Elements, Part A. Academic Press, New York.

Wohlleb, J.C., E. Pollitt, W.H. Mueller, and R. Bigelow. 1983. The Bacon Chow study: maternal supplementation and infant growth. Early Hum. Dev. 9:79-91.

Yudilevich, D.L., and J.H. Sweiry. 1985. Transport of amino acids in the placenta. Biochim. Biophys. Acta 822:169-201.

Ziegler, E.E., A.M. O'Donnell, S.E. Nelson, and S.J. Fomon. 1976. Body composition of the reference fetus. Growth 40:329-341.

20

Substance Use and Abuse During Pregnancy

The use of substances such as tobacco, alcohol and illicit drugs during pregnancy has important general health implications both for the mother and the fetus. A Food and Nutrition Board report entitled *Alternative Dietary Practices and Nutritional Abuses in Pregnancy* (NRC, 1982) considered at length the adverse reproductive effects of cigarette smoking and alcohol abuse as well as the teratogenic potential of caffeine in animals. The present report briefly summarizes the influence of tobacco, alcohol, caffeine, marijuana, and cocaine on the fetus and reviews the data on how these substances may affect dietary intake and nutritional status during pregnancy.

Marijuana use is included because of its relatively common occurrence and because of concern about its possible adverse effect on fetal growth and development. Cocaine is also discussed because of the recent dramatic increase in its use and its potentially devastating effect on the health and well-being of the mother and the fetus. Coverage of other types of substances was considered to be beyond the scope of work of this subcommittee, even though illicit and certain prescription drugs are known to have detrimental effects on nutrition and pregnancy outcome. Use of such substances should be actively assessed when counseling women regarding nutrition and ways to promote a healthy pregnancy.

CIGARETTE SMOKING

Prevalence

Although the prevalence of cigarette smoking in the general U.S. population has declined over the past two decades, it is still a common addiction among pregnant women. The proportion of women of child-bearing age (20 to 44 years) who smoke has decreased from about 40% in 1965 to 30% in 1987 (NCHS, 1989). Smoking rates among girls aged 12 to 17 increased during the mid-1970s but subsequently declined—from 24% in 1974 to 11% in 1988 (NCHS, 1989; NIDA, 1989). Smoking during pregnancy also appears to have decreased. Data from the 1967 and 1980 National Natality Surveys indicate that among married pregnant women aged 20 or older, the proportion of smokers declined from 40 to 25% for white mothers and from 33 to 23% for black mothers (Kleinman and Kopstein, 1987). This decline was limited largely to those who had completed high school; no change was reported in the prevalence of smoking among mothers under age 20. The 1980 National Natality Survey showed that the overall proportion of married mothers who smoked was 25% (Prager et al., 1984), the highest rates occurring among white women, followed by black and Hispanic women. Smoking was also considerably more common among teenage mothers and those who had not completed high school as compared with the older or more educated mothers. Data from the 26 states in the Behavioral Risk Factor Surveillance System in 1985 and 1986 indicate that the overall prevalence of smoking in pregnancy was 21% with higher rates for unmarried (36%) as compared with married (18%) pregnant women (Williamson et al., 1989).

Effects on the Developing Fetus and Child

The effects of maternal smoking on pregnancy and on the developing fetus and child have been reviewed extensively (Abel, 1980b; Berkowitz, 1988; DHEW, 1979; DHHS, 1980). The most consistent observation is the reduction in birth weight (on average 200 g) among infants of smokers. A recent review of the literature on the determinants of low birth weight has, like previous reviews, concluded that cigarette smoking is by far the single most important modifiable factor responsible for fetal growth retardation in developed countries (Kramer, 1987). Other adverse effects include a moderately increased risk of preterm delivery (Fedrick and Anderson, 1976; Meyer et al., 1976; Shiono et al., 1986), perinatal mortality (DHEW, 1979; Meyer and Tonascia, 1977; Meyer et al., 1976), and, possibly, spontaneous abortion (Alberman et al., 1976; Kline et al., 1980b; Kullander and Källén, 1971). A sizable proportion of perinatal deaths and preterm births appears to be mediated through a smoking-related increase in the incidence of placenta previa and abruptio placentae (premature separation of the placenta) (Andrews and McGarry, 1972; DHEW, 1979; Meyer and Tonascia, 1977; Naeye, 1979). In addition, children of mothers who smoke during pregnancy may have slight but measurable deficits in long-term physical growth, intellectual performance, and behavioral development (Butler and Goldstein, 1973; Dunn et al., 1977; Naeye and Peters, 1984; Rantakallio, 1983). Interpreting the long-term effects of maternal smoking is problematic, however, since it is difficult to separate the effect of in utero exposure from postnatal passive exposure and other characteristics of the home environment of smoking parents.

The adverse effects have been found to be proportional to the frequency of smoking and appear to be prevented or reduced if the mother does not smoke during a subsequent pregnancy (Abel, 1980b; DHEW, 1979; DHHS, 1980; Naeye, 1978). The smoking-related effects have also been found to be independent of other factors, such as race, parity, prepregnancy weight, maternal weight gain, and socioeconomic status. These observations support the generally accepted conclusion that the adverse effects of smoking represent a cause-and-effect relationship and are not a reflection of different characteristics of smokers and nonsmokers.

Nutrition-Related Effects of Smoking

Cigarette smoke contains approximately 2,000 different compounds. The exact mechanism behind the detrimental effects of smoking on the fetus and newborn have not been established. The most widely accepted explanation is that smoking causes intrauterine hypoxia through increased carboxyhemoglobin levels or reduced uteroplacental blood flow (Abel, 1980b; Longo, 1982). Other nutrition-related factors may also play a role. Cyanide, a constituent of tobacco smoke, and thiocyanate levels in the blood and urine of smokers and their infants are higher than those of controls (Meberg et al., 1979; Pettigrew et al., 1977). Since vitamin B_{12} and sulfur-containing amino acids are utilized in the detoxification of cyanide, the depletion of these important nutrients may adversely affect the growth and development of the fetuses of smokers. Other studies show statistically significant reductions in the plasma levels of several amino acids and carotene in pregnant women who smoke compared with levels in pregnant nonsmokers (Crosby et al., 1977). The maternal plasma carotene level in smokers has, in turn, been positively associated with birth weight (Metcoff et al., 1989). Cigarette smoking also appears to be related to reduced vitamin C levels. Data from the Second National Health and Nutrition Examination Survey (NHANES II) revealed that serum vitamin C levels in nonpregnant female smokers were lower than in nonsmokers (Woteki et al.,

1986), and serum levels were found to be significantly reduced among smokers after adjusting for vitamin C intake in a small-scale study of adolescent females (Keith and Mossholder, 1986). Smokers have also been reported to have decreased plasma ascorbate levels, which in turn are associated with increased metabolism of vitamin C rather than alterations in absorption or urinary excretion (Kallner et al., 1981). Nonpregnant, adult heavy smokers (≥ 20 cigarettes/day) may require up to twice as much vitamin C to maintain a body pool of vitamin C similar to that in nonsmokers.

In NHANES II (1976-1980), the prevalence of low serum and erythrocyte folate levels was significantly higher for female smokers than for nonsmokers (LSRO, 1984). In addition, hemoglobin concentrations in smokers were found to be higher than those in nonsmokers—a finding that presumably reflects a response to the conversion of hemoglobin to carboxyhemoglobin in smokers. This finding was not confirmed in the data from the Collaborative Perinatal Project, but elevated hemoglobin and hematocrit levels were found in the neonates of smokers (Garn et al., 1978). Because the presence of carboxyhemoglobin in the blood results in elevated hemoglobin concentrations in smokers, the Centers for Disease Control recently recommended higher hemoglobin and hematocrit cutoff values for identifying the risk of anemia for smokers as compared with risk for nonsmokers (CDC, 1989). There is also evidence that smokers may have decreased placental zinc-to-cadmium ratios, which in turn have been related to reduced birth weight (Kuhnert et al., 1987, 1988).

Caloric intake may modify the relationship between smoking and reduced birth weight. Smokers have generally been found to have a somewhat lower prepregnancy weight and weight gain during pregnancy than nonsmokers (Butler et al., 1972; Garn et al., 1979; Rush, 1974). It would therefore be expected that smokers consume less food than nonsmokers; however, data from the National WIC (Supplemental Food Program for Women, Infants, and Children) Evaluation (Rush et al., 1988) and other studies (Haworth et al., 1980a; Picone et al., 1982) have shown that dietary intakes of smokers during pregnancy are higher than those of nonsmokers. Since cigarette smoking has been demonstrated to increase the metabolic rate (Perkins et al., 1989), the lower prepregnancy weight and weight gain in smokers presumably reflect a reduced availability of calories for weight gain. An increase in the nutritional intake of pregnant smokers may counteract some of the smoking-related effects on birth weight (Garn et al., 1979; Metcoff et al., 1985; Rush et al., 1980), but some data show that infants of obese smokers will still weigh significantly less than infants of obese nonsmokers (Haworth et al., 1980b). Thus, it appears that improving the food intake of pregnant smokers does not completely compensate for the negative effect of smoking on birth weight.

In summary, cigarette smoking may affect maternal nutrition (and consequently, fetal nutrition) in two important ways: the increased metabolic rate in smokers can lead to the lower availability of calories, and exposure to tobacco may increase iron requirements and decrease the availability of certain nutrients such as vitamin B_{12}, amino acids, vitamin C, folate, and zinc. In addition, the hypothesized reduction in uteroplacental blood flow in smokers could restrict nutrient and oxygen flow to the fetus.

As a result, mothers who smoke may need special counseling regarding dietary intake and may benefit from multivitamin-mineral supplementation, but this has not been investigated. Furthermore, compensatory intakes should not replace strategies for persuading women to give up smoking. Some smoking cessation programs during pregnancy have been found to be effective in increasing infant birth weight (Sexton and Hebel, 1984), and pregnancy may be a particularly opportune time to introduce antismoking assistance (Sexton and Hebel, 1984; Windsor et al., 1985).

ALCOHOL

Effects on the Developing Fetus and Child

Although the fetal alcohol syndrome (FAS) was not described until 1973 (Jones and Smith, 1973), alcohol is now recognized as a potent teratogen. FAS is estimated to affect approximately one to two infants per 1,000 live births in the United States (Abel and Sokol, 1987) and is characterized by prenatal or postnatal growth retardation, distinct facial anomalies, and mental deficiency (Rosett, 1980). Other potential alcohol-related birth defects include cardiac and genitourinary abnormalities (Ernhart et al., 1985; Hanson et al., 1976), but it is difficult to attribute isolated anomalies to alcohol exposure. In addition to FAS, alcohol has been associated with a spectrum of adverse effects that range from spontaneous abortion (Harlap and Shiono, 1980; Kline et al., 1980a) to subtle behavioral effects in the absence of physical anomalies (Aronson et al., 1985; Shaywitz et al., 1980). The effect of alcohol on central nervous system dysfunction is of particular concern, since some degree of intellectual impairment is frequently reported for children with FAS, especially those having the most severe dysmorphogenesis (Streissguth et al., 1983).

Definitions and Prevalence of Alcohol Use and Abuse

According to national surveys of women aged 18 or older, the proportion who drink alcohol at least occasionally has decreased slightly between 1971 (58%) and 1985 (55%), and the proportion who consume 30 cc (1 oz) or more of pure alcohol per day has dropped from 5 to 3% during the same period (NCHS, 1989). Among women aged 18 to 25, the proportion who reported that they consumed alcohol in the preceding month increased from 58% in 1976 to 68% in 1979 and then declined to 57% in 1988 (NCHS, 1989; NIDA, 1989).

Precise estimates of alcohol abuse cannot easily be obtained because of underreporting of alcohol intake and the difficulty of accurately quantifying alcohol exposure. Nor has any consistent criterion been used for defining alcohol abuse. In the 1980 National Natality Survey, it was found that among 4,405 married women who delivered live infants, 39% consumed some alcohol during the pregnancy and 3% drank three or more servings of alcoholic beverages per week (Prager et al., 1984). Alcohol consumption was highest among white mothers, followed by Hispanic and black mothers. Age and education were both positively related to drinking; i.e., drinking was most prevalent among older and better educated mothers. Other studies have estimated that anywhere from 0.8% (Streissguth et al., 1983) to 9% (Ouellette et al., 1977) of pregnant women are heavy drinkers; most studies report a range of 2 to 3%. Although the definition of heavy use has varied, consumption of two or more drinks per day has commonly been used for identifying heavy alcohol intake. It is not known whether alcohol consumption during pregnancy has declined since the 1977 and 1981 Surgeon General's reports on alcohol and pregnancy, but at least one study found no significant decrease in the relative proportion of heavy drinkers among pregnant women in Seattle, Washington, between 1974-1975 and 1980-1981 (Streissguth et al., 1983).

Although FAS is believed to be limited to chronic alcohol abusers, growth retardation has been observed at lower levels of alcohol consumption (approximately 30 to 60 cc, or 1 to 2 oz, of absolute alcohol daily) (Hanson et al., 1978; Little, 1977; Wright et al., 1983). Another study showed a significantly increased risk of delivering a growth-retarded infant for women who consumed one to two drinks per day (Mills et al., 1984). Still other studies have demonstrated no or inconsistent associations between moderate levels of alcohol consumption and fetal growth (Brooke et al., 1989; Kline et al., 1987; Marbury et al., 1983; Rosett et al., 1983; Tennes and Blackard, 1980). Thus, the evidence concerning the effects of low levels of alcohol consumption is both limited and inconsistent. The possibility that maternal binge drinking may adversely affect the fetus has also been suggested by data on both humans and animals (Clarren et al., 1978, 1988).

Nutrition-Related Effects of Alcohol Use

The exact mechanism by which alcohol adversely affects fetal growth and morphogenesis has not been established. Animal studies have documented direct dose-response effects of alcohol on fetal growth and development and have shown that these effects were not attributable to other factors such as malnutrition (Randall et al., 1981). Alcohol may also affect the fetus indirectly through its effect on maternal nutrition. Since ethanol is a source of energy, chronic alcoholics may have a relatively low intake of proteins, essential fats, vitamins, and minerals. In a prospective study of alcohol use during pregnancy and neonatal outcome in Cleveland, Ohio, investigators compared 24-hour dietary intake histories of patients with positive and negative scores on the Michigan Alcoholism Screening Test (Sokol et al., 1981). Those with positive scores had significantly lower intakes of meat and vegetable protein, dairy foods, cereal and bread, calcium, certain B vitamins, and vitamin D. However, dietary intake was not significantly different among rare, moderate, and heavy drinkers in another study (Ouellette et al., 1977).

There are few data on the effect of alcohol on maternal nutrition. In one study maternal and umbilical cord blood zinc levels were found to be lower in alcoholic than in nonalcoholic pregnant women (Flynn et al., 1981), although the importance of these findings has been questioned (Kiely, 1981). Other studies suggest that alcohol may impair placental transport of amino acids, which in turn may adversely affect fetal nutrition (Fisher et al., 1981). Animal studies have similarly shown that ethanol inhibits placental transport of certain amino acids (Henderson et al., 1981; Lin, 1981) and zinc (Ghishan et al., 1982).

Ethanol can also interfere with the intestinal transport of several essential nutrients including calcium, amino acids, and some vitamins (Wilson and Hoyumpa, 1979). The adverse effects of ethanol on liver function may lead to abnormalities in metabolism and nutrient utilization (Lieber, 1985). However, evidence concerning the adverse effects of alcohol on specific nutritional indices comes largely from studies of nonpregnant hospitalized alcoholics, many of whom had hepatic damage. Specifically, chronic alcohol abuse has been linked to increased urinary zinc excretion and low serum zinc concentrations (Fredricks et al., 1960; McClain and Su, 1983; Vallee et al., 1957), decreased levels of hepatic vitamin A (Leo and Lieber, 1982), impaired uptake and utilization of folate (Halsted et al., 1971), and possibly thiamin malabsorption (Camilo et al., 1981; Hoyumpa, 1983). Thus, zinc, vitamin A, folate, and thiamin deficiencies may occur with chronic alcohol consumption. However, supplementation with fat-soluble vitamins, particularly vitamin A, may not be advisable, partly because of general concerns regarding toxicities, but also because data on animals suggest that vitamin A supplementation combined with ethanol consumption may enhance hepatic toxicity (Leo and Lieber, 1983).

There is evidence from experiments in animals that nutritional factors may act synergistically with alcohol exposure in producing adverse effects. For example, low protein and caloric intakes have been hypothesized to interact with alcohol exposure, leading to higher blood alcohol levels and more severe growth retardation in rats (Wiener et al., 1981). However, inconsistent results have been obtained when the protein content of the diet was increased (Weinberg, 1985; Wiener et al., 1981). Zinc deficiency has also been postulated to be a coteratogen with alcohol. Studies in rats have shown that low zinc intake plus alcohol had more severe effects on the fetus than did either alcohol or low zinc intake alone (Keppen et al., 1985; Ruth and Goldsmith, 1981). Plasma zinc levels and increased urinary zinc excretion were significantly lower in six infants with FAS as compared with levels in controls (Assadi and Ziai, 1986). Zinc supplementation has been suggested as a way to prevent or lessen adverse alcohol-related effects; however, a study in rats produced no evidence that supplementation of a high-ethanol diet with zinc increased the placental transport of zinc (Ghishan and Greene, 1983).

In summary, alcohol may be related to decreased dietary intake, impaired metabolism and absorption of nutrients, and altered nutrient activation and utilization. Interactions between alcohol and deficiencies of such nutrients as protein and zinc may also play a role in the etiology of alcohol-related effects in the fetus. Although there is no convincing evidence that nutritional supplementation will counteract the adverse effects of alcohol, multivitamin-mineral supplementation (excluding vitamin A) may be indicated for women who are known or suspected alcohol abusers. However, since alcohol abuse has clearly been shown to be detrimental to the fetus, nutritional supplementation should not replace efforts to encourage women to limit or eliminate alcohol intake during pregnancy.

CAFFEINE

Caffeine along with theophylline and theobromine are methylxanthines found in coffee, tea, cola, and cocoa beverages. Caffeine is also a common additive in many non-prescription preparations, especially mild analgesics (Graham, 1978). The Food and Nutrition Board's GRAS (Generally Recognized as Safe) Survey Committee estimated in 1977 that 74% of pregnant females consumed some caffeine and that the mean intake for the entire group was 144 mg/day (approximately 1.5 cups of coffee) (NRC, 1977). In a more recent study of pregnant women in Connecticut, the average daily caffeine intake was found to be slightly lower (102 mg) (Bracken et al., 1982).

Pharmacologic Effects of Caffeine and Other Methylxanthines

The three xanthines share several pharmacologic properties; namely, they stimulate the central nervous system and the cardiac muscle, act on the kidney to produce diuresis, and relax smooth muscle (Rall, 1985). Of the three xanthines, caffeine is believed to be the most active central nervous system stimulant and the most extensively studied. Caffeine passes readily to the fetus, but the fetus cannot metabolize caffeine effectively, nor can the infant do so until several months after birth (Aldridge et al., 1979). Maternal consumption of two cups of coffee significantly increases maternal epinephrine concentrations and decreases intervillous placental blood flow (Kirkinen et al., 1983).

Possible Effects on the Developing Fetus

Although there is substantial evidence that caffeine is teratogenic in animals (Bertrand et al., 1965; Collins et al., 1982), there is no convincing evidence that it is associated with birth defects in humans (Heinonen et al., 1977; Kurppa et al., 1982; Linn et al., 1982; Nelson and Forfar, 1971; Rosenberg et al., 1982). Coffee and caffeine consumption have been associated with a reduction in birth weight and an increased risk of low-birth-weight infants, especially among full-term deliveries (Hogue, 1981; Martin and Bracken, 1987; Mau and Netter, 1974; Muñoz et al., 1988; van den Berg, 1977; Watkinson and Fried, 1985), but it is not clear in some of these studies whether the effects were due to caffeine, some other constituent of coffee, or other characteristics of coffee drinkers. Furthermore, most of the studies only assessed coffee consumption (Heinonen et al., 1977; Hogue, 1981; Kurppa et al., 1982; Linn et al., 1982; Mau and Netter, 1974; van den Berg, 1977), while others included additional sources of caffeine (Martin and Bracken, 1987; Nelson and Forfar, 1971; Rosenberg et al., 1982; Watkinson and Fried, 1985). In addition, the level at which adverse effects have been reported ranges from a total daily caffeine intake greater than 150 mg (equivalent to 1.5 or more cups of coffee) (Martin and Bracken, 1987) to seven or more cups of coffee per day (Hogue, 1981). An increased risk of late first- and second-trimester spontaneous abortions in women consuming more than 150 mg of caffeine daily after adjustment for other risk factors has also been reported (Srisuphan and Bracken, 1986). In contrast, other studies have found no significant association between maternal caffeine or coffee consumption and reduced birth weight (Brooke et al., 1989; Hingson et al., 1982; Linn et al., 1982; Tennes and Blackard, 1980) or preterm delivery (Berkowitz et al., 1982; Linn et al., 1982).

Nutrition-Related Effects of Caffeine or Coffee

Little is known about the nutritional status of pregnant women who consume caffeine. One study noted that women who consumed more than 300 mg of caffeine daily during pregnancy had lower weight for height and lower average intakes of calories, protein, calcium, vitamin A, thiamin, riboflavin, and vitamin C than those of women who consumed less than or equal to 300 mg daily (Watkinson and Fried, 1985). The differences, however, were based on a small number of heavy caffeine users and were not statistically significant. Coffee and caffeine intakes have been reported to affect the status of some nutrients in nonpregnant populations. Specifically, caffeine intake has been observed to increase urinary calcium excretion (Massey and Hollingbery, 1988a,b) and coffee consumption has been related to decreased urinary thiamin excretion (Lewis and Inoue, 1981) and depressed zinc and iron absorption (Morck et al., 1983; Pécoud et al., 1975). In a prospective study of pregnant women in Costa Rica, investigators found that consumption of three or more cups of coffee a day was associated with significantly lower maternal and neonatal hemoglobin and hematocrit levels (Muñoz et al., 1988). Since all the women in that study reportedly took prenatal supplements containing iron, supplemental iron did not appear to prevent the hematologic deficits among the coffee consumers. However, coffee consumption may facilitate calcium intake, particularly for Hispanic populations, who tend to dilute the coffee with a substantial amount of milk.

Thus, although there is no convincing evidence that coffee or caffeine causes birth defects in humans, there is some limited evidence that moderate to heavy use of coffee and caffeine may lower infant birth weight. The latter finding has not been reported in all studies and needs to be confirmed by additional investigations. In 1980, the U.S. Food and Drug Administration recommended that the most prudent action for pregnant women and those who may become pregnant was to avoid caffeine-containing products or to use them sparingly (FDA, 1980). Although it appears sensible to limit coffee and caffeine intake during pregnancy, the subcommittee concluded that the data are not sufficient for making a specific recommendation. Information regarding the influence of coffee and caffeine on maternal nutrition is very limited, and it is not known whether nutrient supplements would be necessary or beneficial for those who continue to consume caffeine during pregnancy.

MARIJUANA

Prevalence of Marijuana Use

National surveys estimate that the proportion of women between the ages of 18 and 25 who had used marijuana in the previous month increased from 19% in 1976 to 26% in 1979 and subsequently declined to 11% in 1988 (NCHS, 1989; NIDA, 1989). According to the 1988 survey, the proportions were lower for teenage girls (7%) and for women aged 26 to 34 (7%). In the 1985 survey, usage among the 18 to 25 year olds was substantially higher for whites (18%) and blacks (17%) compared with that for Hispanics (9%) (NIDA, 1987). Although there are no national data on the prevalence of marijuana use during pregnancy, estimates from hospital-based studies have ranged from approximately 10% (Hatch and Bracken, 1986; Linn et al., 1983) to 27% (Zuckerman et al., 1989). Variations in population characteristics as well as differences in methods of ascertaining marijuana use are likely explanations for the wide range. For example, a recent study showed that self-reported maternal marijuana use is lower than the estimate obtained from a combination of interviews and urine assays (Zuckerman et al., 1989). Underreporting was also more common for self-reported marijuana use than for self-reported cigarette or alcohol use during pregnancy (Hingson et al., 1986).

Pharmacologic Effects of Marijuana

The main active ingredient of marijuana, Δ9-tetrahydrocannabinol, crosses the placenta (Indänpään-Heikkilä et al., 1969). Because marijuana is fat-soluble and is excreted at a slow rate (Jones, 1980), the exposure of the fetus to the drug may be prolonged. Marijuana smoking, like tobacco smoking, is also associated with increased carboxyhemoglobin levels (Wu et al., 1988), which in turn may impair fetal oxygenation and, consequently, fetal growth. Indeed, the increase in carboxyhemoglobin levels has been found to be substantially higher for marijuana smoking than for tobacco smoking (Wu et al., 1988). Furthermore, marijuana use tends to increase the heart rate and blood pressure (Foltin et al., 1987), which may lead to reduced uteroplacental blood flow to the fetus.

Effects on the Developing Fetus and Child

Animal experiments indicate that marijuana may have a fetotoxic potential, including increased fetal resorption and reduced birth weight (Harclerode, 1980), but some of these effects may have been related to reductions in food and water consumption (Abel, 1980a). Data on the influence of marijuana on pregnancy outcomes in humans are both limited and inconsistent. Adverse effects that have been reported include decreased birth weight (Hingson et al., 1982; Zuckerman et al., 1989) and body length (Zuckerman et al., 1989), increased frequency of preterm delivery (Gibson et al., 1983), shortened length of gestation (Fried et al., 1984), higher rates of precipitate labor and meconium passage (Greenland et al., 1982), increased risk of infant features compatible with the fetal alcohol syndrome (Hingson et al., 1982), and altered neurobehavioral responses in neonates (Fried, 1980; Scher et al., 1988). Other studies, however, have reported no effect on either birth weight or length of gestation (Linn et al., 1983; Rosett et al., 1983) or produced inconsistent results. For example, one study found that white, but not nonwhite, women who used marijuana at least two to three times monthly during the pregnancy were at an increased risk of delivering a low-birth- weight, small-for-gestational-age, and preterm infant (Hatch and Bracken, 1986). Another investigation, which was based on two pregnancy cohorts followed over different periods, found a reduction in birth weight with increasing frequency of marijuana use during the second, but not the first phase of the study (Kline et al., 1987). Furthermore, a recent study found no association between marijuana use during pregnancy and features compatible with fetal alcohol effects at age 4 (Graham et al., 1988). Possible explanations for the inconsistent findings include differences in the ascertainment and classification of marijuana use, variations in the underreporting of marijuana or other illicit drug use, and the difficulty of controlling for highly interrelated factors such as abuse of other substances.

Possible Nutrition-Related Effects of Marijuana Use

There are few data on the nutritional status of pregnant marijuana users, nor is it known what effect marijuana exposure may have on specific nutrients. Although marijuana reportedly stimulates the appetite (Abel, 1971), studies of women who have consumed marijuana during pregnancy have provided conflicting results regarding their nutritional status. One study found that marijuana users consumed significantly more calories and protein and gained slightly more weight during the pregnancy than did their controls (O'Connell and Fried, 1984). Another study reported that women who had a positive assay for marijuana use weighed slightly less before the pregnancy and gained significantly less weight during the pregnancy as compared with those who had a negative assay (Zuckerman et al., 1989). A third investigation found no consistent relationship between obesity (ponderal index >30) and the frequency of marijuana usage during pregnancy (Linn et al., 1983). Since it appears that prepregnancy weight and maternal weight gain were not controlled for in all investigations (Hatch and Bracken, 1986), it is unclear to what extent nutritional factors may have contributed to some of the reported effects of marijuana.

Despite the relatively high prevalence of marijuana use during pregnancy, no conclusive data are available on the effect of marijuana on the developing fetus. There is, however, suggestive evidence that marijuana use during pregnancy may impair fetal growth.

COCAINE

Prevalence of Cocaine Use

Cocaine use has grown to epidemic proportions during the past decade in the United States. Although cocaine was previously believed to be a relatively safe, nonaddictive euphoriant agent, it is now recognized that cocaine use is associated with substantial morbidity and mortality (Cregler and Mark, 1986; Gawin and Ellinwood, 1988). The National Household Survey on Drug Abuse in 1988 estimated that more than 20 million people in the United States had tried cocaine, including 20% of those between the ages of 18 and 25 (NIDA, 1989). The proportion of women aged 18 to 25 years who had used cocaine in the past month increased from 4.7% in 1982 to 6.3% in 1985 but declined to 3% in 1988 (NCHS, 1989; NIDA, 1989). Among teenage girls, however, the proportion has remained constant between 1985 and 1988 (NIDA, 1987; NIDA, 1989). While earlier surveys have indicated that cocaine usage was more common among whites than nonwhites, rates of recent usage in the 1988 survey were higher for Hispanic and black women as compared with white women (Abelson and Miller, 1985; NIDA, 1989). The subcommittee was unable to find any representative data on the prevalence of cocaine use among pregnant women, but a recent prospective study of consecutive prenatal patients from a poor inner-city population reported that 18% had used cocaine at least once during the pregnancy (Zuckerman et al., 1989). Cocaine addiction is believed to be five times more common than heroin addiction (Gawin and Ellinwood, 1988).

Cocaine is an alkaloid prepared from the plant *Erythroxylon coca*. When used in the free-base form (i.e., crack), it is more potent because it is almost pure cocaine. Cocaine acts as a central nervous system stimulant, causing increased heart rate, hypertension, and vasoconstriction (Cregler and Mark, 1986; Woods et al., 1987). Because of its low molecular weight and high solubility in water and lipids, cocaine readily crosses the placenta (Anonymous, 1988); however, the vasoconstrictive effect of cocaine may reduce placental transport (Fantel and MacPhail, 1982).

Effects on the Developing Fetus and Infant

An association between cocaine exposure and abruptio placentae is fairly well established (Acker et al., 1983; Bingol et al., 1987; Chasnoff and MacGregor, 1987; Chasnoff et al., 1985; Landy and Hinson, 1988; Livesay et al., 1987; Oro and Dixon, 1987). There is also growing evidence that cocaine abuse may be associated with premature labor and intrauterine growth retardation (Chasnoff and MacGregor, 1987; Chouteau et al., 1988; Dixon and Oro, 1987; LeBlanc et al., 1987; Oro and Dixon, 1987; Zuckerman et al., 1989) as well as spontaneous abortion (Chasnoff et al., 1985; Livesay et al., 1987). The teratogenic potential of cocaine is less clear, although there are reports suggesting an increase in congenital anomalies (Bingol et al., 1987; Chasnoff et al., 1988; Kobori et al., 1989). A mild withdrawal syndrome (Chasnoff et al., 1985; Doberczak et al., 1988; Oro and Dixon, 1987) and transient electroencephalogram abnormalities (Doberczak et al., 1988) have been described in some infants born to cocaine-abusing mothers. Of great concern are recent case reports of cerebral infarction in neonates who had been exposed to cocaine in utero (Chasnoff et al., 1986; Ferriero et al., 1988).

Possible Nutrition-Related Effects of Cocaine Use

As is true for marijuana, little is known about the nutrition-related effects of cocaine use. Cocaine's vasoconstrictive ability may lead to fetal hypoxia (Woods et al., 1987) and reduced nutritional supply to the fetus. Since cocaine, like amphetamines, acts as an appetite suppressant (Cregler and Mark, 1986; Gawin and Ellinwood, 1988; Resnick et al., 1977), an inadequate maternal diet may play a role in the growth retardation seen in fetuses of cocaine abusers. In one study, pregnant women with urine assays positive for cocaine weighed significantly less before the pregnancy, had lower hematocrit levels at the time of prenatal registration, and gained slightly less weight during the gestation than did those with negative assays (Frank et al., 1988; Zuckerman et al., 1989). Although the deficit in birth weight did not achieve significance when prepregnancy weight and maternal weight gain were controlled for in the analysis, significant decreases in birth length and head circumference remained (Zuckerman et al., 1989). Thus, these data suggest that the association between cocaine use and growth retardation may be partially but not completely mediated by nutritional factors. Other factors, such as cigarette smoking, alcohol consumption, and other drug abuse, which were not controlled for in all the studies, may also have confounded some of the reported adverse effects.

Since the origin of the current cocaine epidemic is recent, further studies should be conducted to provide more definitive evidence on the effects of cocaine on the course of pregnancy and neonatal outcome. Isolating the influence of cocaine from other factors will nevertheless be difficult, since cocaine use is often accompanied by abuse of other substances as well as other life-style patterns that may be detrimental to the fetus.

SUMMARY AND RECOMMENDATIONS FOR FUTURE RESEARCH

Although the adverse reproductive effects of tobacco, alcohol, and many illicit drugs are well established and there is some, albeit limited and conflicting, evidence that moderate to heavy use of coffee and caffeine may decrease birth weight, the underlying mechanisms responsible for these effects are generally not well understood. Much also remains to be learned concerning critical periods of exposure, dose-response thresholds, factors that modify susceptibility to the adverse effects, and influences of substance abuse on maternal and fetal nutrition. Similarly, little is known about the effects of specific patterns of substance abuse such as binge, as opposed to chronic, alcohol consumption. Furthermore, the factors underlying or associated with substance abuse, including the role of genetic predisposition, need to be delineated.

CLINICAL IMPLICATIONS

• Highest priority should be given to efforts to prevent or stop substance abuse by pregnant women since there is clear evidence that cigarette smoking and alcohol and drug abuse adversely affect the health of the mother and the fetus.

• Since nutritional deficiencies can be expected, especially among heavy substance abusers, diet counseling and other efforts (e.g., referral to a social worker) to improve food intake are recommended.

• Because heavy substance abusers may have difficulty in taking the steps needed to improve their dietary intake, the subcommittee recommends the use of multivitamin-mineral supplements of the type outlined in Chapter 1.

REFERENCES

Abel, E.L. 1971. Effects of marihuana on the solution of anagrams, memory and appetite. Nature 231:260-261.

Abel, E.L. 1980a. Prenatal exposure to cannabis: a critical review of effects on growth, development, and behavior. Behav. Neurol. Biol. 29:137-156.

Abel, E.L. 1980b. Smoking during pregnancy: a review of effects on growth and development of offspring. Hum. Biol. 52:593-625.

Abel, E.L., and R.J. Sokol. 1987. Incidence of fetal alcohol syndrome and economic impact of FAS-related anomalies. Drug Alcohol Depend. 19:51-70.

Abelson, H.I., and J.D. Miller. 1985. A decade of trends in cocaine use in the household population. Natl. Inst. Drug Abuse Res. Monogr. Ser. 61:35-49.

Acker, D., B.P. Sachs, K.J. Tracey, and W.E. Wise. 1983. Abruptio placentae associated with cocaine use. Am. J. Obstet. Gynecol. 146:220-221.

Alberman, E., M. Creasy, M. Elliott, and C. Spicer. 1976. Maternal factors associated with fetal chromosomal anomalies in spontaneous abortions. Br. J. Obstet. Gynaecol. 83:621-627.

Aldridge, A., J.V. Aranda, and A.H. Neims. 1979. Caffeine metabolism in the newborn. Clin. Pharmacol. Ther. 25:447-453.

Andrews, J., and J.M. McGarry. 1972. A community study of smoking in pregnancy. J. Obstet. Gynaecol. Br. Commonw. 79:1057-1073.

Anonymous. 1988. Perinatal toxicity of cocaine. The Med. Lett. 30:59-60.

Aronson, M., M. Kyllerman, K.G. Sabel, B. Sandin, and R. Olegård. 1985. Children of alcoholic mothers. Developmental, perceptual and behavioral characteristics as compared to matched controls. Acta Paediatr. Scand. 74:27-35.

Assadi, F.K., and M. Ziai. 1986. Zinc status of infants with fetal alcohol syndrome. Pediatr. Res. 20:551-554.

Berkowitz, G.S. 1988. Smoking and pregnancy. Pp. 173-191 in J.R. Niebyl, ed. Drug Use in Pregnancy, 2nd ed. Lea & Febiger, Philadelphia.

Berkowitz, G.S., T.R. Holford, and R.L. Berkowitz. 1982. Effects of cigarette smoking, alcohol, coffee and tea consumption on preterm delivery. Early Hum. Dev. 7:239-250.

Bertrand, M., E. Schwan, A. Frandon, A. Vagne, and J. Alary. 1965. Sur un effet tératogène systématique et spécifique de la caféine chez les Rongeurs. C.R. Soc. Biol. 159:2199-2202.

Bingol, N., M. Fuchs, V. Diaz, R.K. Stone, and D.S. Gromisch. 1987. Teratogenicity of cocaine in humans. J. Pediatr. 110:93-96.

Bracken, M.B., C. Bryce-Buchanan, R. Silten, and W. Srisuphan. 1982. Coffee consumption during pregnancy. N. Engl. J. Med. 306:1548-1549.

Brooke, O.G., H.R. Anderson, J.M. Bland, J.L. Peacock, and C.M. Stewart. 1989. Effects on birth weight of smoking, alcohol, caffeine, socioeconomic factors, and psychosocial stress. Br. Med. J. 298:795-801.

Butler, N.R., and H. Goldstein. 1973. Smoking in pregnancy and subsequent child development. Br. Med. J. 4:573-575.

Butler, N.R., H. Goldstein, and E.M. Ross. 1972. Cigarette smoking in pregnancy: its influence on birth weight and perinatal mortality. Br. Med. J. 2:127-130.

Camilo, M.E., M.Y. Morgan, and S. Sherlock. 1981. Erythrocyte transketolase activity in alcoholic liver disease. Scand. J. Gastroenterol. 16:273-279.

CDC (Centers for Disease Control). 1989. CDC criteria for anemia in children and childbearing-aged women. Morbid. Mortal. Week. Rep. 38:400-404.

Chasnoff, I., and S. MacGregor. 1987. Maternal cocaine use and neonatal morbidity. Pediatr. Res. 21:356A.

Chasnoff, I.J., W.J. Burns, S.H. Schnoll, and K.A. Burns. 1985. Cocaine use in pregnancy. N. Engl. J. Med. 313:666-669.

Chasnoff, I.J., M.E. Bussey, R. Savich, and C.M. Stack. 1986. Perinatal cerebral infarction and maternal cocaine use. J. Pediatr. 108:456-459.

Chasnoff, I.J., G.M. Chisum, and W.E. Kaplan. 1988. Maternal cocaine use and genitourinary tract malformations. Teratology 37:201-204.

Chouteau, M., P.B. Namerow, and P. Leppert. 1988. The effect of cocaine abuse on birth weight and gestational age. Obstet. Gynecol. 72:351-354.

Clarren, S.K., E.C. Alvord, Jr., S.M. Sumi, A.P. Streissguth, and D.W. Smith. 1978. Brain malformations related to prenatal exposure to ethanol. J. Pediatr. 92:64-67.

Clarren, S.K., S.J. Astley, and D.M. Bowden. 1988. Physical anomalies and developmental delays in nonhuman primate infants exposed to weekly doses of ethanol during gestation. Teratology 37:561-569.

Collins, T.F.X., J.J. Welsh, T.N. Black, and D.I. Ruggles. 1982. Teratogenic potential of caffeine in rats. Pp. 97-107 in Alternative Dietary Practices and Nutritional Abuses in Pregnancy: Proceedings of a Workshop. Report of the Committee on Nutrition of the Mother and Preschool Child, Food and Nutrition Board, Commission on Life Sciences. National Academy Press, Washington, D.C.

Cregler, L.L., and H. Mark. 1986. Medical complications of cocaine abuse. N. Engl. J. Med. 315:1495-1500.

Crosby, W.M., J. Metcoff, J.P. Costiloe, M. Mameesh, H.H. Sandstead, R.A. Jacob, P.E. McClain, G. Jacobson, W. Reid, and G. Burns. 1977. Fetal malnutrition: an appraisal of correlated factors. Am. J. Obstet. Gynecol. 128:22-31.

DHEW (Department of Health, Education, and Welfare). 1979. Smoking and Health: A Report of the Surgeon General. DHEW Publ. No. (PHS) 79-50066. Office on Smoking and Health, Office of the Assistant Secretary for Health, Public Health Service, U.S. Department of Health, Education, and Welfare, Washington, D.C. (various pagings).

DHHS (Department of Health and Human Services). 1980. The Health Consequences of Smoking for Women: A Report of the Surgeon General. Office on Smoking and Health, Office of the Assistant Secretary for Health, Public Health Service, U.S. Department of Health and Human Services, Washington, D.C. 359 pp.

Dixon, S.Z., and A. Oro. 1987. Cocaine and amphetamine exposure in neonates: perinatal consequences. Pediatr. Res. 21:359A.

Doberczak, T.M., S. Shanzer, R.T. Senie, and S.R. Kandall. 1988. Neonatal neurologic and electroencephalographic effects of intrauterine cocaine exposure. J. Pediatr. 113:354-358.

Dunn, H.G., A.K. McBurney, S. Ingram, and C.M. Hunter. 1977. Maternal cigarette smoking during pregnancy and the child's subsequent development: II. Neurological and intellectual maturation to the age of 6 1/2 years. Can. J. Public Health 68:43-50.

Ernhart, C.B., A.W. Wolf, P.L. Linn, R.J. Sokol, M.J. Kennard, and H.F. Filipovich. 1985. Alcohol-related birth defects: syndromal anomalies, intrauterine growth retardation, and neonatal behavioral assessment. Alcoholism 9:447-453.

Fantel, A.G., and B.J. MacPhail. 1982. The teratogenicity of cocaine. Teratology 26:17-19.

FDA (Food and Drug Administration). 1980. Caffeine and Pregnancy. FDA Drug Bull. 10:19-20.

Fedrick, J., and A.B.M. Anderson. 1976. Factors associated with spontaneous pre-term birth. Br. J. Obstet. Gynaecol. 83:342-350.

Ferriero, D.M., J.C. Partridge, and D.F. Wong. 1988. Congenital defects and stroke in cocaine-exposed neonates. Ann. Neurol. 24:348-349.

Fisher, S.E., M. Atkinson, D.H. Van Thiel, E. Rosenblum, R. David, and I. Holzman. 1981. Selective fetal malnutrition: the effect of ethanol and acetaldehyde upon *in vitro* uptake of alpha amino isobutyric acid by human placenta. Life Sci. 29:1283-1288.

Flynn, A., S.I. Miller, S.S. Martier, N.L. Golden, R.J. Sokol, and B.C. Del Villano. 1981. Zinc status of pregnant alcoholic women: a determinant of fetal outcome. Lancet 1:572-575.

Foltin, R.W., M.W. Fischman, J.J. Pedroso, and G.D. Pearlson. 1987. Marijuana and cocaine interactions in humans: cardiovascular consequences. Pharmacol. Biochem. Behav. 28:459-464.

Frank, D.A., B.S. Zuckerman, H. Amaro, K. Aboagye, H. Bauchner, H. Cabral, L. Fried, R. Hingson, H. Kayne, S.M. Levenson, S. Parker, H. Reece, and R. Vinci. 1988. Cocaine use during pregnancy: prevalence and correlates. Pediatrics 82:888-895.

Fredricks, R.E., K.R. Tanaka, and W.N. Valentine. 1960. Zinc in human blood cells: normal values and abnormalities associated with liver disease. J. Clin. Invest. 39:1651-1656.

Fried, P.A. 1980. Marihuana use by pregnant women: neurobehavioral effects in neonates. Drug Alcohol Depend. 6:415-424.

Fried, P.A., B. Watkinson, and A. Willan. 1984. Marijuana use during pregnancy and decreased length of gestation. Am. J. Obstet. Gynecol. 150:23-27.

Garn, S.M., H.A. Shaw, and K.D. McCabe. 1978. Effect of maternal smoking on hemoglobins and hematocrits of the newborn. Am. J. Clin. Nutr. 31:557-558.

Garn, S.M., K. Hoff, and K.D. McCabe. 1979. Is there nutritional mediation of the "smoking effect" on the fetus. Am. J. Clin. Nutr. 32:1181-1187.

Gawin, F.H., and E.H. Ellinwood, Jr. 1988. Cocaine and other stimulants: actions, abuse, and treatment. N. Engl. J. Med. 318:1173-1182.

Ghishan, F.K., and H.L. Greene. 1983. Fetal alcohol syndrome: failure of zinc supplementation to reverse the effect of ethanol on placental transport of zinc. Pediatr. Res. 17:529-531.

Ghishan, F.K., R. Patwardhan, and H.L. Greene. 1982. Fetal alcohol syndrome: inhibition of placental zinc transport as a potential mechanism for fetal growth retardation in the rat. J. Lab. Clin. Med. 100:45-52.

Gibson, G.T., P.A. Baghurst, and D.P. Colley. 1983. Maternal alcohol, tobacco and cannabis consumption and the outcome of pregnancy. Aust. N.Z.J. Obstet. Gynaecol. 23:15-19.

Graham, D.M. 1978. Caffeine—its identity, dietary sources, intake and biological effects. Nutr. Rev. 36:97-102.

Graham, J.M., Jr., J.W. Hanson, B.L. Darby, H.M. Barr, and A.P. Streissguth. 1988. Independent dysmorphology evaluations at birth and 4 years of age for children exposed to varying amounts of alcohol in utero. Pediatrics 81:772-778.

Greenland, S., K.J. Staisch, N. Brown, and S.J. Gross. 1982. The effects of marijuana use during pregnancy. I. A preliminary epidemiologic study. Am. J. Obstet. Gynecol. 143:408-413.

Halsted, C.H., E.A. Robles, and E. Mezey. 1971. Decreased jejunal uptake of labeled folic acid (^{3}H-PGA) in alcoholic patients: roles of alcohol and nutrition. N. Engl. J. Med. 285:701-706.

Hanson, J.W., K.L. Jones, and D.W. Smith. 1976. Fetal alcohol syndrome: experience with 41 patients. J. Am. Med. Assoc. 235:1458-1460.

Hanson, J.W., A.P. Streissguth, and D.W. Smith. 1978. The effects of moderate alcohol consumption during pregnancy on fetal growth and morphogenesis. J. Pediatr. 92:457-460.

Harclerode, J. 1980. The effect of marijuana on reproduction and development. Pp. 137-166 in R.C. Peterson, ed. Marijuana Research Findings: 1980. NIDA Research Monograph 31. National Institute on Drug Abuse, U.S. Department of Health and Human Services, Rockville, Md.

Harlap, S., and P.H. Shiono. 1980. Alcohol, smoking, and incidence of spontaneous abortions in the first and second trimester. Lancet 2:173-176.

Hatch, E.E., and M.B. Bracken. 1986. Effect of marijuana use in pregnancy on fetal growth. Am. J. Epidemiol. 124:986-993.

Haworth, J.C., J.J. Ellestad-Sayed, J. King, and L.A. Dilling. 1980a. Fetal growth retardation in cigarette-smoking mothers is not due to decreased maternal food intake. Am. J. Obstet. Gynecol. 137:719-723.

Haworth, J.C., J.J. Ellestad-Sayed, J. King, and L.A. Dilling. 1980b. Relation of maternal cigarette smoking, obesity, and energy consumption to infant size. Am. J. Obstet. Gynecol. 138:1185-1189.

Heinonen, O.P., D. Slone, and S. Shapiro. 1977. Caffeine and other xanthine derivatives. Pp. 366-370 in Birth Defects and Drugs in Pregnancy. Publishing Sciences Group, Littleton, Mass.

Henderson, G.I., D. Turner, R.V. Patwardhan, L. Lumeng, A.M. Hoyumpa, and S. Schenker. 1981. Inhibition of placental valine uptake after acute and chronic maternal ethanol consumption. J. Pharmacol. Exp. Ther. 216:465-472.

Hingson, R., J.J. Alpert, N. Day, E. Dooling, H. Kayne, S. Morelock, E. Oppenheimer, and B. Zuckerman. 1982. Effects of maternal drinking and marijuana use on fetal growth and development. Pediatrics 70:539-546.

Hingson, R., B. Zuckerman, H. Amaro, D.A. Frank, H. Kayne, J.R. Sorenson, J. Mitchell, S. Parker, S. Morelock, and R. Timperi. 1986. Maternal marijuana use and neonatal outcome: uncertainty posed by self-reports. Am. J. Public Health 76:667-669.

Hogue, C.J. 1981. Coffee in pregnancy. Lancet 1:554.

Hoyumpa, A.M., Jr. 1983. Alcohol and thiamine metabolism. Alcoholism 7:11-14.

Indänpään-Heikkilä, J., G.E. Fritchie, L.F. Englert, B.T. Ho, and W.M. McIsaac. 1969. Placental transfer of tritiated-1-Δ9-tetrahydrocannabinol. N. Engl. J. Med. 281:330.

Jones, K.L., and D.W. Smith. 1973. Recognition of the fetal alcohol syndrome in early infancy. Lancet 2:999-1001.

Jones, R.T. 1980. Human effects: an overview. Pp. 54-80 in R.C. Petersen, ed. Marijuana Research Findings: 1980. NIDA Research Monograph 31. National Institute on Drug Abuse, U.S. Department of Health and Human Services, Rockville, Md.

Kallner, A.B., D. Hartmann, and D.H. Hornig. 1981. On the requirements of ascorbic acid in man: steady-state turnover and body pool in smokers. Am. J. Clin. Nutr. 34:1347-1355.

Keith, R.E., and S.B. Mossholder. 1986. Ascorbic acid status of smoking and nonsmoking adolescent females. Int. J. Vitam. Nutr. Res. 56:363-366.

Keppen, L.D., T. Pysher, and O.M. Rennert. 1985. Zinc deficiency acts as a co-teratogen with alcohol in fetal alcohol syndrome. Pediatr. Res. 19:944-947.

Kiely, M. 1981. Zinc status and pregnancy outcome. Lancet 1:893.

Kirkinen, P., P. Jouppila, A. Koivula, J. Vuori, and M. Puukka. 1983. The effect of caffeine on placental and fetal blood flow in human pregnancy. Am. J. Obstet. Gynecol. 147:939-942.

Kleinman, J.C., and A. Kopstein. 1987. Smoking during pregnancy, 1967-80. Am. J. Public Health 77:823-825.

Kline, J., P. Shrout, Z. Stein, M. Susser, and D. Warburton. 1980a. Drinking during pregnancy and spontaneous abortion. Lancet 2:176-180.

Kline, J., Z. Stein, M. Susser, and D. Warburton. 1980b. Environmental influences on early reproductive loss in a current New York City study. Pp. 225-240 in I.H. Porter and E.B. Hook, eds. Human Embryonic and Fetal Death. Academic Press, New York.

Kline, J., Z. Stein, and M. Hutzler. 1987. Cigarettes, alcohol and marijuana: varying associations with birthweight. Int. J. Epidemiol. 16:44-51.

Kobori, J.A., D.M. Ferriero, and M. Golabi. 1989. CNS and craniofacial anomalies in infants born to cocaine abusing mothers. Clin. Res. 37:196A.

Kramer, M.S. 1987. Intrauterine growth and gestational duration determinants. Pediatrics 80:502-511.

Kuhnert, B.R., P.M. Kuhnert, S. Debanne, and T.G. Williams. 1987. The relationship between cadmium, zinc, and birth weight in pregnant women who smoke. Am. J. Obstet. Gynecol. 157:1247-1251.

Kuhnert, B.R., P.M. Kuhnert, N. Lazebnik, and P. Erhard. 1988. The effect of maternal smoking on the relationship between maternal and fetal zinc status and infant birth weight. J. Am. Coll. Nutr. 7:309-316.

Kullander, S., and B. Källén. 1971. A prospective study of smoking and pregnancy. Acta Obstet. Gynecol. Scand. 50:83-94.

Kurppa, K., P.C. Holmberg, E. Kuosma, and L. Saxén. 1982. Coffee consumption during pregnancy. N. Engl. J. Med. 306:1548.

Landy, H.J., and J. Hinson. 1988. Placental abruption associated with cocaine use: case report. Reprod. Toxicol. 1:203-205.

LeBlanc, P.E., A.J. Parekh, B. Naso, and L. Glass. 1987. Effects of intrauterine exposure to alkaloidal cocaine ('crack'). Am. J. Dis. Child. 141:937-938.

Leo, M.A., and C.S. Lieber. 1982. Hepatic vitamin A depletion in alcoholic liver injury. N. Engl. J. Med. 307:597-601.

Leo, M.A., and C.S. Lieber. 1983. Hepatic fibrosis after long-term administration of ethanol and moderate vitamin A supplementation in the rat. Hepatology 3:1-11.

Lewis, J.S., and K. Inoue. 1981. Effect of coffee ingestion on urinary thiamin excretion. Fed. Proc., Fed. Am. Soc. Exp. Biol. 40:914.

Lieber, C.S. 1985. Alcohol and the liver: metabolism, metabolic effects and pathogenesis of injury. Acta Med. Scand., Suppl. 703:11-55.

Lin, G.W.J. 1981. Effect of ethanol feeding during pregnancy on placental transfer of alpha-aminoisobutyric acid in the rat. Life Sci. 28:595-601.

Linn, S., S.C. Schoenbaum, R.R. Monson, B. Rosner, P.G. Stubblefield, and K.J. Ryan. 1982. No association between coffee consumption and adverse outcomes of pregnancy. N. Engl. J. Med. 306:141-145.

Linn, S., S.C. Schoenbaum, R.R. Monson, R. Rosner, P.C. Stubblefield, and K.J. Ryan. 1983. The association of marijuana use with outcome of pregnancy. Am. J. Public Health 73:1161-1164.

Little, R.E. 1977. Moderate alcohol use during pregnancy and decreased infant birth weight. Am. J. Public Health 67:1154-1156.

Livesay, S., S. Ehrlich, and L.P. Finnegan. 1987. Cocaine and pregnancy: maternal and infant outcome. Pediatr. Res. 21:238A.

Longo, L.D. 1982. Some health consequences of maternal smoking: issues without answers. Birth Defects 18:13-31.

LSRO (Life Sciences Research Office). 1984. Assessment of the Folate Nutritional Status of the U.S. Population Based on Data Collected in the Second National Health and Nutrition Examination Survey, 1976-1980. Federation of American Societies for Experimental Biology, Bethesda, Md. 96 pp.

Marbury, M.C., S. Linn, R. Monson, S. Schoenbaum, P.G. Stubblefield, and K.J. Ryan. 1983. The association of alcohol consumption with outcome of pregnancy. Am. J. Public Health 73:1165-1168.

Martin, T.R., and M.B. Bracken. 1987. The association between low birth weight and caffeine consumption during pregnancy. Am. J. Epidemiol. 126:813-821.

Massey, L.K., and P.W. Hollingbery. 1988a. Acute effects of dietary caffeine and aspirin on urinary mineral excretion in pre- and postmenopausal women. Nutr. Res. 8:845-851.

Massey, L.K., and P.W. Hollingbery. 1988b. Acute effects of dietary caffeine and sucrose on urinary mineral excretion of healthy adolescents. Nutr. Res. 8:1005-1912.

Mau, G., and P. Netter. 1974. Kaffee-und Alkoholkonsum—Risikofaktoren in der Schwangerschaft? Geburtshilfe Frauenheilkd. 34:1018-1022.

McClain, C.J., and L.C. Su. 1983. Zinc deficiency in the alcoholic: a review. Alcoholism 7:5-10.

Meberg, A., H. Sande, O.P. Foss, and J.T. Stenwig. 1979. Smoking during pregnancy—effects on the fetus and on thiocyanate levels in mother and baby. Acta Paediatr. Scand. 68:547-552.

Metcoff, J., P. Costiloe, W.M. Crosby, S. Dutta, H.H. Sandstead, D. Milne, C.E. Bodwell, and S.H. Majors. 1985. Effect of food supplementation (WIC) during pregnancy on birth weight. Am. J. Clin. Nutr. 41:933-947.

Metcoff, J., P. Costiloe, W.M. Crosby, H.H. Sandstead, and D. Milne. 1989. Smoking in pregnancy: relation of birth weight to maternal plasma carotene and cholesterol levels. Obstet. Gynecol. 74:302-309.

Meyer, M.B., and J.A. Tonascia. 1977. Maternal smoking, pregnancy complications, and perinatal mortality. Am. J. Obstet. Gynecol. 128:494-502.

Meyer, M.B., B.S. Jonas, and J.A. Tonascia. 1976. Perinatal events associated with maternal smoking during pregnancy. Am. J. Epidemiol. 103:464-476.

Mills, J.L., B.I. Graubard, E.E. Harley, G.G. Rhoads, and H.W. Berendes. 1984. Maternal alcohol consumption and birth weight. How much drinking during pregnancy is safe? J. Am. Med. Assoc. 252:1875-1879.

Morck, T.A., S.R. Lynch, and J.D. Cook. 1983. Inhibition of food iron absorption by coffee. Am. J. Clin. Nutr. 37:416-420.

Muñoz, L.M., B. Lönnerdal, C.L. Keen, and K.G. Dewey. 1988. Coffee consumption as a factor in iron deficiency anemia among pregnant women and their infants in Costa Rica. Am. J. Clin. Nutr. 48:645-651.

Naeye, R.L. 1978. Effects of maternal cigarette smoking on the fetus and placenta. Br. J. Obstet. Gynaecol. 85:732-737.

Naeye, R.L. 1979. The duration of maternal cigarette smoking, fetal and placental disorders. Early Hum. Dev. 3:229-237.

Naeye, R.L., and E.C. Peters. 1984. Mental development of children whose mothers smoked during pregnancy. Obstet. Gynecol. 64:601-607.

NCHS (National Center for Health Statistics). 1989. Health United States 1988. DHHS Publ. No. (PHS) 89-1232. National Center for Health Statistics, Public Health Service, U.S. Department of Health and Human Services, Hyattsville, Md. 208 pp.

Nelson, M.M., and J.O. Forfar. 1971. Associations between drugs administered during pregnancy and congenital abnormalities of the fetus. Br. Med. J. 1:523-527.

NIDA (National Institute on Drug Abuse). 1987. National Household Survey on Drug Abuse: Population Estimates 1985. DHHS Publ. No. (ADM) 87-1539. National Institute on Drug Abuse, Public Health Service, U.S. Department of Health and Human Services, Rockville, Md. 73 pp.

NIDA (National Institute on Drug Abuse). 1989. National Household Survey on Drug Abuse: Population Estimates 1988. DHHS Publ. No. (ADM) 89-1636. National Institute on Drug Abuse, Public Health Service, U.S. Department of Health and Human Services, Rockville, Md. 121 pp.

NRC (National Research Council). 1977. Estimating Distribution of Daily Intakes of Caffeine. Report of the Committee on GRAS List Survey—Phase III. Food and Nutrition Board, Division of Biological Sciences, Assembly of Life Sciences. National Academy of Sciences, Washington, D.C. 12 pp.

NRC (National Research Council). 1982. Alternative Dietary Practices and Nutritional Abuses in Pregnancy: Proceedings of a Workshop. Report of the Committee on Nutrition of the Mother and Preschool Child, Food and Nutrition Board, Commission on Life Sciences. National Academy Press, Washington, D.C. 211 pp.

O'Connell, C.M., and P.A. Fried. 1984. An investigation of prenatal cannabis exposure and minor physical anomalies in a low risk population. Neurobehav. Toxicol. Teratol. 6:345-350.

Oro, A.S., and S.D. Dixon. 1987. Perinatal cocaine and methamphetamine exposure: maternal and neonatal correlates. J. Pediatr. 111:571-578.

Ouellette, E.M., H.L. Rosett, N.P. Rosman, and L. Weiner. 1977. Adverse effects on offspring of maternal alcohol abuse during pregnancy. N. Engl. J. Med. 297:528-530.

Pécoud, A., P. Donzel, and J.L. Schelling. 1975. Effect of foodstuffs on the absorption of zinc sulfate. Clin. Pharmacol. Ther. 17:469-474.

Perkins, K.A., L.H. Epstein, B.L. Marks, R.L. Stiller, and R.G. Jacob. 1989. The effect of nicotine on energy expenditure during light physical activity. N. Engl. J. Med. 320:898-903.

Pettigrew, A.R., R.W. Logan, and J. Willocks. 1977. Smoking in pregnancy—effects on birth weight and on cyanide and thiocyanate levels in mother and baby. Br. J. Obstet. Gynaecol. 84:31-34.

Picone, T.A., L.H. Allen, M.M. Schramm, and P.N. Olsen. 1982. Pregnancy outcome in North American women. I. Effects of diet, cigarette smoking, and psychological stress on maternal weight gain. Am. J. Clin. Nutr. 36:1205-1213.

Prager, K., H. Malin, D. Spiegler, P. Van Natta, and P.J. Placek. 1984. Smoking and drinking behavior before and during pregnancy of married mothers of live-born infants and stillborn infants. Public Health Rep. 99:117-127.

Rall, T.W. 1985. Central nervous system stimulants. The methylxanthines. Pp. 589-603 in A.G. Gilman, L.S. Goodman, T.W. Rall, and F. Murad, eds. Goodman and Gilman's The Pharmacological Basis of Therapeutics. MacMillan Publishing, New York.

Randall, C.L., E.A. Lochry, S.S. Hughes, and P.B. Sutker. 1981. Dose-responsive effect of prenatal alcohol exposure on fetal growth and development in mice. Sub. Alcohol Actions Misuse 2:349-357.

Rantakallio, P. 1983. A follow-up study up to the age of 14 of children whose mothers smoked during pregnancy. Acta Paediatr. Scand. 72:747-753.

Resnick, R.B., R.S. Kestenbaum, and L.K. Schwartz. 1977. Acute systemic effects of cocaine in man: a controlled study by intranasal and intravenous routes. Science 195:696-698.

Rosenberg, L., A.A. Mitchell, S. Shapiro, and D. Slone. 1982. Selected birth defects in relation to caffeine-containing beverages. J. Am. Med. Assoc. 247:1429-1432.

Rosett, H.L. 1980. A clinical perpsective of the Fetal Alcohol Syndrome. Alcoholism 4:119-122.

Rosett, H.L., L. Weiner, A. Lee, B. Zuckerman, E. Dooling, and E. Oppenheimer. 1983. Patterns of alcohol consumption and fetal development. Obstet. Gynecol. 61:539-546.

Rush, D. 1974. Examination of the relationship between birthweight, cigarette smoking during pregnancy and maternal weight gain. J. Obstet. Gynaecol. Br. Commonw. 81:746-752.

Rush, D., Z. Stein, and M. Susser. 1980. A randomized controlled trial of prenatal nutritional supplementation in New York City. Pediatrics 65:683-697.

Rush, D., N.L. Sloan, J. Leighton, J.M. Alvir, D.G. Horvitz, W.B. Seaver, G.C. Garbowski, S.S. Johnson, R.A. Kulka, M. Holt, J.W. Devore, J.T. Lynch, M.B. Woodside, and D.S. Shanklin. 1988. The National WIC Evaluation: evaluation of the Special Supplemental Food Program for Women, Infants, and Children. V. Longitudinal study of pregnant women. Am. J. Clin. Nutr. 48:439-483.

Ruth, R.E., and S.K. Goldsmith. 1981. Interaction between zinc deprivation and acute ethanol intoxication during pregnancy in rats. J. Nutr. 111:2034-2038.

Scher, M.S., G.A. Richardson, P.A. Coble, N.L. Day, and D.S. Stoffer. 1988. The effects of prenatal alcohol and marijuana exposure: disturbances in neonatal sleep cycling and arousal. Pediatr. Res. 24:101-105.

Sexton, M., and J.R. Hebel. 1984. A clinical trial of change in maternal smoking and its effect on birth weight. J. Am. Med. Assoc. 251:911-915.

Shaywitz, S.E., D.J. Cohen, and B.A. Shaywitz. 1980. Behavior and learning difficulties in children of normal intelligence born to alcoholic mothers. J. Pediatr. 96:978-982.

Shiono, P.H., M.A. Klebanoff, and G.G. Rhoads. 1986. Smoking and drinking during pregnancy: their effects on preterm birth. J. Am. Med. Assoc. 255:82-84.

Sokol, R.J., S.I. Miller, S. Debanne, N. Golden, G. Collins, J. Kaplan, and S. Martier. 1981. The Cleveland NIAAA prospective alcohol-in-pregnancy study: the first year. Neurobehav. Toxicol. Teratol. 3:203-209.

Srisuphan, W., and M.B. Bracken. 1986. Caffeine consumption during pregnancy and association with late spontaneous abortion. Am. J. Obstet. Gynecol. 154:14-20.

Streissguth, A.P., B.L. Darby, H.M. Barr, J.R. Smith, and D.C. Martin. 1983. Comparison of drinking and smoking patterns during pregnancy over a six-year interval. Am. J. Obstet. Gynecol. 145:716-724.

Tennes, K., and C. Blackard. 1980. Maternal alcohol consumption, birth weight, and minor physical anomalies. Am. J. Obstet. Gynecol. 138:774-780.

Vallee, B.L., W.E. Wacker, A.F. Bartholomay, and F.L. Hoch. 1957. Zinc metabolism in hepatic dysfunction. II. Correlation of metabolic patterns with biochemical findings. N. Engl. J. Med. 257:1055-1065.

van den Berg, B.J. 1977. Epidemiologic observations of prematurity: effects of tobacco, coffee, and alcohol. Pp. 157-176 in D.M. Reed and F.J. Stanley, eds. The Epidemiology of Prematurity. Urban & Schwarzenberg, Baltimore.

Watkinson, B., and P.A. Fried. 1985. Maternal caffeine use before, during and after pregnancy and effects upon offspring. Neurobehav. Toxicol. Teratol. 7:9-17.

Weinberg, J. 1985. Effects of ethanol and maternal nutritional status on fetal development. Alcoholism 9:49-55.

Wiener, S.G., W.J. Shoemaker, L.Y. Koda, and F.E. Bloom. 1981. Interaction of ethanol and nutrition during gestation: influence on maternal and offspring development in the rat. J. Pharmacol. Exp. Ther. 216:572-579.

Williamson, D.F., M.K. Serdula, J.S. Kendrick, and N.J. Binkin. 1989. Comparing the prevalence of smoking in pregnant and nonpregnant women, 1985 to 1986. J. Am. Med. Assoc. 261:70-74.

Wilson, F.A., and A.M. Hoyumpa, Jr. 1979. Ethanol and small intestinal transport. Gastroenterology 76:388-403.

Windsor, R.A., G. Cutter, J. Morris, Y. Reese, B. Manzella, E.E. Bartlett, C. Samuelson, and D. Spanos. 1985. The effectiveness of smoking cessation methods for smokers in public health maternity clinics: a randomized trial. Am. J. Public Health 75:1389-1392.

Woods, J.R., Jr., M.A. Plessinger, and K.E. Clark. 1987. Effect of cocaine on uterine blood flow and fetal oxygenation. J. Am. Med. Assoc. 257:957-961.

Woteki, C., C. Johnson, and R. Murphy. 1986. Nutritional status of the U.S. population: iron, vitamin C, and zinc. Pp. 21-39 in What is America Eating? Proceedings of a Symposium. Food and Nutrition Board, Commission on Life Sciences. National Academy Press, Washington, D.C.

Wright, J.T., E.J. Waterson, I.G. Barrison, P.J. Toplis, I.G. Lewis, M.G. Gordon, K.D. MacRae, N.F. Morris, and I.M. Murray-Lyon. 1983. Alcohol consumption, pregnancy, and low birthweight. Lancet 1:663-665.

Wu, T.C., D.P. Tashkin, B. Djahed, and J.E. Rose. 1988. Pulmonary hazards of smoking marijuana as compared with tobacco. N. Engl. J. Med. 318:347-351.

Zuckerman, B., D.A. Frank, R. Hingson, H. Amaro, S.M. Levenson, H. Kayne, S. Parker, R. Vinci, K. Aboagye, L.E. Fried, H. Cabral, R. Timperi, and H. Bauchner. 1989. Effects of maternal marijuana and cocaine use on fetal growth. N. Engl. J. Med. 320:762-768.

21
Periconceptional Vitamin Supplementation and Neural Tube Defects

Very early in pregnancy, the developing embryo is susceptible to malformations from a variety of causes. Animal studies suggest that these causes may include certain maternal nutrient deficiencies or excesses if they occur during embryogenesis (i.e., during the first 2 months of gestation). The implications of this for human nutrition are uncertain. Evidence that excessive intake of vitamin A may be teratogenic (i.e., may cause birth defects) is covered in Chapter 17. This chapter considers evidence relating to periconceptional micronutrient status and supplementation to neural tube defects. The periconceptional period is a term that lacks a tight definition. The subcommittee suggests that it be used to denote a period from 1 to 3 months before conception to week 6 of gestation. The critical period for the formation of the neural tube is from 17 to 30 days gestation.

NEURAL TUBE DEFECTS

Neural tube defects such as spina bifida have been linked by several investigators to periconceptional nutrient intake. The seriousness and the frequency with which neural tube defects occur warrant careful consideration of evidence from studies that address nutrition-related approaches for reducing their incidence.

Occurrence

Despite a recent decline in the occurrence rate, 2,500 to 3,000 infants are born with neural tube defects in the United States each year. It is estimated that 30,000 living Americans have spina bifida. Many other cases of neural tube defects are aborted, stillborn, or die early in life. The magnitude of the problem on a worldwide basis is estimated at 300,000 to 400,000 births per year.

Occurrence rates for neural tube defects vary widely according to geographic area, socioeconomic status, and ethnic background. Rates are relatively low in the United States, the highest rates being found in the Southeast and lowest rates in the West. In each area, rates are much lower for blacks than for whites. Marked changes in the occurrence rate of neural tube defects have been observed; the rate peaked in the middle of this century and has progressively declined over the past 40 years in North America and Western Europe. The risk of a recurrent neural tube defect, i.e., more than one affected child born to the same parents, is much greater than the risk of occurrence. Recurrence rates have been estimated to be as high as 2 to 10%, compared with an occurrence rate of <0.04% in a low-risk area. However, the absolute number of first occurrences to parents greatly exceeds that of recurrent events.

Possible Causes

Neural tube defects result from genetic-environmental interactions. The genetic component, which probably involves several genes, is complex and not well understood. The sum of epidemiologic and other evidence indicates a strong environmental component. The nature of the environmental factors, especially the supposed role of micronutrient nutrition and metabolism, has become the focus of intense scientific interest and debate. To reduce the risk of neural tube defects, periconceptional vitamin supplementation has been recommended, especially for all women who have had a previous pregnancy complicated by a neural tube defect (International Conference on Prepregnancy Nutrition, 1987) but also for all pregnant women (Holmes, 1988; International Conference on Prepregnancy Nutrition, 1987). However, most researchers have been cautious about overinterpreting their data.

Evidence of Effects of Nutrients

The subcommittee examined evidence from studies in animal models and in humans addressing the possible value of folate and multivitamin supplementation commencing prior to conception. The human studies reported to date have involved laboratory assays, supplementation studies, and case-control studies, but no randomized controlled clinical trials.

Studies in Animal Models

Animal models provide some support for the hypothesis that vitamin deficiencies may be one etiologic factor in the multifactorial etiology of human neural tube defects (Kalter and Warkany, 1959). However, folate deficiency produced neural tube defects in rats only when folate antagonists were given (Nelson et al., 1955).

The therapeutic use of the anticonvulsant drug valproic acid during pregnancy is associated with a 20-fold excess risk of neural tube defects (Lammer et al., 1987). A similar teratogenic effect of valproic acid has been demonstrated in mice (Trots et al., 1987). When folinic acid, the metabolically active form of folic acid, is administered, the rate of valproate-induced neural tube defects is reduced. A recent preliminary report indicates that valproate impairs the activity of the enzyme glutamate formyltransferase (EC 2.1.2.6), which catalyzes the conversion of tetrahydrofolate to folinic acid (Wegner and Nau, 1989). These observations indicate that neural tube defects can result from disturbed folate metabolism.

Laboratory Assays

The results of laboratory assays suggest that maternal folate status may be abnormal in subjects whose offspring have neural tube defects. Smithells et al. (1976) observed significantly lower levels of red cell folate and white cell ascorbate during the first trimester in mothers who delivered an infant with a neural tube defect. Similarly, Yates et al. (1987) reported that mothers with an affected pregnancy had lower red cell folate levels than those of controls. Moreover, red cell folate levels were lowest in the group with three or more neural tube defect pregnancies. No differences were found for serum folate or for other serum vitamin measurements. Molloy et al. (1985) observed no difference in maternal serum folate or vitamin B_{12} levels between those with neural tube defect pregnancies and controls. These observations suggest that a change in maternal folate metabolism may be associated with neural tube defect pregnancies, but they do not necessarily suggest that a low intake of folate was involved.

Epidemiologic Observations

Epidemiologic observations indicate that poor maternal nutrition could be important in the etiology of neural tube defects (Laurence et al., 1980). These observations were not sufficiently detailed to indicate any specific nutrient deficiency.

Periconceptional Vitamin Supplementation Studies

In 1981, Laurence and colleagues reported the outcome of a folate supplementation study (4 mg of folate per day) in South Wales. Subjects and controls were women who had a previous neural tube defect pregnancy. They reported a statistically significant higher incidence of recurrence rates in the placebo group, but only after the folate group was adjusted for noncompliers, as determined from blood analyses (Laurence et al., 1981). The study group was very small ($N = 111$) with a total of six neural tube defects occurring in test and control groups combined.

Smithells et al. (1983) reported the combined results of studies on two cohorts of women with previous neural tube defect pregnancies included in the United Kingdom Multicenter Trial. The trial was a nonrandomized study of periconceptional multivitamin and mineral supplementation. The recurrence rate among subjects receiving the multivitamin preparation was 0.7% (3 out of 454) in comparison with a recurrence rate for the nonsupplemented group of 4.8% (24 out of 519). This apparent sevenfold protective effect is extremely unlikely to be attributable to chance. However, bias in this nonrandomized trial cannot be excluded (Wald and Polani, 1984), especially since predictors of neural tube defects are still poorly understood. For example, willingness to collaborate in a study involving administration of a capsule three times a day for several months or the initiative to consult with a doctor prior to conception may be factors associated with a relatively low risk of a recurrent neural tube defect. The marked and unexplained decrease in the overall rate of recurrence during the study period has added further to the complexities of interpreting the data. The confusion and controversy associated with this study are a direct consequence of an inadequate design that did not include appropriate controls. Although the presumptive evidence for a beneficial effect of the multivitamin mineral preparation is quite strong, Smithells and colleagues have stated that "further studies are a prerequisite for policy decisions designed to reduce the occurrence of neural tube defects" (Smithells et al., 1983).

Case-Control and Cohort Studies of Periconceptional Multivitamin Use

The results of three case-control studies and one cohort study of multivitamin or folate supplements or dietary folate intake in relation to the occurrence of neural tube defects were reported in 1988 and 1989. In one of these studies (Mulinare et al., 1988), the use of a folic acid-containing multivitamin during the periconceptional period was associated with a reduced prevalence of neural tube defects as compared with the prevalence among nonusers (0.9 compared with 3.3 per 1,000, respectively).

The precise composition of the multivitamin preparations in this study were not available; the mothers were interviewed between 2.5 and 16 years after the relevant pregnancy. The investigators emphasized that they could not exclude the possibility that a factor associated with the use of multivitamins rather than the vitamin intake per se was the real determinant of the observed decrease. Such factors might involve socioeconomic status, since poor women and women with relatively few years of formal education are not as likely to take multivitamins as their more advantaged counterparts (Block et al., 1988; Koplan et al., 1986).

Milunsky and colleagues (1989) reported that the use of folic acid–containing multivitamins during the first 6 weeks of pregnancy was associated with a 73% reduction in the prevalence of neural tube defects. No protective effect of multivitamins without folate was observed, nor was there any apparent benefit of folate supplements started after 6 weeks of gestation. Among women not taking folate supplements, the prevalence of neural tube defects was lower among those with dietary folate intakes exceeding 100 μg/day than among those with lower intakes. (The estimated mean daily folate intake of women aged 19 to 44 in the United States is approximately 220 μg [Subar et al., 1989; USDA, 1985]). The cohort in this study consisted of 23,500 women undergoing maternal serum α-fetoprotein screening or amniocentesis at approximately week 16 of gestation, 49 of whom had an affected fetus. Several biases are possible in the study. For example, some of the subjects knew the results of their screening before being interviewed. Furthermore, women who elected to take folate supplements before week 6 of gestation may have had characteristics different from those of women who did not take supplements or who started their supplements later in gestation.

Bower and Stanley (1989) found a reduction in the occurrence of neural tube defects with increasing dietary intake of free folate during the first 6 weeks of pregnancy. Similar but weaker trends were seen when the effect of total folate intake was examined. These investigators concluded that dietary folate deficiency in early pregnancy is associated with the occurrence of neural tube defects but that confirmation is required before the issue of prevention can be addressed.

In a large population-based case-control study conducted in California and Illinois, Mills et al. (1989) found no evidence of a protective effect from the use of a multivitamin preparation during the periconceptional period. Although these investigators attempted to minimize recall bias by using two control groups (one consisting of mothers who had delivered stillborn infants or infants with other abnormalities and one comprising women who had given birth to normal infants), the possibility of recall error or misclassification of multivitamin use cannot be discounted.

Although the results of these studies are not consistent, they do, however, point clearly to the need for more definitive studies of maternal vitamin intake, especially folate intake, in the periconceptional period.

Limitations of the Evidence

Data associating the periconceptional use of multivitamin or folate preparations with protection against neural tube defects are inconsistent. Although the findings of some key studies; e.g., the United Kingdom Multicenter Trial (nonrandomized) (Smithells et al., 1983), the Centers for Disease Control case-control study (Mulinare et al., 1988), and the Boston cohort study (Milunsky et al., 1989), were very unlikely to be due to chance, factors other than periconceptional vitamin use cannot be excluded as possible explanations for the results. For example, there is evidence that the average diets consumed by women who take vitamin supplements have a higher nutrient density than the diets of nonusers (Kurinij et al., 1986). Furthermore, dietary factors other than vitamins may provide protection.

In animal models, maternal zinc deficiency has produced lesions similar to anencephaly (another type of neural tube defect) in humans, and neural tube defects are produced more readily by zinc deficiencies than by deficiency of any other micronutrient (Hurley, 1980). Other evidence from studies in humans suggests that maternal zinc deficiency is potentially teratogenic, including neural tube defects as one of the adverse outcomes (see the review by Hambidge et al., 1975).

Well-designed randomized, prospective studies of periconceptional vitamin supplementation are needed to examine the putative protection against neural tube defects. Two major studies are in progress—one organized by the Medical Research Council in the United Kingdom and the other in Hungary. Additional studies will be necessary.

Although the daily administration of a multivitamin preparation may appear superficially to be simple, relatively inexpensive, safe, and possibly beneficial, there are persuasive reasons for caution. The quantities of vitamins in a standard multivitamin preparation are unlikely to be harmful, but the possibility of side effects cannot be overlooked. For example, inadvertent overuse of vitamins may damage the fetus. Furthermore, a recommendation to take multivitamins during the periconceptional period will divert attention from other factors that may be the true causative factors of neural tube defects.

CONCLUSION

The subcommittee concluded that the scientific evidence does not provide a sufficient basis for making recommendations concerning the periconceptional use of vitamins and minerals for the prevention of neural tube defects. However, it recognizes the importance of the questions that have been raised and the critical need for adequate, carefully designed research to provide definitive answers as soon as possible. Meanwhile, since one or more nutritional factors are likely to play a role in the etiology of human neural tube defects, it would be desirable for women of childbearing age to follow dietary guidelines. Guidelines that encourage increased consumption of fruits, vegetables, whole grain breads and cereals, and legumes—all of which are good sources of folate and other micronutrients— may be found in publications of both the public and private sector (e.g., ACS [1984]; AHA [1988]; AICR [1985]; NCI [1987]; NRC [1989]; and USDA/DHHS [1985]).

REFERENCES

ACS (American Cancer Society). 1984. Nutrition and Cancer: Cause and Prevention. American Cancer Society Special Report. American Cancer Society, New York. 10 pp.

AHA (American Heart Association). 1988. Dietary guidelines for healthy American adults: a statement for physicians and health professionals by the Nutrition Committee, American Heart Association. Circulation 77:721A-724A.

AICR (American Institute for Cancer Research). 1985. Dietary Guidelines to Lower Cancer Risk. American Institute for Cancer Research, Washington, D.C. 14 pp.

Block, G., C. Cox, J. Madans, G.B. Schreiber, L. Licitra, and N. Melia. 1988. Vitamin supplement use, by demographic characteristics. Am. J. Epidemiol. 127:297-309.

Bower, C., and F.J. Stanley. 1989. Dietary folate as a risk factor for neural-tube defects: evidence from a case-control study in Western Australia. Med. J. Aust. 150:613-619.

Hambidge, K.M., K.H. Neldner, and P.A. Walravens. 1975. Zinc, acrodermatitis enteropathica, and congenital malformations. Lancet 1:577-578.

Holmes, L.B. 1988. Does taking vitamins at the time of conception prevent neural tube defects? J. Am. Med. Assoc. 260:3181.

Hurley, L.S. 1980. Trace elements II: manganese and zinc. Pp. 199-227 in Developmental Nutrition. Prentice-Hall, Englewood Cliffs, N.J.

International Conference on Prepregnancy Nutrition. 1987. Report from the International Conference on Prepregnancy Nutrition. March of Dimes Birth Defects Foundation, White Plains, N.Y. 4 pp.

Kalter, H., and J. Warkany. 1959. Experimental production of congenital malformations in mammals by metabolic procedure. Physiol. Rev. 39:69-115.

Koplan, J.P., J.L. Annest, P.M. Layde, and G.L. Rubin. 1986. Nutrient intake and supplementation in the United States (NHANES II). Am. J. Public Health 76:287-289.

Kurinij, N., M.A. Klebanoff, and B.I. Graubard. 1986. Dietary supplement and food intake in women of childbearing age. J. Am. Diet. Assoc. 16:1536-1540.

Lammer, E.J., L.E. Sever, and G.P. Oakley, Jr. 1987. Teratogen update: valproic acid. Teratology 35:465-473.

Laurence, K.M., N. James, M. Miller, and H. Campbell. 1980. Increased risk of recurrence of pregnancies complicated by fetal neural tube defects in mothers receiving poor diets, and possible benefit of dietary counselling. Br. Med. J. 281:1592-1594.

Laurence, K.M., N. James, M.H. Miller, G.B. Tennant, and H. Campbell. 1981. Double-blind randomised controlled trial of folate treatment before conception to prevent recurrence of neural-tube defects. Br. Med. J. 282:1509-1511.

Mills, J.L., G.G. Rhoads, J.L. Simpson, G.C. Cunningham, M.R. Conley, M.R. Lassman, M.E. Walden, O.R. Depp, H.J. Hoffman, and the National Institute of Child Health and Human Development Neural Tube Defects Study Group. 1989. The absence of a relation between the periconceptional use of vitamins and neural-tube defects. N. Engl. J. Med. 321:430-435.

Milunsky, A., H. Jick, S.S. Jick, C.L. Bruell, D.S. MacLaughlin, K.J. Rothman, and W. Willett. 1989. Multivitamin/folic acid supplementation in early pregnancy reduces the prevalence of neural tube defects. J. Am. Med. Assoc. 262:2847-2852.

Molloy, A.M., P. Kirke, I. Hillary, D.G. Weir, and J.M. Scott. 1985. Maternal serum folate and vitamin B_{12} concentrations in pregnancies associated with neural tube defects. Arch. Dis. Child. 60:660-665.

Mulinare, J., J.F. Cordero, J.D. Erickson, and R.J. Berry. 1988. Periconceptional use of multivitamins and the occurrence of neural tube defects. J. Am. Med. Assoc. 260:3141-3145.

NCI (National Cancer Institute). 1987. Diet, Nutrition, and Cancer Prevention: A Guide to Food Choices. NIH Publ. No. 87-2878. National Institutes of Health, Public Health Service, U.S. Department of Health and Human Services. U.S. Government Printing Office. Washington, D.C. 39 pp.

Nelson, M.M., H.V. Wright, C.W. Asling, and H.M. Evans. 1955. Multiple congenital abnormalities resulting from transitory deficiency of pteroylglutamic acid during gestation in the rat. J. Nutr. 56:349-370.

NRC (National Research Council). 1989. Diet and Health: Implications for Reducing Chronic Disease Risk. Report of the Committee on Diet and Health, Food and Nutrition Board, Commission on Life Sciences. National Academy Press, Washington, D.C. 749 pp.

Smithells, R.W., S. Sheppard, and C.J. Schorah. 1976. Vitamin deficiencies and neural tube defects. Arch. Dis. Child. 51:944-950.

Smithells, R.W., N.C. Nevin, M.J. Seller, S. Sheppard, R. Harris, A.P. Read, D.W. Fielding, S. Walker, C.J. Schorah, and J. Wild. 1983. Further experience of vitamin supplementation for prevention of neural tube defect recurrences. Lancet 1:1027-1031.

Subar, A.F., G. Block, and L.D. James. 1989. Folate intake and food sources in the US population. Am. J. Clin. Nutr. 50:508-516.

Trotz, M., C. Wegner, and H. Nau. 1987. Valproic acid-induced neural tube defects: reduction by folinic acid in the mouse. Life Sci. 41:103-110.

USDA (U.S. Department of Agriculture). 1985. Nationwide Food Consumption Survey. Continuing Survey of Food Intakes by Individuals. Women 19-50 Years and Their Children 1-5 Years, 1 Day, 1985. Report No. 85-1. Nutrition Monitoring Division, Human Nutrition Information Service, U.S. Department of Agriculture, Hyattsville, Md. 102 pp.

USDA/DHHS (U.S. Department of Agriculture/Department of Health and Human Services). 1985. Nutrition and Your Health. Dietary Guidelines for Americans, 2nd ed. Home and Garden Bulletin No. 232. U.S. Department of Agriculture/Department of Health and Human Services. Washington, D.C. 24 pp.

Wald, N.J., and P.E. Polani. 1984. Neural-tube defects and vitamins: the need for a randomized clinical trial. Br. J. Obstet. Gynaecol. 91:516-523.

Wegner, C.H.R., and H. Nau. 1989. Valproic acid-induced neural tube defects: disturbance of the folate metabolism in day 9 mouse embryo. Teratology 39:488

Yates, J.R.W., M.A. Ferguson-Smith, A. Shenkin, R. Guzman-Rodriguez, M. White, and B.J. Clark. 1987. Is disordered folate metabolism the basis for the genetic predispostion to neural tube defects? Clin. Genet. 31:279-287.

APPENDIXES

Appendix
A

Considerations in Constructing
Gestational Weight Gain Charts

Gestational weight gain charts have been used in clinical practice for many years. In Chapter 4, the subcommittee reviews the characteristics of some of the wide variety of charts currently in use in the United States. The lack of standardization across charts is due primarily to the lack of appropriate data on which to base the weight gain curves used in these charts. In this appendix, the subcommittee outlines research and development issues it believes should be considered in the construction of gestational weight gain charts.

RECOMMENDED CHARACTERISTICS OF
GESTATIONAL WEIGHT GAIN CHARTS

The subcommittee recommends that a new gestational weight gain chart be developed with the following characteristics and supporting materials:

1. **Gestational age, i.e., weeks from last normal menstrual period, on the horizontal axis, and achieved weight, i.e., total body weight in kilograms or pounds, on the vertical axis.** There should be some provision for adjusting the gestational age scale for any early-second-trimester ultrasound assessment suggesting that previous estimates of gestational age might be in error. The weight scale (vertical axis) should include both metric and American units. The vertical axis on the weight gain chart should be

calibrated for the woman's weight at the initial prenatal visit by entering prepregnancy weight at zero weeks of gestation and then adding a specified increment to the prepregnancy weight at each tick mark—similar to the approach used by Dimperio (1988) and shown in Figure 4-5, Chapter 4.

2. **Different charts for different classifications of prepregnancy weight for height, i.e., underweight, moderate weight, overweight, and obese, and possibly for short women,** similar to that shown in Figure 4-4, Chapter 4.

3. **A normative or average curve to represent the pattern of weight gain by week of gestation for each classification of prepregnancy weight for height.**

4. **Lines drawn to show upper and lower limits around the average curve,** similar to those shown in Figure 4-4, Chapter 4. These limits should be based on epidemiologic evidence. They could be percentiles or standard deviations of the observed representative (normative) population. Alternatively, they could be cutoff values established by comparison of two overlapping distributions: a distribution of maternal weight at any gestational age for healthy women with good outcomes and a comparable distribution of maternal weight for the abnormal population, i.e., the population with unfavorable pregnancy outcomes. A method for determining these cutoff values is presented below. The general methodology originally developed for application to postnatal child growth curves has been described by Galen and Gambino (1975) and by Haas and Habicht (1990). A chart incorporating cutoff values would allow estimation of the probability that a woman would have a poor pregnancy outcome given her weight gain to a specific week of pregnancy. However, it would not be useful in the evaluation of a woman's rate of weight gain measured over repeated prenatal visits.

5. **Criteria for evaluating the rate of weight gain and patterns of gain, either as a part of the chart itself or in accompanying instructions.** To a certain degree, the curve of average gain in the normative population provides guidance to the practitioner. Data-based guidelines for normal rates (kilograms or pounds per week) and acceptable upper and lower limits should be developed so that the subcommittee's recommendation of a linear gain during the second and third trimesters (Chapter 1) can be validated. Such guidelines should be established in the same way as the upper and lower limits of achieved weight, i.e., as either statistical measures of the normative population or as empirically derived cutoff values to discriminate favorable from unfavorable outcomes. The criteria may best be presented as a table of acceptable rates of gain to accompany the gestational weight gain chart. One alternative would be to include three different slopes or inclinations representing excessive (steep slope), desirable, or inadequate (shallow or negative slope) rates of weight gain. The slopes of the three curves may need to be changed for different trimesters of pregnancy if

research shows different desirable or normative rates for different stages of pregnancy.

6. **Clear, consistent criteria based on adequate research for assessing prepregnancy weight status as part of the chart or supporting documentation.** These should include the appropriate way to express prepregnancy weight (i.e., a body mass index or as a percentage of desirable body weight), the appropriate reference standard to use, whether or not frame size should be considered, and cutoff values to apply to the reference standard. The research needed to establish the prepregnancy weight-for-height classification scheme ideally should focus on establishing cutoff values for underweight and overweight women based on data regarding unfavorable and favorable pregnancy outcomes (as well as other short-term and long-term maternal health risks such as postpartum obesity) for women with different weights for height.

7. **Easy to use, i.e., requiring only a few simple measurements, and including indices that are easy to calculate or determine from tables or nomograms**, as well as an unambiguous classification scheme.

These and other design issues should be based on adequate research, much of which has not yet been undertaken. The instrument needs to be validated and evaluated in clinical settings. Consideration should be given not only to its diagnostic capabilities but also to the training effort needed, intra- and interobserver reliability of the measurements, acceptability to the clinic staff, utility as an instructional tool for the patient, and, if relevant, usefulness as a data collection instrument for research or surveillance.

RESEARCH NEEDS

To develop a chart with most of the characteristics described above, new research will be needed, specifically, large-scale studies to establish normative or desirable values for prepregnancy weight for height and incremental and total weight gain patterns. The sample sizes should be large enough to establish precise values for weight gain at the extremes (5th and 95th percentiles). The limits of the range of normative or desirable gestational weight gain should be established by examining the distribution of prepregnancy weight for height in relation to gestational weight gain among women with good as compared to poor pregnancy outcomes.

To establish an optimal or ideal range of prepregnancy weight and gestational weight gain, one needs to sample a population that experiences both desirable and undesirable pregnancy outcomes. Most of the current reference curves for gestational weight gain are based on data for women who had favorable outcomes, i.e., healthy, full-term infants with normal birth weights. As Figure A-1 shows, these women represent a subset (subpopulation B) of the total gestational weight gain distribution for the general

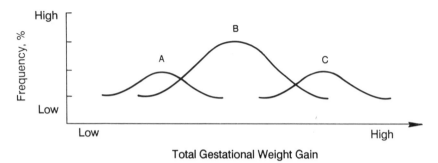

FIGURE A-1   Hypothetical distributions of gestational weight gain in three subpopulations of women.

population. There are women at the extremes of the gestational weight gain distribution who have less favorable outcomes, such as intrauterine growth retardation (subpopulation A) or fetal macrosomia (subpopulation C). Similar subpopulations are likely to exist for other maternal measures (horizontal axis), such as prepregnancy weight, accumulated weight gain to a specific stage of pregnancy, or rate of weight gain during specific trimesters of pregnancy. Moreover, the distribution of gestational weight gain in the three subpopulations representing the range of fetal growth is likely to be different for women with different prepregnancy weights. One could also subdivide the distribution of gestational weight gain in Figure A-1 to represent other outcomes. For example, subpopulation A could be women who deliver preterm infants, and population C could be women who retain the fat accumulated during pregnancy and are thus at risk of later obesity. (In this case, the distribution of gestational weight gain for subpopulations A and C would likely overlap.) Subpopulation B could be women who deliver full-term infants and do not retain pregnancy-acquired adipose tissue after delivery.

The Society of Actuaries (1959, 1960; Society of Actuaries/Association of Life Insurance Medical Directors of America, 1980) applied this scheme to obtain the 1959 and 1983 Metropolitan Life Insurance Company's tables of ideal body weight. To distinguish the subgroups, it used mortality data during a specified period following the measurement of weight. It examined the distributions of body weight for those who died and for those who survived during the period of observation: subpopulation B would represent the weights of those who survived. Since the Metropolitan Life

Insurance Company's ranges are based on postreproductive mortality and not pregnancy outcomes, they may be inappropriate for classifying mothers by prepregnancy weight for height.

A better criterion for establishing the desirable range of prepregnancy weights in gestational weight gain charts might be the risk of poor pregnancy outcomes, such as extremes in fetal growth, risk of obstetric complications, or development of postpartum obesity. However, an analysis that considers prepregnancy weight in identifying an optimal range for gestational weight gain requires application of sophisticated statistical methods, because prepregnancy weight plays two roles in the causal chain leading to some outcomes: it has an independent effect on fetal growth, and it modifies the effect of gestational weight gain on fetal growth (Figure 2-2, Chapter 2).

The degree of overlap among the three distributions illustrated in Figure A-1 is relatively easy to analyze, if it is not necessary to assume complex relationships of prepregnancy weight and gestational weight gain to outcomes. Such an analysis can yield important information on the appropriate cutoff values for gestational weight gain or prepregnancy weight. These values can then be used as the upper and lower limits of the gestational weight gain charts or for classification of underweight and overweight prior to pregnancy. The analytic methods were described in detail by Galen and Gambino (1975) and elaborated by Habicht et al. (1982), Swets and Pickett (1982), and Swets (1988).

An analysis of this type could be applied to incremental gestational weight gain data as well. Results of analysis of gestational weight gain rates could lead to recommendations for optimal rates at different stages of pregnancy.

To be useful to the clinician, the status or course of a patient's weight gain must be assessed accurately early enough in the pregnancy to allow for intervention. The determination of desirable total weight gain is useful in that it provides the end point through which a gestational weight gain curve should pass. However, the pattern of gain by trimester of pregnancy and the rate of gain between prenatal visits are more informative to the clinician. Therefore, future research should be longitudinal, allowing for frequent (at least monthly) measurements of weight beginning as early as possible in gestation and continuing throughout pregnancy. This type of research could yield essential information on the variation in rates of weight gain but would require a large sample size to evaluate effectively the relationship of these rates to the occurrence of relatively infrequent outcomes such as preterm delivery, intrauterine growth retardation, macrosomia, or perinatal death.

Data on normative rates of weight gain throughout pregnancy would allow for the construction of improved incremental weight gain charts and also of weight gain velocity charts, which display gestational duration on the horizontal axis and rate of gain on the vertical axis. Weight gain velocity graphs are powerful research tools but are infrequently used by clinicians to study postnatal growth of children (Tanner, 1986). There are no weight velocity curves for monitoring pregnancy in healthy adult women, but some have been developed for the assessment of pregnancies in teenagers (Hediger et al., 1989).

The research proposed here would provide the basic information needed to construct clinically useful gestational weight gain charts. Research should also be encouraged in the development of simplified assessment tools, such as those described by Rosso (1985) (Chapter 4, Figure 4-8), but the assumptions on which they are based need to be scrutinized and the instruments properly validated.

REFERENCES

Dimperio, D. 1988. Prenatal Nutrition: Clinical Guidelines for Nurses. March of Dimes Birth Defects Foundation, White Plains, N.Y. 134 pp.

Galen, R.S., and S.R. Gambino. 1975. Beyond Normality: The Predictive Value and Efficiency of Medical Diagnoses. John Wiley & Sons, New York. 237 pp.

Haas, J.D., and J.P. Habicht. 1990. Growth and growth charts in the assessment of preschool nutritional status. Pp. 160-183 in G.A. Harrison and J.C. Waterlow, eds. Diet and Disease in Traditional and Developing Societies. Cambridge University Press, Cambridge.

Habicht, J.P., L.D. Meyers, and C. Brownie. 1982. Indicators for identifying and counting the improperly nourished. Am. J. Clin. Nutr. 35:1241-1254.

Hediger, M.L., T.O. Scholl, D.H. Belsky, I.G. Ances, and R.W. Salmon. 1989. Patterns of weight gain in adolescent pregnancy: effects on birth weight and preterm delivery. Obstet. Gynecol. 74:6-12.

Rosso, P. 1985. A new chart to monitor weight gain during pregnancy. Am. J. Clin. Nutr. 41:644-652.

Society of Actuaries. 1959. Build and Blood Pressure Study 1959, Vol. I. Society of Actuaries, Chicago. 268 pp.

Society of Actuaries. 1960. Build and Blood Pressure Study 1959, Vol. II. Society of Actuaries, Chicago. 240 pp.

Society of Actuaries/Association of Life Insurance Medical Directors of America. 1980. Build Study 1979. Society of Actuaries/Association of Life Insurance Medical Directors of America, Chicago. 255 pp.

Swets, J.A. 1988. Measuring the accuracy of diagnostic systems. Science 240:1285-1293.

Swets, J.A., and R.M. Pickett. 1982. Evaluation of Diagnostic Systems: Methods from Signal Detection Theory. Academic Press, New York. 253 pp.

Tanner, J.M. 1986. Use and abuse of growth standards. Pp. 95-109 in F. Falkner and J.M. Tanner, eds. Human Growth: A Comprehensive Treatise, 2nd ed., Vol. 3. Methodology: Ecological, Genetic, and Nutritional Effects on Growth. Plenum Press, New York.

Appendix
B

Provisional Weight Gain Charts by Prepregnancy Body Mass Index (BMI).

A. For Normal Weight Women with BMI
of 19.8 to 26.0 (Metric)[a]

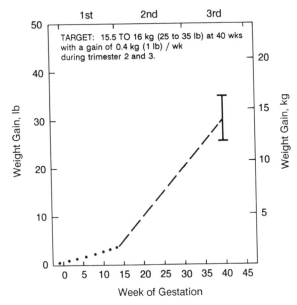

[a] Assumes a 1.6-kg (3.5-lb) gain in first trimester and the remaining gain at a rate of 0.44 kg (0.97 lb) per week.

[b] Assumes a 2.3-kg (5-lb) gain in first trimester and the remaining gain at a rate of 0.49 kg (1.07 lb) per week.

[c] Assumes a 0.9-kg (2-lb) gain in first trimester and the remaining gain at a rate of 0.3 kg (0.67 lb) per week.

B. For Underweight Women with BMI
Less Than 19.8 (Metric)[b]

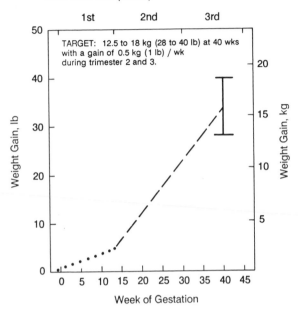

C. For Overweight Women with BMI
of >26.0 to 29.0 (Metric)[c]

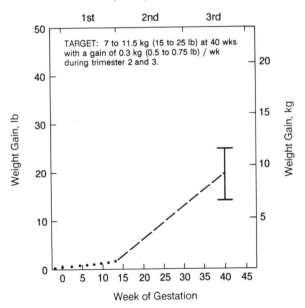

Appendix
C

Table for Estimating Body Mass Index (Metric)[a] by Using Either Metric or English Measurements of Prepregnancy Weight and Height; BMIs < 19.8 = low; BMIs 26.1 – 29.0 = high; BMIs > 29.0 = obesity (see shaded area above heavy line).

(Table follows on pages 434 and 435.)

Weight		Height, in. (and cm)																								
		55.9	56.7	57.5	58.3	59.1	59.8	60.6	61.4	62.2	63.0	63.8	64.6	65.4	66.1	66.9	67.7	68.5	69.3	70.1	70.9	71.7	72.4	73.2	74.0
lb	kg	(142)	(144)	(146)	(148)	(150)	(152)	(154)	(156)	(158)	(160)	(162)	(164)	(166)	(168)	(170)	(172)	(174)	(176)	(178)	(180)	(182)	(184)	(186)	(188)
220	100	49.6	48.2	46.9	45.7	44.4	43.3	42.2	41.1	40.1	39.1	38.1	37.2	36.3	35.4	34.6	33.8	33.0	32.3	31.6	30.9	30.2	29.5	28.9	28.3
218	99	49.1	47.7	46.4	45.2	44.0	42.8	41.7	40.7	39.7	38.7	37.7	36.8	35.9	35.1	34.3	33.5	32.7	32.0	31.2	30.6	29.9	29.2	28.6	28.0
216	98	48.6	47.3	46.0	44.7	43.6	42.4	41.3	40.3	39.3	38.3	37.3	36.4	35.6	34.7	33.9	33.1	32.4	31.6	30.9	30.2	29.6	28.9	28.3	27.7
213	97	48.1	46.8	45.5	44.3	43.1	42.0	40.9	39.9	38.9	37.9	37.0	36.1	35.2	34.4	33.6	32.8	32.0	31.3	30.6	29.9	29.3	28.7	28.0	27.4
211	96	47.6	46.3	45.0	43.8	42.7	41.6	40.5	39.4	38.5	37.5	36.6	35.7	34.8	34.0	33.2	32.4	31.7	31.0	30.3	29.6	29.0	28.4	27.7	27.2
209	95	47.1	45.8	44.6	43.4	42.2	41.1	40.1	39.0	38.1	37.1	36.2	35.3	34.5	33.7	32.9	32.1	31.4	30.7	30.0	29.3	28.7	28.1	27.5	26.9
207	94	46.6	45.3	44.1	42.9	41.8	40.7	39.6	38.6	37.7	36.7	35.8	34.9	34.1	33.3	32.5	31.8	31.0	30.3	29.7	29.0	28.4	27.8	27.2	26.6
205	93	46.1	44.8	43.6	42.5	41.3	40.3	39.2	38.2	37.3	36.3	35.4	34.6	33.7	33.0	32.2	31.4	30.7	30.0	29.4	28.7	28.1	27.5	26.9	26.3
202	92	45.6	44.4	43.2	42.0	40.9	39.8	38.8	37.8	36.9	35.9	35.1	34.2	33.4	32.6	31.8	31.1	30.4	29.7	29.0	28.4	27.8	27.2	26.6	26.0
200	91	45.1	43.9	42.7	41.5	40.4	39.4	38.4	37.4	36.5	35.5	34.7	33.8	33.0	32.2	31.5	30.8	30.1	29.4	28.7	28.1	27.5	26.9	26.3	25.7
198	90	44.6	43.4	42.2	41.1	40.0	39.0	37.9	37.0	36.1	35.2	34.3	33.5	32.7	31.9	31.1	30.4	29.7	29.1	28.4	27.8	27.2	26.6	26.0	25.5
196	89	44.1	42.9	41.8	40.6	39.6	38.5	37.5	36.6	35.7	34.8	33.9	33.1	32.3	31.5	30.8	30.1	29.4	28.7	28.1	27.5	26.9	26.3	25.7	25.2
194	88	43.6	42.4	41.3	40.2	39.1	38.1	37.1	36.2	35.3	34.4	33.5	32.7	31.9	31.2	30.4	29.7	29.1	28.4	27.8	27.2	26.6	26.0	25.4	24.9
191	87	43.1	42.0	40.8	39.7	38.7	37.7	36.7	35.7	34.9	34.0	33.2	32.3	31.6	30.8	30.1	29.4	28.7	28.1	27.5	26.9	26.3	25.7	25.1	24.6
189	86	42.7	41.5	40.3	39.3	38.2	37.2	36.3	35.3	34.4	33.6	32.8	32.0	31.2	30.5	29.8	29.1	28.4	27.8	27.1	26.5	26.0	25.4	24.8	24.3
187	85	42.2	41.0	39.9	38.8	37.8	36.8	35.8	34.9	34.0	33.2	32.4	31.6	30.8	30.1	29.4	28.7	28.1	27.4	26.8	26.2	25.7	25.1	24.6	24.0
185	84	41.7	40.5	39.4	38.3	37.3	36.4	35.4	34.5	33.6	32.8	32.0	31.2	30.5	29.8	29.1	28.4	27.7	27.1	26.5	25.9	25.4	24.8	24.3	23.8
183	83	41.2	40.0	38.9	37.9	36.9	35.9	35.0	34.1	33.2	32.4	31.6	30.9	30.1	29.4	28.7	28.1	27.4	26.8	26.2	25.6	25.1	24.5	24.0	23.5
180	82	40.7	39.5	38.5	37.4	36.4	35.5	34.6	33.7	32.8	32.0	31.2	30.5	29.8	29.1	28.4	27.7	27.1	26.5	25.9	25.3	24.8	24.2	23.7	23.2
178	81	40.2	39.1	38.0	37.0	36.0	35.1	34.2	33.3	32.4	31.6	30.9	30.1	29.4	28.7	28.0	27.4	26.8	26.1	25.6	25.0	24.5	23.9	23.4	22.9
176	80	39.7	38.6	37.5	36.5	35.6	34.6	33.7	32.9	32.0	31.3	30.5	29.7	29.0	28.3	27.7	27.0	26.4	25.8	25.2	24.7	24.2	23.6	23.1	22.6
174	79	39.2	38.1	37.1	36.1	35.1	34.2	33.3	32.5	31.6	30.9	30.1	29.4	28.7	28.0	27.3	26.7	26.1	25.5	24.9	24.4	23.9	23.3	22.8	22.4
172	78	38.7	37.6	36.6	35.6	34.7	33.8	32.9	32.1	31.2	30.5	29.7	29.0	28.3	27.6	27.0	26.4	25.8	25.2	24.6	24.1	23.5	23.0	22.5	22.1
169	77	38.2	37.1	36.1	35.2	34.2	33.3	32.5	31.6	30.8	30.1	29.3	28.6	27.9	27.3	26.6	26.0	25.4	24.9	24.3	23.8	23.2	22.7	22.3	21.8
167	76	37.7	36.7	35.7	34.7	33.8	32.9	32.0	31.2	30.4	29.7	28.9	28.3	27.6	26.9	26.3	25.7	25.1	24.5	24.0	23.5	22.9	22.4	22.0	21.5
165	75	37.2	36.2	35.2	34.2	33.3	32.5	31.6	30.8	30.0	29.3	28.6	27.9	27.2	26.6	26.0	25.4	24.8	24.2	23.7	23.1	22.6	22.2	21.7	21.2
163	74	36.7	35.7	34.7	33.8	32.9	32.0	31.2	30.4	29.6	28.9	28.2	27.5	26.9	26.2	25.6	25.0	24.5	23.9	23.4	22.8	22.3	21.9	21.4	20.9
161	73	36.2	35.2	34.2	33.3	32.4	31.6	30.8	30.0	29.2	28.5	27.8	27.1	26.5	25.9	25.3	24.7	24.1	23.6	23.0	22.5	22.0	21.6	21.1	20.7
158	72	35.7	34.7	33.8	32.9	32.0	31.2	30.4	29.6	28.8	28.1	27.4	26.8	26.1	25.5	24.9	24.3	23.8	23.2	22.7	22.2	21.7	21.3	20.8	20.4
156	71	35.2	34.2	33.3	32.4	31.6	30.7	29.9	29.2	28.4	27.7	27.1	26.4	25.8	25.2	24.6	24.0	23.5	22.9	22.4	21.9	21.4	21.0	20.5	20.1
154	70	34.7	33.8	32.8	32.0	31.1	30.3	29.5	28.8	28.0	27.3	26.7	26.0	25.4	24.8	24.2	23.7	23.1	22.6	22.1	21.6	21.1	20.7	20.2	19.8

Weight (lb)	Weight (kg)																									Body Mass Index [a]	
152	69	34.2	33.3	32.4	31.5	30.7	29.9	29.1	28.4	27.6	27.0	26.3	25.7	25.0	24.4	23.9	23.3	22.8	22.3	21.8	21.3	20.8	20.4	19.9	19.5
150	68	33.7	32.8	31.9	31.0	30.2	29.4	28.7	27.9	27.2	26.6	25.9	25.3	24.7	24.1	23.5	23.0	22.5	22.0	21.5	21.0	20.5	20.1	19.7	19.2
147	67	33.2	32.3	31.4	30.6	29.8	29.0	28.3	27.5	26.8	26.2	25.5	24.9	24.3	23.7	23.2	22.6	22.1	21.6	21.1	20.7	20.2	19.8	19.4	19.0
145	66	32.7	31.8	31.0	30.1	29.3	28.6	27.8	27.1	26.4	25.8	25.1	24.5	24.0	23.4	22.8	22.3	21.8	21.3	20.8	20.4	19.9	19.5	19.1	18.7
143	65	32.2	31.3	30.5	29.7	28.9	28.1	27.4	26.7	26.0	25.4	24.8	24.2	23.6	23.0	22.5	22.0	21.5	21.0	20.5	20.1	19.6	19.2	18.8	18.4
141	64	31.7	30.9	30.0	29.2	28.4	27.7	27.0	26.3	25.6	25.0	24.4	23.8	23.2	22.7	22.1	21.6	21.1	20.7	20.2	19.8	19.3	18.9	18.5	18.1
139	63	31.2	30.4	29.6	28.8	28.0	27.3	26.6	25.9	25.2	24.6	24.0	23.4	22.9	22.3	21.8	21.3	20.8	20.3	19.9	19.4	19.0	18.6	18.2	17.8
136	62	30.7	29.9	29.1	28.3	27.6	26.6	26.1	25.5	24.8	24.2	23.6	23.1	22.5	22.0	21.5	21.0	20.5	20.0	19.6	19.1	18.7	18.3	17.9	17.5
134	61	30.3	29.4	28.6	27.8	27.1	26.4	25.7	25.1	24.4	23.8	23.2	22.7	22.1	21.6	21.1	20.6	20.1	19.7	19.3	18.8	18.4	18.0	17.6	17.3
132	60	29.8	28.9	28.1	27.4	26.7	26.0	25.3	24.7	24.0	23.4	22.9	22.3	21.8	21.3	20.8	20.3	19.8	19.4	18.9	18.5	18.1	17.7	17.3	17.0
130	59	29.3	28.5	27.7	26.9	26.2	25.5	24.9	24.2	23.6	23.0	22.5	21.9	21.4	20.9	20.3	19.8	19.4	19.0	18.6	18.2	17.8	17.4	17.1	16.7
128	58	28.8	28.0	27.2	26.5	25.8	25.1	24.5	23.8	23.2	22.7	22.1	21.6	21.0	20.5	19.9	19.5	19.0	18.7	18.3	17.9	17.5	17.1	16.8	16.4
125	57	28.3	27.5	26.7	26.0	25.3	24.7	24.0	23.4	22.8	22.3	21.7	21.2	20.7	20.2	19.6	19.2	18.7	18.4	18.0	17.6	17.2	16.8	16.5	16.1
123	56	27.8	27.0	26.3	25.6	24.9	24.2	23.6	23.0	22.4	21.9	21.3	20.8	20.3	19.8	19.3	18.9	18.4	18.1	17.7	17.3	16.9	16.5	16.2	15.8
121	55	27.3	26.5	25.8	25.1	24.4	23.8	23.2	22.6	22.0	21.5	21.0	20.4	20.0	19.5	19.0	18.6	18.1	17.8	17.4	17.0	16.6	16.2	15.9	15.6
119	54	26.8	26.0	25.3	24.7	24.0	23.4	22.8	22.2	21.6	21.1	20.6	20.1	19.6	19.1	18.6	18.2	17.8	17.4	17.0	16.7	16.3	15.9	15.6	15.3
117	53	26.3	25.6	24.9	24.2	23.6	22.9	22.3	21.8	21.2	20.7	20.2	19.7	19.2	18.8	18.3	17.8	17.4	17.1	16.7	16.4	16.0	15.7	15.3	15.0
114	52	25.8	25.1	24.4	23.7	23.1	22.5	21.9	21.4	20.8	20.3	19.8	19.3	18.9	18.4	17.9	17.5	17.1	16.7	16.4	16.0	15.7	15.4	15.0	14.7
112	51	25.3	24.6	23.9	23.3	22.7	22.1	21.5	21.0	20.4	19.9	19.4	19.0	18.5	18.1	17.6	17.2	16.8	16.4	16.1	15.7	15.4	15.1	14.7	14.4
110	50	24.8	24.1	23.5	22.8	22.2	21.6	21.1	20.5	20.0	19.5	19.1	18.6	18.1	17.7	17.3	16.9	16.5	16.1	15.8	15.4	15.1	14.8	14.5	14.1
108	49	24.3	23.6	23.0	22.4	21.8	21.2	20.7	20.1	19.6	19.1	18.7	18.2	17.8	17.4	16.9	16.6	16.2	15.8	15.5	15.1	14.8	14.5	14.2	13.9
106	48	23.8	23.1	22.5	21.9	21.3	20.7	20.2	19.7	19.2	18.7	18.3	17.8	17.4	17.0	16.6	16.2	15.9	15.5	15.1	14.8	14.5	14.2	13.9	13.6
103	47	23.3	22.7	22.0	21.5	20.9	20.3	19.8	19.3	18.8	18.3	17.9	17.5	17.1	16.7	16.3	15.9	15.5	15.2	14.8	14.5	14.2	13.9	13.6	13.3
101	46	22.8	22.2	21.6	21.0	20.4	19.9	19.4	18.9	18.4	17.9	17.5	17.1	16.7	16.3	15.9	15.5	15.2	14.9	14.5	14.2	13.9	13.6	13.3	13.0
99	45	22.3	21.7	21.1	20.5	20.0	19.5	19.0	18.5	18.0	17.6	17.1	16.7	16.3	15.9	15.6	15.2	14.9	14.5	14.2	13.9	13.6	13.3	13.0	12.7
97	44	21.8	21.2	20.6	20.1	19.6	19.0	18.6	18.1	17.6	17.2	16.8	16.4	16.0	15.6	15.2	14.9	14.5	14.2	13.9	13.6	13.3	13.0	12.7	12.4
95	43	21.3	20.7	20.2	19.6	19.1	18.6	18.1	17.7	17.2	16.8	16.4	16.0	15.6	15.2	14.9	14.5	14.2	13.9	13.6	13.3	13.0	12.7	12.4	12.2
92	42	20.8	20.3	19.7	19.2	18.7	18.2	17.7	17.3	16.8	16.4	16.0	15.6	15.2	14.9	14.5	14.2	13.9	13.6	13.3	13.0	12.7	12.4	12.1	11.9
90	41	20.3	19.8	19.2	18.7	18.2	17.7	17.3	16.8	16.4	16.0	15.6	15.2	14.9	14.5	14.2	13.9	13.6	13.3	13.0	12.7	12.4	12.1	11.9	11.6
88	40	19.8	19.3	18.8	18.3	17.8	17.3	16.9	16.4	16.0	15.6	15.2	14.9	14.5	14.2	13.8	13.5	13.2	13.0	12.7	12.4	12.1	11.8	11.6	11.3

[a] BMI (metric) = (kg/m^2) × 100; BMI (English) = (lb/in.^{2}) × 100.
BMI (metric) × 0.142 = BMI (English); BMI (English) × 7 = BMI (metric).

Appendix D

Biographical Sketches of Committee Members

Barbara Abrams, Dr.P.H., R.D., is assistant professor in the Departments of Social and Administrative Health Sciences, School of Public Health, University of California, Berkeley, and the Department of Obstetrics, Gynecology and Reproductive Sciences, School of Medicine, University of California, San Francisco. She worked as a perinatal nutritionist for more than a decade and has conducted several epidemiologic studies on maternal weight gain, nutrition, and pregnancy outcome.

Lindsay Allen, Ph.D., is professor in the Department of Nutritional Sciences at the University of Connecticut, Storrs. She has conducted research on relationships between nutrition and the outcome of human pregnancy and lactation in the United States as well as in other countries. In recent years, her special interest has been the effect of marginal malnutrition on the function of women and children in Mexico.

Gertrud S. Berkowitz, Ph.D., is perinatal epidemiologist and associate professor in the Department of Obstetrics, Gynecology, and Reproductive Science and the Department of Community Medicine at Mount Sinai School of Medicine, New York. She has conducted various research studies on preterm delivery and intrauterine growth retardation and has written about the role of environmental and occupational hazards during pregnancy.

Nancy F. Butte, Ph.D., is assistant professor of pediatrics at Baylor College of Medicine. She has conducted research on infant nutrition, lactation, and energy metabolism.

Ronald A. Chez, M.D., is professor of obstetrics and gynecology at the University of South Florida School of Medicine in Tampa. He previously held positions as chief of the Pregnancy Research Branch and clinical director of the National Institute of Child and Human Development as well as chair of the Department of Obstetrics and Gynecology at Pennsylvania State University. His research has focused on aspects of fetal physiology, including the exchange of substrates across the placenta.

Peter R. Dallman, M.D., is professor of pediatrics at the University of California, San Francisco. His research deals with the manifestations, diagnosis, and prevalence of iron deficiency. He has served on national and international committees and panels to establish iron requirements and to devise strategies for preventing iron deficiency.

Jere D. Haas, Ph.D., is professor of nutritional sciences at Cornell University. He has conducted research on the maternal, fetal, and infant responses to stresses at extreme high altitudes as well as on relationships between maternal nutritional status and fetal growth, postnatal growth, and postnatal development and morbidity in Bolivia, Peru, Guatemala, Indonesia, and the United States.

Michael Hambidge, M.D., Sc.D., is professor of pediatrics at the University of Colorado Health Sciences Center. He is also director of both the Center for Human Nutrition and the Pediatric Clinic Research Center in the School of Medicine at the university. His major interest is human nutrition, including research, training, education, and improving nutrition practices in the community.

Margit Hamosh, Ph.D., is professor in the Department of Pediatrics and chief of the department's Division of Developmental Biology and Nutrition at Georgetown University Medical Center. She has conducted research on lung development and on fat digestion and absorption, emphasizing the ontogeny of digestive enzymes and compensatory digestive function in pancreatic insufficiency, lipid clearance, the composition of human milk, and the function of its components in the neonate. Dr. Hamosh has served on several committees of the National Institutes of Health and is president of the International Society of Research on Human Milk and Lactation.

Francis E. Johnston, Ph.D., is professor and chairman of the Department of Anthropology of the University of Pennsylvania. His research focuses on the growth, development, and body composition of children and youth, especially in relationship to nutritional status.

Janet C. King, Ph.D., is professor of nutrition and chair of the Department of Nutritional Sciences at the University of California, Berkeley. She has conducted research on nutritional needs during pregnancy and has published on the protein, energy, and zinc requirements of pregnant women. She has served on many national committees involved in establishing policies relating to prenatal care.

Avanelle Kirksey, Ph.D., is Meredith Distinguished Professor of Nutrition at Purdue University. She has published widely in the area of vitamin B_6 in pregnancy and lactation. She has been a collaborator in maternal and infant nutrition research in Egypt and presently serves as facilitator for Midwest Universities Consortium for International Activities for graduate nutrition programs in Indonesia.

Joel C. Kleinman, Ph.D., is director of the Division of Analysis, National Center for Health Statistics, Centers for Disease Control. He has published extensively on statistical and epidemiologic issues related to low birth weight and infant mortality. He has been a member of the U.S. Public Health Service Work Group on Maternal and Infant Health Objectives for the Year 2000 and the Subcommittee on Infant Mortality and Low Birth Weight of the Department of Health and Human Services Secretary's Task Force on Minority Health.

Michael S. Kramer, M.D., is professor of pediatrics and of epidemiology and biostatistics at the McGill University Faculty of Medicine in Montreal. He has been a career research scholar of the National Health Research and Development Program, Health and Welfare Canada, and is currently a senior career investigator of the Fonds de la Recherche en Santé du Québec. His primary research interests are the determinants and consequences of preterm birth and intrauterine growth retardation and the diagnostic and therapeutic management of the young febrile child.

Sally Ann Lederman, Ph.D., is assistant professor of public health and nutrition at Columbia University's Faculty of Medicine. In animals, she has studied the effect of dietary changes on pregnancy outcome and lactation performance, focusing on changes in maternal body composition. In humans, she has studied the relationship of birth weight to maternal body weight and pregnancy weight changes in teenage mothers and in mothers bearing twins. She has also studied demographic factors influencing low birth weight in New York City and psychosocial predictors of pregnancy outcome in several ethnic groups and of lactation success among poor women in Brazil.

Charles S. Mahan, M.D., is deputy secretary for health and state health officer for Florida, director of the Robert Wood Johnson Healthy Futures Program, and professor of obstetrics and gynecology at the University of Florida College of Medicine. His special interests have been preterm birth prevention, food supplementation in pregnancy, family-centered maternity care, prevention of unnecessary cesarean deliveries, infant mortality, improved care for low-income women, and out-of-hospital birth centers.

Jennifer Niebyl, M.D., is professor and head of the Department of Obstetrics and Gynecology at the University of Iowa, Iowa City. Earlier in her career, she was director of the Division of Maternal-Fetal Medicine in the Department of Gynecology and Obstetrics at the Johns Hopkins University. Her major research interest is the use of medications during pregnancy.

Roy M. Pitkin, M.D., is professor and chair of the Department of Obstetrics and Gynecology at the University of California, Los Angeles. Before assuming this post in 1987, he was professor and head of the Department of Obstetrics and Gynecology at the University of Iowa, Ames. He previously chaired the Committee on Nutrition of the Mother and Preschool Child of the Food and Nutrition Board, National Academy of Sciences.

Kathleen M. Rasmussen, Sc.D., R.D., is associate professor of nutrition at Cornell University and program director of a National Institutes of Health training grant in maternal and child nutrition. Her research has focused on the effects of maternal malnutrition on reproductive performance, with an emphasis on lactation.

John W. Sparks, M.D., is associate professor in the Department of Pediatrics at the University of Colorado. A neonatologist, he has served as director of Newborn Services and medical director of the Neonatal Intensive Care Unit at University Hospital, Denver. Scientific interests include the physiology, metabolism, and nutrition of the fetus and newborn.

Mervyn Susser, M.B., B.Ch., D.P.H., is Sergievsky Professor of Epidemiology and founder and director of the Sergievsky Center at Columbia University in New York. The Center is endowed for the study of the epidemiology of neurodevelopmental disorders. He has also been head of epidemiology in the Columbia University School of Public Health. His work covers several specific fields, including prenatal development and prenatal nutrition, as well as such general topics as causality and the social sciences in epidemiology.

Acronyms

ACOG   American College of Obstetricians and Gynecologists
BMI   body mass index
BMR   basal metabolic rate
CSFII   Continuing Survey of Food Intake by Individuals
DNA   deoxyribonucleic acid
EP   erythrocyte protoporphyrin
FAS   fetal alcohol syndrome
Fe/TIBC   ratio of serum iron to total iron binding capacity
FNB   Food and Nutrition Board
GA   gestational age
HES   national Health Examination Survey, Cycle I (1960-1962)
HHANES   Hispanic Health and Nutrition Examination Survey
IU   international unit
IUGR   intrauterine growth retardation
LBW   low birth weight
LMP   last menstrual period
MCV   mean corpuscular volume
MLI   Metropolitan Life Insurance Company
NCHS   National Center for Health Statistics
NE   niacin equivalent
NFCS   Nationwide Food Consumption Survey
NHANES I   first National Health and Nutrition Examination Survey
   (1971-1974)

NHANES II   second National Health and Nutrition Examination Survey
   (1976-1980)
NNS   National Natality Survey
PIH   pregnancy-induced hypertension
PLP   pyridoxal phosphate
PTH   parathyroid hormone
PUFA   polyunsaturated fatty acids
RBP   retinol binding protein
RDA   Recommended Dietary Allowances
RE   retinol equivalent
RMR   resting metabolic rate
RNA   ribonucleic acid
SD   standard deviation
SEM   standard error of the mean
SGA   small for gestational age
U.S. RDA   U.S. Recommended Daily Allowances
USDA   U.S. Department of Agriculture
VLBW   very low birth weight
WIC   Special Supplemental Food Program for Women, Infants, and
   Children

Glossary

Abruptio placentae   premature detachment of the placenta.

Balance study   a method for estimating nutrient requirements by measuring all dietary intake and physiologic loss of the nutrient and comparing intake with loss.

Bioavailability   proportion of a nutrient absorbed from food and available for physiologic function.

Body mass index (BMI)   an expression of body weight for height used for children and adults. In this report, metric units are used, namely, BMI $= [(kg/m^2) \times 100]$

Carotene   a precursor of vitamin A, sometimes called provitamin A.

Case-control study   a study in which individuals with a particular condition (the cases) are selected for comparison with a series of individuals in whom the condition is absent (the controls). Cases and controls are compared with respect to exposures believed to be relevant to the development of the condition being studied.

Ceruloplasmin   a protein that carries the majority of the copper in the blood.

Chelator   a substance that binds metals (e.g., trace elements such as copper).

Confounding variable   a variable that biases the apparent relationship between an exposure (putative cause) and outcome (putative effect) under study. To qualify as a confounder, a variable must itself be a cause of the outcome and associated with the exposure but must not lie on the causal path between exposure and outcome.

Congenital anomalies   birth defects.

Consequences   health outcomes (effects) caused by the determinants.

Determinants   causal (etiologic) factors.

Disproportionality   the condition of having a low ponderal index (defined below).

Dizygotic twins   twins who are the product of two ova, often called fraternal twins; cf **monozygotic twins.**

Effect modifier   a factor that increases or decreases the magnitude of the effect of a determinant on a particular consequence.

Embryo   the developing organism from 1 week after conception to the end of the second month of gestation.

Embryogenesis, period of   the period during which the embryo develops, i.e., from the first week through the second month of gestation. See **embryo.**

Essential amino acids   amino acids with essential functions that cannot be synthesized by humans. See **nonessential amino acids.**

Estrus   the period of ovulation and sexual activity in nonhuman female animals.

Etiologic fraction   population attributable risk, that is, the proportion of all cases of a disease or other condition in a specified population that is attributable to an exposure.

Factorial approach   a method for estimating nutrient requirements by summing the estimated amounts of nutrient required for each of several purposes, e.g., replacement of endogenous loss and growth.

Fetal alcohol syndrome   a syndrome related to alcohol use during pregnancy and characterized by prenatal or postnatal growth retardation, distinct facial anomalies, and mental deficiency.

Fetopelvic disproportion   a disparity between the size of the mother's pelvis and the size, shape, or position of the head of the fetus. This can result in prolonged labor and inability to deliver vaginally. Often called cephalopelvic disproportion.

Fetus   the developing organism in the human uterus after the second month of gestation.

Functional measurements of nutritional status   tests to determine the adequacy of nutritional status to support the functions of subcellular constituents, cells, tissues, organs, biologic systems, or the whole body.

Gestational duration   the duration of pregnancy, usually calculated from the first day of the last normal menstrual period to delivery. Normal gestational durations average approximately 280 days.

Gestational weight gain   weight gained between conception and delivery. Ordinarily it includes maternal body weight and the weight of the products of conception. See discussion in Chapter 4.

Goitrogens   substances that cause goiters or enlargement of the thyroid gland.

High birth weight   infant birth weight greater than 4,000 g.

Homeostatic   pertaining to a stable state of the internal environment of the body that is maintained by dynamic processes of feedback and regulation.

Hyperemesis gravidarum   severe and prolonged vomiting during pregnancy.

Hypocalciuria   a low concentration of calcium in the urine.

Infant mortality rate   deaths during the first year of life per 1,000 live births.

Intrauterine growth retardation   lower-than-expected birth weight for a given gestational age. Usually defined as a birth weight below the 10th percentile for gestational age based on a given reference population and, hence, often used synonymously with small-for-gestational age.

Keshan disease   a serious, often fatal cardiomyopathy resulting from selenium deficiency.

Lactation performance   degree of success of breastfeeding, as determined by measurements such as milk volume, milk composition, duration of breastfeeding, and infant growth.

Lactose intolerance   a condition in which the intestinal enzyme lactase, which breaks down lactose to glucose plus galactose, is lacking; this may lead to cramps and diarrhea after consumption of certain lactose-containing foods (e.g., milk).

Large-for-gestational age   usually defined as birth weight above the 90th percentile for gestational age, based on a given reference population.

Low birth weight   infant birth weight less than 2,500 g.

Menarche   the initiation of menstruation.

Menorrhagia   excessive menstrual blood loss (>80 ml of menstrual blood per month).

Micronutrients   vitamins and minerals.

Monozygotic twins   originating from a single fertilized ovum, applied to identical twins; cf **dizygotic**.

Multiple pregnancy   carrying more than one fetus, e.g., twins or triplets.

Neonatal   during the first 28 days after birth.

Net weight gain   total gestational weight gain minus the infant's birth weight.

Nonessential amino acids   amino acids with essential functions that can be synthesized by humans if suitable sources of carbon, nitrogen, and energy are available.

Odds ratio   the ratio of the odds of a condition occurring in exposed individuals compared with the odds in unexposed persons; generally used as an approximation of the relative risk.

Optimally grown infants   defined in this report as an infant born at week 39 to 41 of gestation with a birth weight between 3,000 and 4,000 grams.

Parity   the number of children previously born to a woman.

Periconceptional period   a period from 1 to 3 months prior to gestation through the first 6 weeks of gestation.

Pica   ingestion of nonfood substances such as laundry starch and clay.

Ponderal index   an expression of weight for height used mainly for infants. In newborns, the index is usually expressed as birth weight in grams × 100 divided by the birth length in centimeters cubed.

Postterm birth   birth occurring after a gestation of 42 or more weeks.

Preeclampsia   hypertension accompanied by generalized pitting edema or proteinuria after the twentieth week of gestation.

Preterm birth   birth occurring after a gestation of less than 37 weeks.

Primigravida   a woman during her first pregnancy.

Primipara   a woman who has produced one 500-g infant (or after week 20 of gestation), regardless of the infant's viability.

Rate of weight gain per week   weight gained over a specified period divided by the duration of that period in weeks.

Recurrent neural tube defect   more than one child with a neural tube defect born to the same parents.

Retinol   preformed vitamin A.

Reverse causality the erroneous inference that a factor under study causes a given outcome when, in fact, the factor is an effect (consequence) of that outcome. The error arises because of failure to ensure that exposure to the factor actually preceded development of the outcome.

Shoulder dystocia difficulty in delivering the shoulders of the fetus through the birth canal after its head has emerged.

Small-for-gestational age see **Intrauterine growth retardation**.

Spontaneous abortion miscarriage.

Stadiometer a device for measuring height.

Static measurements of nutritional status determination of overt signs of clinical deficiency and of nutrient or metabolite levels in blood or tissues.

Teratogenic causing deformities in the fetus.

Thermogenesis heat production (energy expenditure) following the ingestion of food or exposure to cold above that produced by basal metabolism.

Toxemia (eclampsia) coma and convulsive seizures occurring between approximately the twentieth week of pregnancy and the end of the first week postpartum.

Turnover utilization and replacement (of nutrients).

Very low birth weight infant birth weight less than 1,500 g.

Vitamer any one of a number of compounds that have specific vitamin activity.

Index

posture changes during pregnancy, 65
recalled, 87
research needs on, 112
trends in, 42, 57
see also Weight for height, prepregnancy
Hemoglobin
concentration, and criteria for anemia,
284–285
impaired production, 274, 283–284
normal values during pregnancy, 275
High birth weight, 52, 55–56, 58, 178, 180,
187, 192, 201, 204, 227–230
High-risk groups, research
recommendations, 22
Hispanic Health and Nutrition
Examination Survey (HHANES),
278, 279
Hispanics
birth weight trends among, 46, 54–55
weight gain and obesity, 4
see also Race and ethnic origin
Hormonal levels, in twin pregnancies, 219
Human chorionic somatomammotropin,
108
Human placental calcium-binding protein,
324
Human placental lactogen, 108
Hydrocephalus, 340
Hypercalcemia, 327
Hyperemesis gravidarum, 192, 352
Hyperparathyroidism, 319
Hypertension
and birth weight, 53
calcium supplementation and, 321–322,
331
gestational weight gain and, 9, 200, 201,
204
maternal mortality from, 200
in twin pregnancies, 213, 215
zinc deficiency and, 301–303
Hypocalcemia, 181, 229, 325
Hypocalciuria, 321
Hypoglycemia, 181, 229, 326
Hypoparathyroidism, 327
Hypothyroidism, 308

I

India
cumulative increase in maternal weight,
102, 104
energy intake, maternal weight gain, and
birth weight, 152, 153
malnutrition and calcium balance in, 321
vitamin D supplementation studies, 328
Indonesia

energy intake, maternal weight gain, and
birth weight, 154
energy supplementation and lactation
performance, 202
weight gain rates of pregnant women,
102, 104, 105
Industrialized countries
body fat content changes in pregnant
women, 133, 202
energy intake, maternal weight gain, and
birth weight in, 138–143, 149–150,
156–159, 163
energy supplementation of pregnant
women in, 161–164
folate deficiency in, 18
iron deficiency in, 272–273, 278
maternal mortality in, 199
resting metabolic rate in pregnant
women, 165
see also specific countries
Infant mortality
anemia and, 274, 275
birth weight and, 4, 28, 51, 178, 180,
181, 215, 218
fetal deaths, 178, 180, 181
gestational age and, 181, 229
gestational weight gain and, 8, 97,
177–179, 204, 228, 229
high-protein supplements and, 163
IUGR and, 182, 204, 229
preterm births and, 28
by race, 180
in twin pregnancies, 212, 215, 218, 220
trends in, 50, 51, 58
Insulin resistance, 108
Interactions among nutrients
calcium, 254, 288
copper, 254, 300, 303, 307, 311
folate, 366
iron, 254, 288, 290, 300, 303, 304, 310,
330
magnesium, 254, 288, 330
manganese, 310
molybdenum, 311
protein, 254
phosphorus, 254
potential for, 16, 242, 255, 373
research needs on, 21
vitamin B_6, 254
zinc, 254, 290, 300, 303, 304–305, 307
Intrauterine devices, 280
Intrauterine growth retardation (IUGR)
birth length and head circumference,
194, 229
and child health problems, 181, 182, 229
energy supplementation and, 8–9
factors contributing to decrease in, 55

Y

Z